NEW GENE THERAPY AND CANCER RESEARCH

NEW GENE THERAPY AND CANCER RESEARCH

WILMA B. GUSTAFSSON
EDITOR

Nova Biomedical Books
New York

For permission to use material from this book please contact us:
Telephone 631-231-7269; Fax 631-231-8175
Web Site: http://www.novapublishers.com

LIBRARY OF CONGRESS CATALOGING-IN-PUBLICATION DATA

New gene therapy and cancer research / Wilma B. Gustafsson (editor).
p. ; cm.
Includes bibliographical references.
ISBN-13: 978-1-60021-969-6 (hardcover)
ISBN-10: 1-60021-969-1 (hardcover)
1. Cancer--Gene therapy. I. Gustafsson, Wilma B.
[DNLM: 1. Neoplasms--therapy. 2. Gene Therapy. QZ 266 N5317 2007]
RC271.G45N49 2007
616.99'40695--dc22

2007034868

Published by Nova Science Publishers, Inc. ✦ New York

CONTENTS

PREFACE

Genes, which are carried on chromosomes, are the basic physical and functional units of heredity. Genes are specific sequences of bases that encode instructions on how to make proteins. Although genes get a lot of attention, it's the proteins that perform most life functions and even make up the majority of cellular structures. When genes are altered so that the encoded proteins are unable to carry out their normal functions, genetic disorders can result. Gene therapy is an experimental treatment that involves introducing genetic material into a person's cells to fight disease. Gene therapy is being studied in clinical trials for many different types of cancer and for numerous other diseases. This book offers important research from around the globe dedicated to this dynamic subject.

Chapter I - Breast cancer research has developed at a rapid pace over the past few decades, leading to longer survival times for breast cancer patients and opening up the possibility of developing curative treatments for advanced breast cancer. Hopes for individualized treatments have been raised by recent discoveries related to the cancer multistep process, characterized by genetic alterations of normal host cells and by non-genetic changes in the behaviors of malignant cells and of host cells interacting with the tumor. While most subsequent changes may result in cell death, some can affect key genes involved in cell survival, proliferation, invasiveness, motility, drug resistance and other malignant characteristics. Our increasing knowledge of the specific proteins, genes and biological pathways associated with the progression and development of breast cancer, alongside the failure of conventional treatments, has prompted us to explore gene therapy as an alternative therapeutic strategy. In this review, the authors summarize trends in the different approaches to breast cancer treatment, classified as: 1. Corrective gene therapy, which aims to restore normal function of a deleted or mutated gene; 2. Proapoptotic gene therapy, in which restoration or enhancement of the capacity to undergo apoptosis may be a crucial event, rendering tumors sensitive to classical anticancer agents; 3. Immunomodulatory gene therapy, in which gene delivery to tumor or normal tissue enhances the ability of the immune system to mount an effective cytotoxic response; 4. Genetic modulation of resistance or sensitivity, since conventional therapy fails in many breast cancer patients because their tumours are resistant to DNA-damaging agents, e.g., chemotherapy; 5. antiangiogenic gene therapy to block tumor growth through regression of neovascularisation, and 6. Suicide gene therapy, in which delivery of an exogenous gene results in cancer cell death. These genes may express a toxic molecule that affects cellular viability or express enzymes that selectively activate specific prodrugs. Gene therapy is expected to play an increasing role in clinical breast cancer treatment, and combined modality therapy with gene therapy and chemotherapy or radiation therapy has already shown promising results.

Chapter II - In this chapter the potential of using pulsed-high intensity focused ultrasound (HIFU), a type of therapeutic ultrasound, will be discussed. A short review of other physical means for enhanced gene delivery will first be presented. This will be followed by an overview of therapeutic ultrasound, including a description of the primary ultrasound mechanisms for producing bio-effects, as well as a short summary of the different therapeutic ultrasound applications, most of which deal with enhancing the delivery of drugs. Next, a more detailed description of the ultrasound mechanisms for enhancing gene delivery will be presented, followed by a review of the manner by which pulsed-HIFU exposures can be combined with various modes of administration of genes (local, intravascular, and systemic) *in vivo*. The last two short sections will deal with using pulsed-HIFU to remotely control the expression of delivered genes, and some safety considerations involved with employing these exposures.

Chapter III - Discovery of the pathways involved in the molecular regulation of angiogenesis has made it possible to test the hypothesis that blocking the angiogenic switch may keep tumor growth in check, and has added a new investigational arm to the field of cancer therapy. Angiogenesis inhibitors are heterogeneous in origin and potency; pre-clinical studies have clearly indicated that these factors are essentially cytostatic and need long-term administration in order to obtain prolonged anti-tumor effects. The experimental approaches attempted to date with endogenous factors, reviewed herein, indicate overall that delivery of anti-angiogenic factors or their cDNA by gene therapy approaches is mainly effective in the preventive setting. Meanwhile, anti-angiogenic drugs have entered the clinical arena, usually in combination with chemotherapy, to treat patients with advanced solid tumors with encouraging results in terms of survival. On the other hand, resistance to angiogenesis inhibitors has rapidly emerged and the current hypothesis formulated to explain this clinically relevant phenomenon will also be presented in this chapter. Decoding the biological mechanisms underlying resistance to angiogenesis inhibition, along with the identification of useful biomarkers of response and the design of appropriate combined treatments, will eventually allow for the achievement of durable control of advanced tumors.

Chapter IV - Over two-thirds of clinical trials in gene therapy are directed against cancer. Suicide gene therapy, or gene directed enzyme prodrug therapy (GDEPT), has been tested in 98 clinical trials worldwide, has reached phase III trials and makes up almost 8% of all current gene therapy trials. GDEPT aims to improve the selectivity of chemotherapy by gene transfer, thus enabling target cells to convert non-toxic prodrugs to cytotoxic drugs. A recent, but as yet clinically untested, development is the targeting of tumour blood vessels using gene therapy. Endothelial cells lining tumour blood vessels are an attractive target, since they are readily accessible for systemic administration and relatively minor vascular damage can amplify into macro-regional tumour infarction. This chapter will review the literature on the heterogeneity of endothelial cells, concentrating on tumour-endothelial factors. The authors will give an update on gene directed enzyme prodrug systems that have reached clinical trials, as well as those that are in the early phase of development, followed by an overview of approaches to target GDEPT to tumour vessels.

Chapter V - Bladder cancer (transitional cell carcinoma) has been treated with traditional therapeutic alternatives, including transurethral resection, cystectomy, chemotherapy and radiation. Despite these recommended modalities, the therapeutic effect is often insufficient particularly in advanced, recurred, or metastasized diseases. Recently, with the great development of molecular biology with gene transfer methods, cancer gene therapy has become a reality for clinical application. The authors reviewed the background of and explore gene therapy for bladder cancer and performed a comprehensive literature search with publications.

Gene therapy strategies were broadly categorized as cytotoxic, corrective and immune-modulating gene transfer. A suppressive / corrective gene transfer such as cell cycle regulators is effective in cell culture and animal models, but the clinical realization of specific corrective gene transfer affecting each and every target cell without any detrimental influence on expression of other genes remains a challenge. Cytotoxic gene therapy represents a straightforward approach and is an attractive choice as either monotherapy or in combination with other anticancer therapies. Although this approach showed efficacy in animal models, limitations are the current inability to transduce large percentages of tumor cells and unwanted induction of host immunity to repeat application particularly using viral vector systems. Immunomodulation / cytokine gene therapy has the potential of inducing antitumor immunity with possible prevention of metastasis. As most patients ultimately die of metastatic disease, this would represent a major step ahead in anticancer therapy.

Therapeutic gene transfer has proven to be safe and efficacious in pre-clinical studies of bladder cancer using cell cultures and animal models in the previous literatures. Clinical gene therapy trials offer a safe and feasible therapy in an actual clinical scenario; however, it demonstrates only modest antitumor efficacy. Given the current limitations of cancer gene therapy, this progress is promising because of especially considering that the current developments and applications were impossible approximately two decades ago. Further research is warranted for overcoming limitations.

Chapter VI - Gliomas are the most common form of primary intracranial malignancy, with glioblastoma multiforme (GBM) carrying the worst prognosis. Among all of the novel therapies being explored for this disease, gene and viral oncolytic therapies are becoming a promising alternative. To achieve either a robust transgene expression or efficient viral replication with limited toxicity, a variety of delivery systems are being developed and tested. These include stem cells, viral vectors, liposomes and synthetic polymers. This chapter explores gene therapy and oncolytic viral therapy for malignant gliomas. The rationale for vector development and transgene selection is explored. Special attention is placed on modifications made to adenoviral oncolytic vectors in order to render them specific for gliomas. In addition, the authorsdiscuss the results of novel treatment strategies, with a special emphasis on the results obtained in human clinical trials.

Chapter VII - In the present work the authors have developed several models of cancer vaccines, employing a murine melanoma and nonviral procedures for gene transfer. Many efforts have been made in relation to cancer vaccines, attempting to elucidate the best way to induce correct activation of the immune system in order to achieve proper antitumor response. Engineered cells seem to be the most successful approach, since they better reproduce the processes that occur in real patients, including events that today still escape our understanding. However, purified antigens represent an easier approach in terms of their preparation, reproducibility and facility to become a commercial medicine. This is why they continue to center attention, though their results are still not particularly satisfactory. In an attempt to establish the best approach for stimulating the immune response and also securing the simplest treatment, the authors have tested different preventive vaccination models such as: a) purified antigens from irradiated B16 melanoma tumor cells (Tumor Membrane Proteins, TMP); b) such antigens encapsulated in liposomes; c) lipopolyplexes formed by cationic liposomes bearing antigens plus the cationic polymer polyethyleneimine (PEI), carrying DNA; d) freshly transfected and irradiated B16 cells, producing cytokines; and e) a very reduced number of transfected cells, selected by means of magnetic bead procedures. The results obtained show different rates of tumor growth inhibition - performance improving when adjusting the combinations of plasmid bearing the cytokine gene and TMP antigens in the lipopolyplexes. The best inhibition (total) was obtained with freshly transfected (not selected) cells, which allowed us to perform further experiments consisting of a vaccine with only the truly transfected (cytokine-producing) cells. On this occasion, reducing the cell number to only 20% that of the prior doses, the authors achieved about 80% of tumor growth inhibition. All these results encourage the conduction of further studies of this kind, with the purpose of increasing accuracy and optimizing cancer vaccine procedures.

Chapter VIII - The availability of human genome sequence has revolutionalized the ability of medical science to manipulate genes either by inducing or silencing specific gene expression which modulates many grave diseases and disorders including cancer. Vectors are being developed based on the capacity of polymers or lipids to mediate appropriate interactions with the cellular environment or to interface with specific cellular processes. Number of novel delivery strategies has been proposed to improve the efficiency of *in vivo* plasmid DNA or siRNA tansfection. However, only few of these strategies have been shown to enhance the expression of injected plasmid DNA or siRNA. Non-viral delivery methods, especially ones that focus on the use of biodegradable synthetic polymers represent the persistent future of polynucleotide based therapy. This chapter describes recent success of poly (β-amino ester)s (PAE)s as non-viral vectors and highlights their future in the development of polynucleotide based cancer therapy. Among non-viral vectors, PAEs received high attention owing to their safety and high transfection efficiency *in vitro* and *in vivo*. Ease of synthesis and efficient manipulation of physicochemical properties have made PAEs polymer of choice for gene delivery studies. Purpose of this chapter is to provide novel insight with respect to this type of gene delivery system. It primarily reports the chemical structure of frequently studied PAE backbones along with the classification on the basis of their chemical nature. Secondly, the influence on transfection by polymer backbones is described. Thirdly, important properties such as surface properties, molecular weight, dissociation and degradation, structural chemistry and charge density of polyplexes are considered. Fourthly, chapter highlights potential of PAEs in the siRNA delivery for cancer therapy and finally, chapter gives a very brief look at success of PAEs *in vivo* gene and siRNA delivery.

Chapter IX - Targeted therapy is a novel approach towards treatment of cancer either by improving drug delivery from the site of application into the tumour cell or by switching the site of the activation of a prodrug from the liver to the site of tumour growth, thereby enhancing the loco-regional anti tumour effect. Furthermore, regional application and activation of a prodrug allow a reduction of dosage of the prodrug and minimizes systemic distribution and thus systemic side effects of the drug.

Liposomes were among the first experimental carriers of cytotoxic agents. However, both doxorubicin-loaded streptavidin liposomes and 111In-DTPA-labelled pegylated liposomes failed to demonstrate a significant tumour-specific accumulation of active agents.

Nitrogen mustard N-Oxide dissolved in lipiodol was given in animals with metastatic VX2 tumours by simultaneous intra-arterial and intraperitoneal administration resulting in complete tumour remission in almost all rabbits. Antibodies too were employed for targeting peritoneal tumour either using specific cytotoxic monoclonal antibodies or by trying to impart site-specific alterations in the disposition of drug molecules using anti-drug antibodies.

Finally microencapsulated cells containing a prodrug converting enzyme (Capcell™) were introduced in 1998. These Capcell™ served as a site specific prodrug converter when administered intraperitoneally and have shown promising treatment results in experimental models of peritoneal cancer of pancreatic and colorectal origin and went further into clinical evaluation.

L293 cells were genetically modified to express the cytochrome P450 enzyme 2B1 under the control of a cytomegalovirus immediate early promoter. This CYP2B1 enzyme converts ifosfamide to its active cytotoxic compounds. The cells are encapsulated in a cellulose sulfate formulation. By using GFP-transfected colon 26 tumour cells in mice the authors established a well reproducible animal model of metastatic peritoneal cancer. Fluorescent imaging of GFP-transfected tumour was used to demonstrate tumour distribution in the peritoneal cavity and to estimate tumour growth and tumour response to treatment in this model. The application of Capcell™ and ifosfamide into the peritoneal cavity as a gene directed enzyme prodrug therapy is a safe and well tolerated procedure in animal models and may help to target chemotherapeutic agents specifically at metastatic peritoneal cancer.

Chapter X - Despite the important progress obtained in the treatment of many malignancies, the need to develop new treatments to fight cancer is compelling.

Artificially created tumor models can be useful in the early stages of basic and applied research. The laboratory controlled disease, based on heterotopically grafted tumors in genetically identical small rodents that usually are young and healthy at the beginning of the trial, usually differs from human cancer in patients that spontaneously contracted the disease. Such patients are genetically heterogeneous and predominantly aged people whose immune system failed in fighting against the disease. These disparate situations can explain the failure of the translation to the field of some successful trials conducted in the laboratory. On the other hand, millions of pet dogs and cats will have cancer diagnosed every year. In many of those animals, the malignancy will look and behave as much as it would in humans, spreading to the same organs. In this context, spontaneous tumors appearing in large animals (especially companion animals) could offer a unique opportunity for both: (i) to develop new therapies for inherent pathologies and (ii) as models for human cancer biology and translational cancer therapeutics. With a potentially large population of cases for investigation, veterinary clinical trials can be completed faster and at significantly lower expense than similar human clinical trials. The successful trials could be easily translated to humans being benefited both humans and animal patients.

This review discusses the outcomes of different assayed gene therapy approaches reported by many research centers on a variety of tumors such as melanoma, soft tissue sarcoma, fibrosarcoma and osteosarcoma, as well as the authors own experience on spontaneous canine and equine melanoma.

The encouraging results obtained by means of these spontaneous cancer models in large animals supports not only their ready application in veterinary clinical oncology, but also as preclinical proof of concept and safety assay for forthcoming human gene therapy trials.

In: New Gene Therapy and Cancer Research
Editor: Wilma B. Gustafsson, pp. 1-7

ISBN: 978-1-60021-969-6

Expert Commentary

CD40 Ligand-Based Cancer Therapy

Angelica Loskog[1] and Aristides G. Eliopoulos[2]
[1]Clinical Immunology Division, Uppsala University, Uppsala, Sweden;
[2]Molecular and Cellular Biology Laboratory, University of Crete Medical School, Heraklion, Greece.

Abstract

Immunotherapy of cancer has intrigued the scientific community ever since it became clear that the immune system could eradicate tumor cells. To gain full capacity of immunotherapy it is important to activate tumor-specific cytotoxic T lymphocytes (CTLs) and defeat the suppressive actions of regulatory T (Treg) cells present in the tumor microenvironment. In experimental models of cancer, CD40 ligand (CD40L)-based therapy has reached these two goals. In addition to its immunostimulatory properties, CD40L can trigger apoptosis of tumor cells by mechanisms that are now beginning to emerge. Because of its dual properties as an immune activator and apoptosis inducer, CD40L is an attractive candidate for cancer therapy. It is currently under evaluation for its effect on human cancer.

CD40 Ligand

The CD40 ligand (CD40L) is a member of the tumor necrosis factor (TNF) gene family and is expressed by a variety of cells including lymphoid, endothelial, and smooth muscle cells. However, it is the expression of CD40L on activated T helper (Th) cells of both Th1 and Th2 type that has been at major focus. CD40L binds to its receptor, CD40. Similar to CD40L, CD40 is expressed on a variety of lymphoid, endothelial, and smooth muscle cells but can also be found on fibroblasts, neuronal cells, keratinocytes and carcinomas [1]. CD40L submit signals as a single molecule but it is most potent as a trimer, binding to trimerized CD40. The action of CD40L-signaling depends on the interacting cell types and includes diverse events such as apoptosis, proliferation, differentiation, cytokine production, and Ig class switch [2]. Mutations in the CD40L gene cause hyper IgM conditions and reduced capacity to defeat infections. On the other hand, overexpression of CD40L has been associated with several autoimmune diseases [1]. If CD40L expression causes autoimmunity or is merely a symptom of disease remains unknown. Indeed, in disease models of cancer, CD40L therapy does not appear to induce autoimmunity [2].

Induction of Apoptosis in Tumor Cells via CD40 Stimulation

The ability of CD40L to trigger apoptosis is intriguing given the absence of 'death domain' sequences in the cytoplasmic tail of CD40. However, apoptosis may occur indirectly via induction of death ligands such as TNFα, Fas ligand (FasL) and TNF-related apoptosis-inducing ligand (TRAIL) in stimulated cells. These death ligands may then promote apoptosis in an autocrine/paracrine manner [3-5]. Importantly, it is malignant cells (mainly CD40-positive tumor cells of epithelial origin) and not normal cells that undergo CD40L-dependent apoptosis. It has been demonstrated that CD40-stimulation of normal B lymphocytes or urothelial cells induces the rapid downregulation of the CD40-interacting proteins TRAF2 and TRAF3 thereby 'dampening' signals which promote apoptosis [6-8]. In contrast, CD40-stimulation of the malignant counterparts does not downregulate TRAF expression but utilizes TRAF3 to transduce signals leading to inhibition of proliferation [9] and induction of apoptosis [6]. The aforementioned in vitro studies led to the evaluation of CD40L as an apoptosis-induction therapy for human tumors. In SCID mouse models xenotransplanted with human ovarian carcinoma, breast cancer, or multiple myeloma cells CD40L administration induced significant inhibition of tumor growth [10-12]. Similarly, SGN-40, a humanized α-CD40 agonistic antibody, has demonstrated potent anti-proliferative and pro-apoptotic effects on B cell lymphomas and is currently under evaluation in a phase I clinical trial [13,14]. CD40L therapy, however, largely depends on functional immune system for effective tumor eradication. In a syngeneic mouse bladder cancer model, CD40L therapy has been thoroughly investigated. CD40L cured aggressively growing tumors in these mice but in an immunodeficient model, the tumor growth was only delayed [15,16]. These data clearly demonstrate the importance of the engagement of the immune system in CD40L-mediated therapy. Apoptosis induction may also contribute to this effect through antigen presentation to tumor-specific T cells. Several strategies are under development to enhance apoptosis upon CD40-stimulation. It has been demonstrated, for example, that CD40 ligation results in the engagement of the anti-apoptotic PI3 kinase signaling pathway and that PI3 kinase inhibition sensitizes tumor cells to CD40L-induced apoptosis. PI3 kinase pathway inhibitors could therefore be interesting drugs to use in combination with CD40-directed tumor therapies. Moreover, strong synergy between CD40L administration and chemotherapeutic agents such as 5FU and cis-platin has been observed in vitro and in mouse tumor models [9,10,17].

CD40L-Stimulation of the Immune System

Platelets have been considered as cell fragments only important for blood clot formation during vessel damage. However, platelets release preformed CD40L molecules within seconds after stimulation at the site of injury [18]. Potential targets are antigen-engulfing tissue residing DCs that upon CD40-activation will differentiate into a mature stage and migrate to local lymph nodes for contact with lymphocytes. Hence, platelets are very important for the initiation of adaptive responses. Immature DCs have high capacity of engulfing antigens in their surroundings. They express low to medium levels of antigen presenting molecules e.g. the major histocompatibility complex (MHC) molecules I and II. They also express low amounts or lack expression of the costimulatory molecules CD80/86 and the cytokines IL1β, IL6, IL12, and IFNγ [19]. Upon CD40L/CD40 interaction, however, the DCs decrease their capacity for antigen uptake and up-regulate the antigen processing and presentation machinery. Thus, MHC I and II molecules as well as the costimulatory molecules CD80/CD86 increases on the cell surface. CCR7 is upregulated to ensure DC migration to lymph nodes [20]. The DCs will produce a variety of cytokines upon activation including IL1β, IL6, IL12 and IFNγ [19]. The T cells receive the so-called 'activation signal 1' via MHC interactions with the T cell receptor (TcR) and 'signal 2' via costimulation (B7/CD28) and CD40/CD40L interactions. The first signal provides activation of antigen-specific T cells. Without costimulation, the antigen-stimulated T cells would undergo anergy or even apoptosis [21]. Continuous CD40-stimulation of the DCs will prolong their IL12 producing phase and, hence, their capacity to drive Th1 type responses [2]. IL12 enhances activation of both T cells and NK cells which produce IFNγ. Release of IFNγ will in turn promote MHC-I upregulation on target cells and enhance the activation of macrophages that will participate as effector cells in the Th1 response. Although B lymphocytes (Th2 response) are dependent on CD40 for full differentiation, Ig-class switch and proliferation, they do not appear to significantly participate in the anti-tumor effects of CD40L [2].

The CD40L/Tumor Cycle

The role of CD40L in tumor therapy is multifaceted (Figure 1). First, engagement of CD40 can directly trigger apoptosis and inhibition of proliferation in CD40-positive tumor cells. Apoptosis induction may also enhance uptake of tumor material by DCs. CD40-activation of DCs dramatically enhances tumor antigen presentation and costimulation to CTLs. CD40L may also upregulate MHC-I, B7, and death receptors such as Fas and TNFR on the tumor cell surface [19,22], thus enhancing their recognition and killing by tumor-specific CTLs. CD40L-based therapies have shown potent effects in various murine models of cancer including neuroblastoma, mastocytoma, fibrosarcoma, colon,, ovarian, lung, prostate and bladder cancer, malignant melanoma, myeloma and pre-B lymphoma [2]. The main effector mechanism has shown to be dependent on a functional specific immune system as discussed above. Cell depletion studies have shown that CTLs are crucial for the effects of CD40L administration on tumor cell lysis and memory induction. In an orthotopic bladder cancer model, immunosuppressive regulatory T cells (Treg) were present in the tumors of

CD40L treated as well as control treated mice. However, the number of Treg in lymph nodes was decreased upon CD40L therapy. Further, T cells from these mice were not able to inhibit proliferation of T cells from naïve mice as opposed to T cells from control treated, tumor-bearing mice. CD40L therapy may, hence, both activate the immune system as well as play a key role in the inhibition of Treg cells [15].

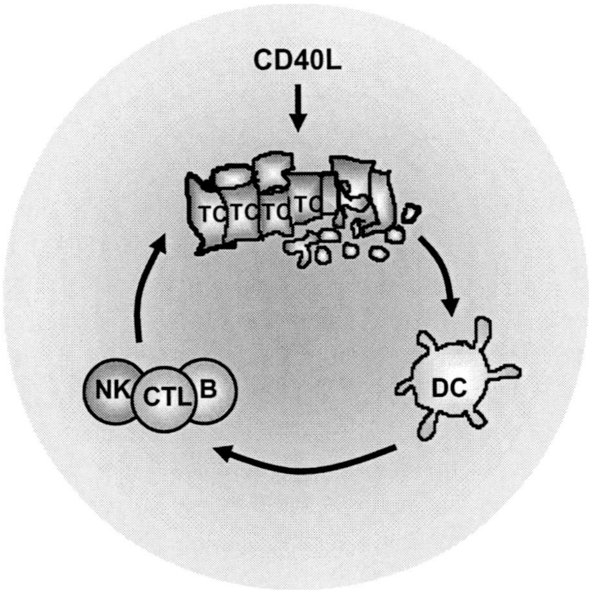

Figure 1. The CD40L/tumor cycle. CD40L therapy of tumors will induce apoptosis of CD40+ tumor cells (TC). This will enhance antigen uptake by DCs. CD40L will also stimulate the DCs to mature, migrate to lymph nodes and activate immune cells to mount responses against the tumor. Upon CD40L-stimulation, tumor cells may enhance their expression of MHC-I and death receptors making them better targets for CTLs.

CD40L in Clinical Cancer Trials

Soluble trimerized CD40L has been investigated in 32 patients with advanced solid tumors including renal cell carcinoma, head and neck cancer, cervical cancer, sarcoma, rectal carcinoma, esophageal carcinoma, breast carcinoma, peritoneal carcinomatosis, adenocarcinoma (unknown primary tumor) and non-Hodgkin's lymphoma. Patients received daily subcutaneous injections for 5 days/dose. Toxicity, maximum tolerated dose (MTD) and pharmacokinetics were evaluated. In one patient with breast carcinoma, grade 4 elevations of hepatic transaminases (AST, ALT) were seen. Otherwise, only a few cases of anemia (not dose dependent), neutropenia, lymphopenia and pain were observed. Dyspnea, asthenia, dyspepsia and pneumonia were seen in one patient each at the MTD level. Two patients had partial responses. Twelve patients had stable disease, however, only 6 of them remained stable during the final two treatment courses [23].

Two studies have been done on B cell chronic lymphocytic leukemia (B-CLL). In the first study, 11 patients were infused with their own ex vivo treated (AdCD40L gene transfer) B-CLL cells. No dose-limiting toxicity was seen in these patients. However, general flu-like symptoms were seen such as fever, fatigue, arthralgia, myalgia, nausea and anorexia by 12 hours post infusion. Less common adverse reactions included headache, edema, dehydration and diarrhea. In a few patients increased, but transient, levels of transaminases were seen. All abnormalities resolved within a few days post treatment. As expected, IL12 and IFNγ were increased upon treatment demonstrating Th1 responses and their importance as biological markers of CD40L therapy. Most patients demonstrated decreased lymphocyte numbers (>97% were B-CLL cell prior therapy) and lymph node size post treatment. The effect could be sustained weeks to months after treatment [24]. In the second study on B-CLL, 9 patients received 3-8 subcutaneous vaccinations with cells activated by IL2 and CD40L gene therapy. Local pain, redness and swelling were observed at the vaccination site. In this study, no hepatic dysfunction was observed. A third of the patients had >50% decrease in lymph node size at 6-week evaluation. This effect was not sustained longer than 12 weeks [25].

Adenovirus-mediated CD40L therapy is currently under evaluation for bladder cancer in humans and malignant melanoma in dogs, both studies taking place at Uppsala University in Sweden.

Conclusions

The anti-tumor effects of CD40L are intriguing. The mechanism by which CD40 activation exerts these effects includes inhibition of tumor cell proliferation, induction of apoptosis, sensitization to other anti-cancer agents and stimulation of potent anti-tumor immune responses. Apoptosis induced by CD40L in CD40-positive carcinomas not only directly reduce tumor burden, but also increase antigen uptake and presentation by dendritic cells, thereby amplifying CTL and NK cell responses. Despite the theoretical risk of autoimmunity by this potent immune activator, no such adverse effect has been observed in experimental animal models or in phase-I/II clinical trials in humans. The absence of severe side-effects further supports the therapeutical potential of CD40L for the treatment of cancer. This potential is currently under evaluation in phase I clinical trials.

Acknowledgments

Research in the authors' laboratory is funded by the European Commission grant 'Apotherapy' (contract no 037344) to A.L and A.G.E, and by an Association for International Cancer Research (AICR, UK) grant to A.G.E.

References

[1] Schönbeck, U., & Libby, P. (2001) The CD40/CD154 receptor/ligand dyad. *Cell. Mol. Life Sci., 58*, 4-43.

[2] Loskog, A., & Tötterman, T.H. (2007) CD40L – a multipotent moleculer for tumor therapy. *Endocr Metab Immune Disord Drug Targets. 7*,23-8.

[3] Grell, M., Zimmermann, G., Gottfried, E., Chen, C.M., Grunwald, U., Huang, D.C., Wu Lee, Y.H., Durkop, H., Engelmann, H., Scheurich, P., Wajant, H., & Strasser, A. (1999) Induction of cell death by tumour necrosis factor (TNF) receptor 2, CD40 and CD30: a role for TNF-R1 activation by endogenous membrane-anchored TNF. *EMBO J. 18*, 3034-3043.

[4] Eliopoulos, A.G., Davies, C., Knox, P.G., Gallagher, N.J., Afford, S.C., Adams, D.H., & Young, L.S. (2000) CD40 induces apoptosis in carcinoma cells through activation of cytotoxic ligands of the tumor necrosis factor superfamily. M*ol. Cell. Biol. 20*, 5503-5515.

[5] Afford, S.C., Ahmed-Choudhury, J., Randhawa, S., Russell, C., Youster, J., Crosby, H.A., Eliopoulos, A., Hubscher, S.G., Young, L.S., & Adams, D.H. (2001) CD40 activation-induced, Fas-dependent apoptosis and NF-kappaB/AP-1 signaling in human intrahepatic biliary epithelial cells. *FASEB J. 15*, 2345-2354.

[6] Georgopoulos, N.T., Steele, L.P., Thomson, M.J., Selby, P.J., Southgate, J., & Trejdosiewicz L.K. (2006) A novel mechanism of CD40-induced apoptosis of carcinoma cells involving TRAF3 and JNK/AP-1 activation. *Cell. Death. Differ. 13*, 1564-1576.

[7] Grech, A.P., Amesbury, M., Chan, T., Gardam, S., Basten, A., & Brink, R. (2004) TRAF2 differentially regulates the canonical and noncanonical pathways of NF-kappaB activation in mature B cells. *Immunity. 21*, 629-642.

[8] Hostager, B.S., Haxhinasto, S.A., Rowland, S.L., & Bishop, G.A. (2003) Tumor necrosis factor receptor-associated factor 2 (TRAF2)-deficient B lymphocytes reveal novel roles for TRAF2 in CD40 signaling. *J. Biol. Chem. 278*, 45382-45390.

[9] Eliopoulos, A.G., Dawson, C.W, Mosialos, G., Floettmann, J.E., Rowe, M., Armitage, R.J., Dawson, J., Zapata, J.M., Kerr, D.J., Wakelam, M.J., Reed, J.C., Kieff, E., & Young, L.S. (1996) CD40-induced growth inhibition in epithelial cells is mimicked by Epstein-Barr virus-encoded LMP1: Involvement of TRAF3 as a common mediator. *Oncogene 13*: 2243-2254.

[10]Ghamande, S., Hylander, B.L., Oflazoglu, E., Lele, S., Fanslow, W., & Repasky, E.A. (2001) Recombinant CD40 ligand therapy has significant antitumor effects on CD40-positive ovarian tumor xenografts grown in SCID mice and demonstrates an augmented effect with cisplatin. *Cancer Res. 61*:7556-7562.

[11]Tong, A.W., Papayoti, M.H., Netto, G., Armstrong, D.T, Ordonez, G., Lawson, J.M., & Stone, M.J. (2001) Growth-inhibitory effects of CD40 ligand (CD154) and its endogenous expression in human breast cancer. *Clin Cancer Res. 7*:691-703.

[12]Tong, A.W., Seamour, B., Chen, J., Su, D., Ordonez, G., Frase, L., Netto, G., & Stone, M.J. (2000) CD40 ligand-induced apoptosis is Fas-independent in human multiple myeloma cells. *Leuk Lymphoma. 36:*543-558.

[13]Law, C.L., Gordon, K.A., Collier, J., Klussman, K., McEarchern, J.A., Cerveny, C.G., Mixan, B.J., Lee, W.P., Lin, Z., Valdez, P., Wahl, A.F., & Grewal, I.S. (2005) Preclinical antilymphoma activity of a humanized anti-CD40 monoclonal antibody, SGN-40. *Cancer Res. 65*:8331-8338.

[14]Kelley, S.K., Gelzleichter, T., Xie, D., Lee, W.P., Darbonne, W.C., Qureshi, F., Kissler, K., Oflazoglu, E., & Grewal, I.S. (2006) Preclinical pharmacokinetics, pharmacodynamics, and activity of a humanized anti-CD40 antibody (SGN-40) in rodents and non-human primates. *Br J Pharmacol. 148*:1116-1123.

[15]Loskog, A.S.I, Fransson, M.E., & Tötterman, T.H. (2005) AdCD40L gene therapy counteracts T regulatory cells and cures aggressive tumors in an orthotopic bladder cancer model. *Clin. Cancer Res. 11*, 8816-8821.

[16]Loskog, A., Totterman, T.H., Bohle, A., & Brandau, S. (2002) In vitro activation of cancer patient-derived dendritic cells by tumor cells genetically modified to express CD154. *Cancer Gene Ther 9*, 846-853.

[17]Davies C.C., Mason, J., Wakelam, M.J, Young, L.S. & Eliopoulos, A.G. (2004) Inhibition of phosphatidylinositol 3 kinase and ERK MAPK regulated protein synthesis reveals the pro-apoptotic properties of CD40 ligation in carcinoma cells. *J. Biol. Chem. 279*: 1010-1019.

[18]Elzey, B.D., Sprague, D.L., & Ratliff, T.L (2005) The emerging role of platelets in adaptive immunity. *Cell Immunol 238*, 1-9.

[19]Loskog, A., Ninalga, C., & Tötterman, T.H. (2006) Dendritic cells engineered to express CD40L continuously produce IL12 and resist negative signals from Tr1/Th3 dominated tumors. *Cancer Immunol. Immunother 55*, 588-597.

[20]Hill, S.C., Youde, S.J., Man, S., Teale, G.R., Baxendale, A.J., Hislop, A., Davies, C.C., Luesley, D.M., Blom, A.M., Rickinson, A.B., Young, L.S., & Eliopoulos, A.G. (2005) Activation of CD40 in cervical carcinoma cells facilitates CTL responses and augments chemotherapy-induced apoptosis. *J Immunol. 174*: 41-50.

[21]Del Prete, A., Shao, W.H., Mitola, S., Santoro, G., Sozzani, S., & Haribabu, B. (2007) Regulation of dendritic cell migration and adaptive immune response by leukotriene B4 receptors: a role for LTB4 in up-regulation of CCR7 expression and function. *Blood 109*, 626-631.

[22]Appleman, L.J., Tzachanis, D., Grader-Beck, T., van Puijenbroek, A.A., & Boussiotis, V.A. (2001) Helper T cell anergy: from biochemistry to cancer pathophysiology and therapeutics. *J Mol Med 78*, 673-683.

[23]Vonderheide, R.H., Dutcher, J.P., Anderson, J.E., Eckhardt, G.S., Stephans, K.F., Razvillas, B., Garl, S., Butine, M.D., Perry, V.P., Armitage, R.J., Ghalie, R., Caron, D.A., & Gribben, J.G. (2001) Phase I study of recombinant human CD40 ligand in cancer patients *J. Clin. Oncol 19*, 3280-3287.

[24]Wierda, W.G., Cantwell, M.J., Woods, S.J., Rassenti, L.Z., Prussak, C.E., & Kipps, T.J. (2000) CD40-ligand (CD154) gene therapy for chronic lymphocytic leukemia. *Blood 96*, 2917-2924.

[25]Biagi, E., Rousseau, R., Yvon, E., Schwartz, M., Dotti, G., Foster, A., Havlik-Cooper, D., Grilley, B., Gee, A., Baker, K., Carrum, G., Rice, L., Adreeff, M., Popat, U., & Brenner, M. (2005) Responses to human CD40 ligand/human interleukin-2 autologous cell vaccine in patients with B-cell chronic lymphocytic leukemia. *Clin. Cancer Res 11*, 6916-6923.

In: New Gene Therapy and Cancer Research
Editor: Wilma B. Gustafsson, pp. 9-66
ISBN: 978-1-60021-969-6

Chapter I

NEW TRENDS IN GENE THERAPY FOR BREAST CANCER

J. Prados[1,], C. Melguizo[2], R. Ortiz[1], H. Boulaiz[1], E. Carrillo[1], J. A. Marchal[1], C. Vélez[3], A. R. Rama[1], F. Rodríguez-Serrano[3], O. Caba[3], A. Mártinez[3], F. Hita[3], M. Peran[3], R. Madeddu[4] and A. Aránega[1]

[1]Biopathology and Medicine Regenerative Institute (IBIMER), Department of Human Anatomy and Embriology, School of Medicine, University of Granada, Granada E-18071, Spain;
[2]Department of Health Sciences, University of Almería, Almería E-04002, Spain;
[3]Department of Health Sciences, University of Jaén, Jaén E-23071, Spain;
[4]Department of Biomedical Science, University of Sassary, Sassary 07100, Italy.

ABSTRACT

Breast cancer research has developed at a rapid pace over the past few decades, leading to longer survival times for breast cancer patients and opening up the possibility of developing curative treatments for advanced breast cancer. Hopes for individualized treatments have been raised by recent discoveries related to the cancer multistep process, characterized by genetic alterations of normal host cells and by non-genetic changes in the behaviors of malignant cells and of host cells interacting with the tumor. While most subsequent changes may result in cell death, some can affect key genes involved in cell survival, proliferation, invasiveness, motility, drug resistance and other malignant characteristics. Our increasing knowledge of the specific proteins, genes and biological pathways associated with the progression and development of breast cancer, alongside the failure of conventional treatments, has prompted us to explore gene therapy as an alternative therapeutic strategy. In this review, we summarize trends in the different approaches to breast cancer treatment, classified as: 1. Corrective gene therapy, which aims to restore normal function of a deleted or mutated gene; 2. Proapoptotic gene therapy, in which restoration or enhancement of the capacity to undergo apoptosis may be a crucial event, rendering tumors sensitive to classical anticancer agents; 3. Immunomodulatory gene therapy, in which gene delivery to tumor or normal tissue enhances the ability of the immune system to mount an effective cytotoxic response; 4. Genetic modulation of resistance or sensitivity, since conventional therapy fails in many breast cancer patients because their tumours are resistant to DNA-damaging agents, e.g., chemotherapy; 5. antiangiogenic gene therapy to block tumor growth through regression of neovascularisation, and 6. Suicide gene therapy, in which delivery of an exogenous gene results in cancer cell death. These genes may express a toxic molecule that affects cellular viability or express enzymes that selectively activate specific prodrugs. Gene therapy is expected to play an increasing role in clinical breast cancer treatment, and combined modality therapy with gene therapy and chemotherapy or radiation therapy has already shown promising results.

Keywords: breast cancer, gene therapy, RNAi, immunotherapy, apoptosis, resistance chemotherapy, suicide gene, angiogenesis.

INTRODUCTION

Breast cancer represents the most common tumor of females in many industrialized countries (O'Shaughnessy, 2005). Breast cancer is the first cause of death by neoplasia among women and represents nearly 25% of non-accidental deaths of 35 to 54-yr-old females (Ursin et al., 1997). The frequency of breast cancer increases with age until menopause, after which it continues to rise but at a slower rate (Guinee, 2000).

Although breast cancer has long been considered a single entity with a common management and treatment, it is actually an extremely heterogeneous disease. Classically, human breast carcinoma has been classified for therapeutic purposes into two distinct categories: hormone-correlated and hormone-uncorrelated. Recent advances in the application of genomic and proteomic analyses to molecular biology have revealed that many more factors may be involved in breast cancer growth and progression and that some clusters of these factors can distinguish subgroups of patients with different prognoses. From a biological point of view, breast cancer is correlated with multiple histopathological forms, growth rates, variations in metastatic capacity, and responses to hormonal therapy. All of these variations are a reflection (phenotype) of numerous genomic modifications that take place during tumor transformation (Szyf et al., 2004; Hodgson et al., 2004). Uncontrolled cellular proliferation and/or apoptosis can lead to breast cancer as a consequence of the accumulation of genetic lesions, giving rise to alterations that activate protooncogenes and inactivate tumor suppressor genes (Green and Streuli, 2004). Genetic alterations may be inherited, e.g., germline mutations or as somatic mutations acquired by exposure to environmental carcinogens. The hormonal (especially estrogenic) factor plays a major role in breast cancer genesis. Estrogens act as promoters or inductors of breast cancer only when malignant transformation has started (Jones and Buzdar, 2004; Guinee, 2000).

The etiology of breast cancer includes a heterogeneous and complex set of genetic alterations: amplifications, deletions and gene mutations of the previously kind of genes can all take place in the genome of breast cancer. Mutated or inactivated *p53* is present in approximately 50% of metastatic breast cancer case and is related to a poor prognosis, even in patients with negative lymph nodes. The level of its expression is also elevated in preinvasive cancerous lesions, indicating that this antioncogene is inactivated in early stages of breast oncogenesis. *p53* is located in chromosome 17p13 and encodes p53, a 53 Kea nuclear protein that is present in its wild form at very low concentrations and plays an important role in tumor suppression by controlling transcription, cell cycle, and apoptosis (Vogelstein et al., 2000; Vousden and Lu, 2002). Levels of p53 protein are downregulated by the binding of proteins that promote p53 degradation via the ubiquitin/proteasome pathway, e.g., MDM2, COP1, PIRH2 or JNK. Because most of these genes are upregulated by p53, this leads to a regulation loop that maintains a very low level of p53 in normal cells. *p53* activation is a two-step process that starts after genotoxic or non-genotoxic stresses. First, p53 protein level is increased by inhibition of its interaction with negative regulators, e.g., *mdm2*. Overtranslation of p53 RNA is a complementary mechanism that ensures p53 accumulation. Second, various modulators (kinases, acetylases) activate *p53* transcriptional activity. A plethora of proteins have been found to bind various regions of p53 in order to regulate the specificity of its activity (Toledo and Wahl, 2006). The transactivating properties of p53 are responsible for downstream signaling, which includes a large series of genes. The p53 protein specifically binds to the DNA of the p53 response element (p53 RE), located either in the promoter or in the intron of target genes (El-Deiry, 2003; Tokino and Nakamura, 2000). The mechanism leading to the choice between either cell cycle arrest and DNA repair or apoptosis has not yet been elucidated but is independent of the type of stress that activates p53 (Vousden and Lu, 2002) (Figure 1). The various p53 pathways have been divided into five parts by Levine et al. (2006): 1) Stress signals that activate the p53 pathway. 2) Upstream mediators that detect and interpret upstream signals. 3) Core regulation of p53 via its interaction with several proteins that modulate its stability. 4) Downstream events, mainly transcriptional activation or protein-protein interactions. 5) Final outcome: growth arrest, apoptosis, or DNA repair. There is a risk of an accumulation of genomic instability and mutations in other genes due to the failure of *p53* normal function. Li-Fraumeni syndrome patients showed germline mutations and a higher risk of several cancer types, including breast cancer (Royds and Iacopetta, 2006).

On the other hand, both *BRCA1* and *BRCA2* are tumor suppressor genes involved in breast, ovarian, and prostate cancers (Levy-Lahad and Friedman, 2007) and are responsible for 40-45% of familial breast cancer (Rosen et al., 2003). *BRCA1* gene is located at 17q21 and encodes for an 1863 amino acid protein involved in DNA repair, transcriptional transactivation, cell cycle control, and apoptosis. This gene binds to several regulating proteins, including DNA repair protein Rad 51, tumor suppressor gene p53, c-myc, BRCA1-associated RING domain protein (BARD1), RNA polymerase II holoenzyme, RNA helicase A, CtBP-interacting protein, and BRCA2 protein (Rosen et al., 2006) (Figure 2). BRCA1 also associates with E2F, cyclins, and cyclin dependent kinases, suggesting that may be an important negative regulator of cell cycle via interaction with E2F transcriptional factors and phosphorylation by cyclins/cdk complexes (Mullan et al., 2006). *BRCA2* is another highly penetrant autosomal dominant susceptibility gene responsible for familial breast cancer susceptibility. This gene located at chromosome 13q12-13 and encodes for 3418 amino acids and 26 coding exons. The BRCA2 protein plays a role in transcriptional regulation and DNA repair *via* its amino terminal third exon. BRCA2 also has intrinsic HAT activity, which maps at its aminoterminal region, and acetylates primarily H3 and H4 of free histones, suggesting that HAT activity of BRCA2 may play a major in transcription regulation and tumor suppressor functions.

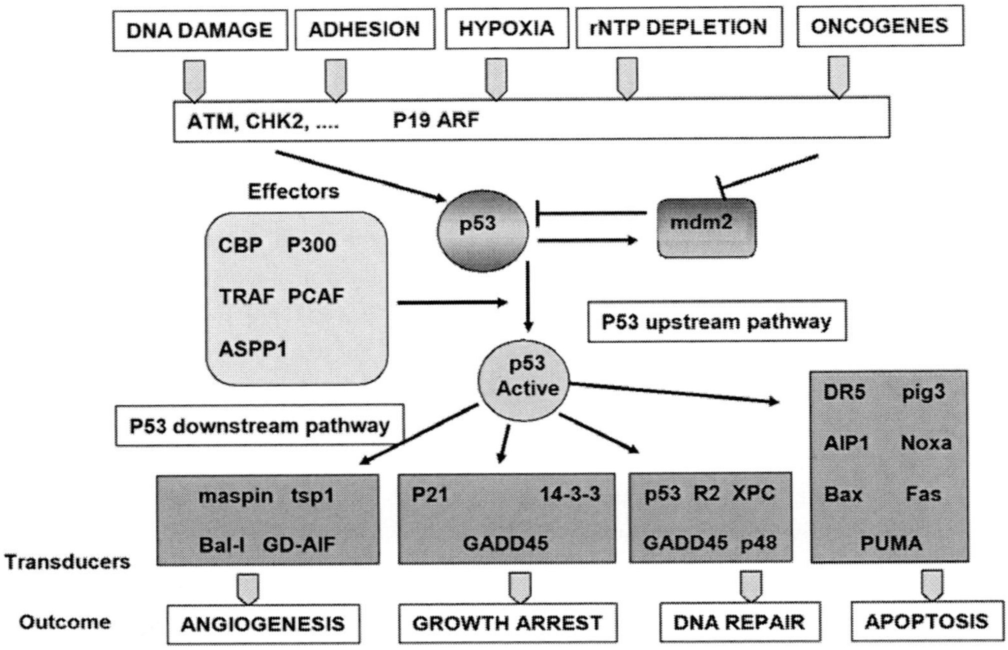

Figure 1. A simplified model of some of the p53 components upstream and downstream pathway. Under normal conditions, p53 pathway operates on 'standby' mode. Activation occurs in response to a variety of cellular stresses such as DNA damage, adhesion, hypoxia, rNTP depletion and expression of activated oncogenes. Post-translational modifications (such as phosphorylation) activate the protein for DNA binding. Some transcriptional coactivators may promote specific cellular responses such as apoptosis, angiogenesis, growth arrest and DNA repair. MDM2 acts as a negative feedback regulator of the pathway by promoting the degradation of p53. Other important constituents of the pathway have been omitted.

The ataxia-telangiectasia mutated gene (*ATM* gene) is located at 11q22–23 and encodes a 350 kDa amino acid protein. ATM belongs to a family of proteins involved in cell cycle control and DNA-damage recognition. The mechanism of ATM activation involves a modification in response to a post-irradiation alteration in chromatin structure (Shiloh, 2003). These proteins then phosphorylate several substrates (including p53) in response to DNA damage and activate radiation signal transduction pathways and/or recruit proteins to sites of DNA repair (Khanna and Chenevix-Trench, 2004). It has been shown that ATM is also involved directly in the regulation of the breast cancer gene product BRCA1 (Ahmed and Rahman, 2006). At ATM, a leucine zipper consensus sequence can also be found in the N-terminus, although there is no clear-cut evidence that this motif is responsible for the interaction of ATM with itself or with other proteins. There is also a praline-rich region that is a site for interaction with c-Abl, which could act as a positive regulator of p53 by relieving the inhibitory effect of the mdm2 protein (Shafman et al., 1997). ATM is also required for c-Abl-mediated assembly of the Rad51 repair protein complex after ionizing radiation. c-Abl directly phosphorylates Rad51, resulting in an enhanced association between Rad51 and Rad52 that may lead to DNA repair (Morrison et al., 2000).

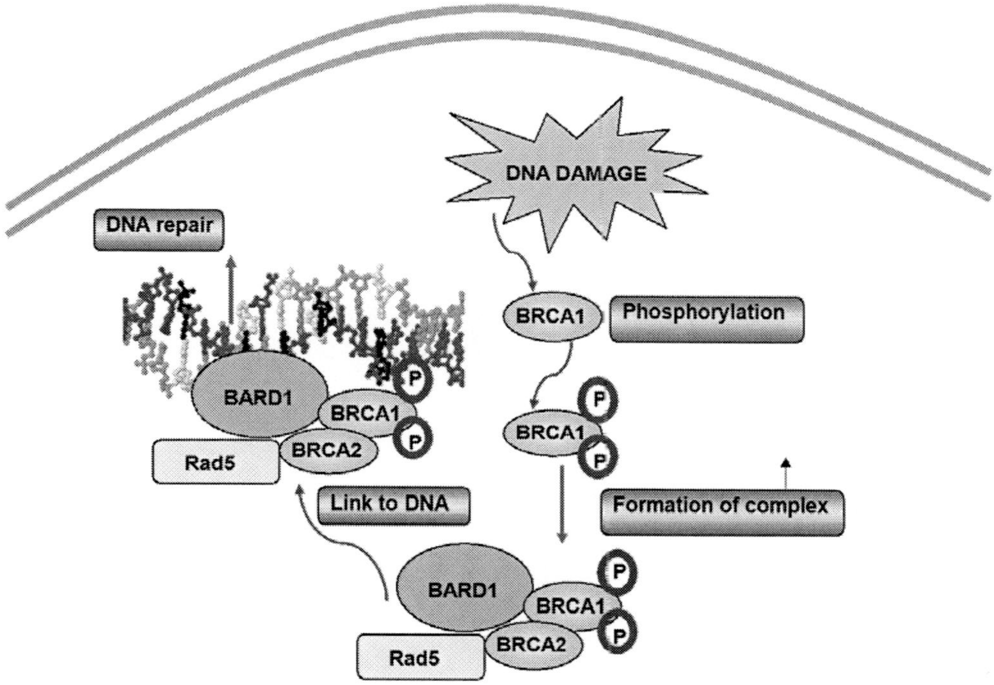

Figure 2. BCRA1 and BCRA2 function through its interaction with several proteins. In response to DNA damage and after the phosphorylation of BRCA1, a macromolecular complex consisting of BRCA1, BRCA2, BARD1 and Rad51 functions to repair DNA.

The estrogen receptor gene (*ESR*) contributes to the development of the top five cancers of women (Service, 1998). The primary role of ESR is to regulate the transcription rate of certain genes by binding as a hormone receptor complex to specific sequences of DNA designated hormone response elements (HREs). This interaction results in the up- or down-regulation of transcription, depending on the action of specific auxiliary factors (Bjornstrom and Sjoberg, 2005). The pathological function of variant ESR remains unclear. It has been suggested that it contributes to hormone resistance but there is no direct association (Hudelist et al., 2003) and studies of ESR germ-line mutations have not supported this hypothesis. Therefore, certain mutations in ESR appear to have little relevance in *in vivo* models (Anderson et al., 1997), although they have shown large effects in some breast cancer models.

Finally, PTEN is a phosphatase that echibits high homology with tensin. Mapped on human chromosome 10q23, its target is not a protein but a lipid tucked into the cell membrane. The target lipid is phosphatidylinositol-3,4,5-triphosphate (PIP3), a key component that stimulates cell growth and blocks apoptosis. PTEN loss maintains the PIP3 pathway activated, allowing the uncontrolled growth of mutated cells (Sansal and Sellers,

2004). Somatic mutations in *PTEN* gene are rare in breast tumors (Petrocelli and Slingerland, 2001), whereas germline mutations predispose to this type of cancer in association with Cowden disease (Liaw et al., 1997).

Extensive research currently under way in molecular biology and pathology and cancer genomics and proteomics will hopefully contribute to further elucidation of all genetic and environmental factors involved in the development, differentiation, and involution of the mammary gland. This may afford insights into the etiopathogenesis, early detection, potential prevention and treatment of breast cancer. The limited success of available treatment modalities for breast cancer means that new strategies need to be developed, and the possibility of modifying the breast cancer cell by the introduction of genetic material opens the way to a new approach based on gene therapy. In recent years, various gene therapy approaches to breast carcinoma have been developed, including corrective and propaoptotic gene therapy, immunomodulatory gene therapy, genetic modulation of resistance or sensitivity, antiangiogenic gene therapy, and suicide gene therapy. Initial clinical trials in breast cancer on the use of a combined approach, i.e., gene therapy with chemotherapy or radiation, have shown promising results.

Corrective and Proapoptotic Gene Therapy

Ablation of Gene Function using RNAi and Antisense Molecules

Knowledge of molecular mechanisms in breast cancer opens up the possibility of specific interventions using gene therapy. As commented above, there is a need for gene-therapy approaches to complement classical therapies, which have had only limited success. The use of RNAi and antisense oligonucleotides may modulate dysregulated genes altered by mutation, gene amplification, gene rearrangement or overexpression, which contribute to oncogenesis by removing controls on normal cell cycle regulation. However, these systems must be evaluated in *in vivo* and *in vitro* studies to determine their applicability in breast cancer.

RNAi Therapy in Breast Cancer

Since its discovery in 1998 (Fire et al., 1998), RNA interference has emerged as a powerful "gene-silencing" technique. RNA interference (RNAi) is a biological process, in which double-stranded RNA inhibits gene expression in a highly specific fashion similar to or better than antisense sequences. dsRNAs induce specific degradation of the target mRNA. Since this process takes place after the transcription of DNA, it is known as post-transcriptional gene silencing (PTGS). It has been shown that this mechanism works in almost all higher organisms and is therefore thought to be a natural regulatory system in cells for protection against viral attacks. RNAi is initiated by an enzyme called Dicer, which cuts long double-stranded RNA molecules into dsRNA duplexes consisting of 21 to 23 nucleotides with 3'-overhangs of two or three nucleotides. These molecules are subsequently incorporated into the RNA-induced silencing complex (RISC), which must be activated from its latent form to the activated state of RISC. The single-stranded antisense strand then presumably guides RISC to its target mRNA (Tuschl et al., 1999), cutting the m-RNA at the complementary segment. The cut mRNA is very unstable and rapidly breaks down, thereby inhibiting the expression of a specific gene (Figure 3).

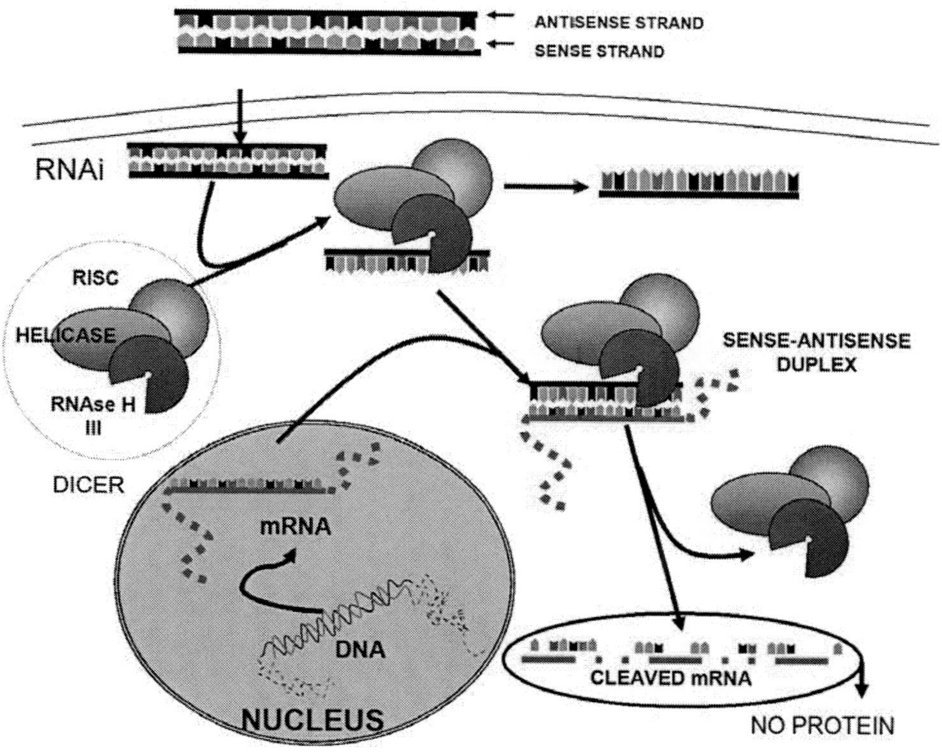

Figure 3. RNAi mechanism of action. RNAi is transported across the plasma membrane. Once in the cytoplasm, the double-stranded RNA oligonucleotide is recognized and bound by a protein complex termed RISC. A helicase activity unwinds the two RNA strands and facilitates binding of the antisense strand to the target RNA. Once bound to the target RNA, a ribonuclease cleaves the targeted RNA.

Breast Cancer-Related Genes as a Potential Targets for RNAi

Protein tyrosine kinase (PTK) receptor is an important intracellular signal transduction regulator in which mutations occur frequently. Hence, genes related to this pathway (*Her2*, *c-myc*, *cyclin D1*, etc) are good targets for RNAi. Studies on the breast cancer cell line SKBR-3 showed that Her2 iRNA, alone or in combination with anthracycline, could suppress cellular growth *in vitro* and *in vivo* (Hu et al., 2006). Similar results were obtained in MCF-7 cells with the c-myc RNAi. This oncogene has a pivotal function in breast cancer. A decrease in the level of c-Myc protein may significantly inhibit tumor growth and be a potential therapeutic target in human breast cancer (Wang et al., 2005). Molecules related to p53 pathways are others possible targets. Recent studies (Grillo et al., 2006) showed that inhibition of endogenous cyclin D1 or CDK4 expression by RNAi resulted in hypophosphorylation of the Rb gene and accumulation of cells in G1. These results support the prevailing view that pharmacological inhibition of cyclin D1/CDK4 complexes is a useful strategy to inhibit tumor growth.

On the other hand, terminal ends of linear chromosomes are organized into telomeres to prevent their recognition as DNA breaks (Patry et al., 2003). During successive cycles of DNA replication, telomere repeats are continuously shortened, and the synthesis of new repeats by telomerase is required to prevent cellular senescence. Although telomerase levels are usually very low in normal, slowly dividing cells, telomere length in rapidly dividing human cancers is maintained by elevated levels of telomerase. Chang et al. (2007) demonstrated detection and knockdown telomerase expression in human breast cancer cells mediating RNAi. This offers a new approach to RNAi target validation that is not currently possible in live cells and holds promising potential for biological applications in therapy based on mRNA expression. Id1, a member of the Id family of helix–loop–helix transcriptional regulatory proteins, is implicated in cellular senescence and can suppress p16 (INK4a) expression. Suppression of Id1 expression in breast cancer cells by RNAi resulted in downregulation inhibition of c-Myc level and premature cellular senescence (Swarbrick et al., 2005). Tang et al. (2005) demonstrated that inhibition of β-TrCP (related to proteosome pathway) by RNAi suppresses growth of human breast cancer cells and increases the antiproliferative effects of anticancer drugs such as doxorubicin, tamoxifen, and paclitaxel on human mammary tumor cells.

Another possible use of RNAi technology is to target the molecules involved in angiogenesis, invasion/metastasis, and immune evasion and resistance. Wang et al. (2006) showed that RNAi for HIF-1-α (an anti-apoptotic protein) can promote cell apoptosis, inhibit VEGF expression, and delay cell cycle progression in MCF-7. Some experiments on the RNAi targeting of molecules related to tumor cell mobility, e.g., CXC chemokine receptor 4 (CXCR4), found a decrease in MDA-MB-231 breast cancer cell expansion (Lapteva et al., 2004). Direct injection of a pool of RNAi targeting CXCR4 prevented tumorigenesis of a breast cancer cell line in an animal model (Liang et al., 2005). Therefore, RNAi targeting of CXCR4 may represent a potentially novel preventive and therapeutic strategy for breast cancer management. In relation to metastasis, silencing epithelial adhesion molecule (EpCAM) gene expression with RNAi decreased cell proliferation in several different breast cancer cell lines due to involvement of this glycoprotein in intercellular adhesion (Osta et al., 2004). Finally, genes that encode the multidrug-resistance protein are another possible target for RNAi action. In fact, RNAi against the breast cancer resistance protein (BCRP), which confers resistance to various anticancer drugs like mitoxantrone, may be effective in reversing resistance in breast cancer and has shown promise in therapeutic applications (Lv et al., 2007). Although a number of important breast oncogenic targets have been identified and RNAi-mediated gene silencing of these targets has produced favorable effects *in vitro* and in preclinical animal models, the translation of these findings to the more complex clinical arena remains a formidable challenge. RNAi therapy probably has a clinical role in conjunction with chemotherapy, radiotherapy and/or immunotherapy.

RNAi In Vivo Application: Problems and Perspectives

The main obstacle for the application of RNAi technology in the clinical setting remains the efficient delivery of these small molecules to the targeted cell. The RNAi used for gene silencing in cancer can derive from dsRNA, DNA vectors, or viral vectors. The efficacy of the direct introduction of chemically synthesized RNAis into cells is limited by the following factors: 1) the short-lived nature of their transient gene silencing effects, 2) their instability (extracellular degradation occurs at around 36–48 h), and 3) the duration of gene silencing in tumor cells (at around 3 days for approximately 1 week). In order to overcome this last limitation RNAis can be coupled with fusogenic peptides, linked to antibodies to cell surface receptor ligands for cell-specific delivery, or encased in lipid complexes, cationic liposomes or other types of particles (Shankar et al., 2005). The transient action of RNAi may also be avoided by using vectors that constitutively express RNAi (Shi, 2003). An interesting advance is the generation of plasmids that allow inducible expression of shRNA with the tetracycline operator (Czauderna et al., 2003). However, efficient and stable silencing has most effectively been obtained by using retroviral and lentiviral vectors, which can integrate the new RNAi gene into the breast cancer cell line genome in a stable manner.

Although experiments to elucidate the underlying mechanism are progressing rapidly, we are still at the beginnings of our understanding of the molecular processes responsible for RNAi and the extent of their biological function. However, practical applications have already allowed rapid surveys of gene functions and may result in novel therapeutic interventions.

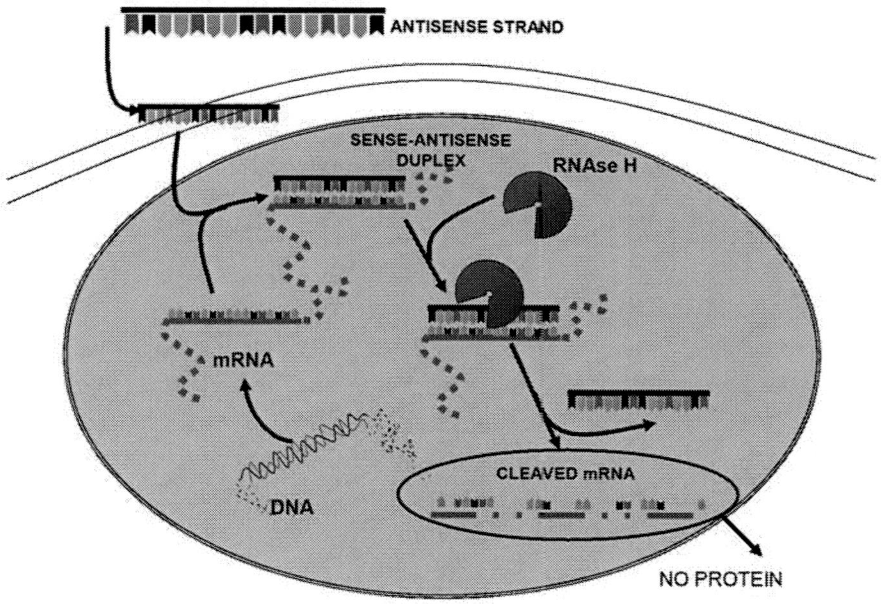

Figure 4. Antisense mechanism of action. Singlestranded oligonucleotides are transported across the plasma membrane. Once in the cytoplasm, single-stranded oligonucleotides accumulate in the cell nucleus, where they bind to their targeted mRNA. Once bound to the RNA, RNase H recognizes the oligonucleotide/RNA duplex as a substrate, cleaving the RNA strand and releasing the antisense oligonucleotide.

Antisense Therapy in Breast Cancer

Antisense therapy in oncology involves the use of approximately 20 nucleotides (oligonucleotide) that are synthesized to be complementary to the specific "sense" (5' to 3'orientation) mRNA sequence responsible for encoding the targeted protein. Once introduced into a cell, the "antisense" oligonucleotide (ASO) hybridizes to the corresponding mRNA sequence (Kurreck, 2003) and activates RNase H, which cleaves the RNA moiety of a DNA/RNA heteroduplex or binds to an mRNA and inhibits translation by steric blockade of the ribosome. The specificity of this approach is based on the estimation that any sequence of at least 13 bases in RNA and 17 bases in DNA is represented only once within the human genome. While small molecules designed for therapeutic use generally recognize a specific protein target based on its molecular domain structure, an ASO recognizes a specific mRNA based on its sequence. Hence, antisense drugs have high selectivity and affinity for their targets, show rapid effects and their destination is readily evaluated. These characteristics make antisense an attractive strategy for breast cancer treatment (Figure 4).

Breast Cancer Related Genes as Potential Targets for Antisense Oligonucleotides

The Bcl-2 protein family includes proteins that can promote either cell survival (Bcl-2, Bcl-XL, Mcl-1, A1, Bcl-W) or apoptosis (Bax, Bak, Bcl-XS, Bok). The relative amounts and the balance between these pro- and anti-apoptotic proteins influence the susceptibility of cells to a death signal. Expression of Bcl-2 and Bcl-XL (anti-apoptotic proteins) is significantly higher in primary breast cancers, where they might play a pivotal role in tumor initiation, progression, and resistance to chemotherapy and radiotherapy (Zinkel, 2006).

Antisense Bcl-2 (G3139, oblimersen sodium, Genasense, Genta, Berkeley Heights, NJ), an ASO designed to bind to the first six codons of the human Bcl-2 mRNA (Tolcher, 2005), caused increased apoptosis in MDA435/LCC6 human breast cancer cells (Chi et al., 2000). Moreover, combined treatment with G3139 and cytotoxic agents resulted in additive cytotoxicity in both cell lines. The initial clinical results of G3139 were also encouraging (Jansen et al., 1999). After 21 patients with Bcl-2-positive relapsed NHL received a 14-d sc infusion of G3139, Bcl-2 protein was reduced in 7 of 16 assessable patients, indicating its potential antitumor activity. Antisense oligonucleotide 4259, which targets the coding region of bcl-xL mRNA, can induce a decrease in Bcl-XL mRNA/protein levels in MCF-7, T-47D, ZR-75-1 and MDA-MB-231 breast cancer cells, inducing cell apoptosis (Simoes-Wust et al., 2000). Emi et al. (2005) reported an increase in the chemosensitivity of human breast cancer cell lines BT-474, ZR-75-1, MDA-MB-231 and MDA-MB-453 after their treatment with AS Bcl-2 (corresponding to the first six codons of the human Bcl-2 open reading frame) and AS Bcl-x in combination with anticancer drugs (doxorubicin, mitomycin C, paclitaxel and docetaxel). Bcl-2 antisense-based therapy is a viable strategy for inducing apoptosis and enhancing the chemosensitivity of breast cancers. Similar chemotherapeutic effects have been observed with activation of mitochondria-dependent apoptosis pathway by downregulation of Bcl-2. In addition, paclitaxel phosphorylates Bcl-2 and inactivates its antiapoptotic function, thereby sensitizing tumor cells to the treatment (Sawada et al., 2003). A randomized phase III study is required to demonstrate the expected survival benefit in combination with ASO Bcl-2.

The protooncogene *HER-2/neu* (*C-erbB-2* or human epidermal growth factor receptor-2 - HER-2-) encodes a 185 kDa transmembrane glycoprotein with intrinsic tyrosine kinase activity. HER-2 can homodimerize or heterodimerize with HER-1, HER-3 and HER-4 and leads to phosphorylation of the intracellular region of the receptor, triggering a signal transduction pathway that increases cell growth. Two major downstream signaling pathways of the ErbB family include the Ras-Raf-MAPK pathway and the Akt-phosphatidylinositol 3-kinase (PI3K) pathway (Mendelson and Baselga, 2003). *HER-2* gene is overexpressed in approximately 30% of breast cancer patients, indicating a poor prognosis, and is associated with drug resistance (Mendelson and Baselga, 2003). HER-2 downregulation is accompanied by an accumulation of SK-BR-3 cell in G1 phase. The use of ASO sequence with drugs such as doxorubicin hydrochloride cis-platinum and 5-fluorouracil reduces breast carcinoma cell growth. Some studies showed that systemic treatment with HER-2 ASO also significantly inhibited the growth of BT-474 xenografts in nude mice and that the combination of HER-2 ASO and doxorubicin resulted in an enhanced antitumor effect *in vivo* (Roh et al., 1999). These results suggest that antisense therapy targeting HER-2 may be a new strategy for enhancing chemotherapeutic efficacy in breast cancer patients.

Protein kinase A (PKA) is present in mammalian cells with two distinct isoforms (PKAI and PKA-II) that differ only in their regulatory subunits (termed RI in PKA-I and RII in PKA-II, respectively). Four isoforms of R subunits /RIa, RIb, RIIa, and RIIb) have been identified. Differential expression of PKA-I and PKA-II has been correlated with cell differentiation and neoplastic transformation. In fact, preferential expression of PKA-II is found in normal nonproliferating tissues and in growth-arrested cells, whereas PKA-I and/or its regulatory subunit RI-α is generally overexpressed in human cancer cell lines and primary tumors. Moreover, RI-α/PKA-I overexpression is associated with a worse prognosis in patients affected by breast cancer (Miller et al., 1993), and PKA-I has been directly implicated in the acquisition of the multidrug-resistant (MDR) phenotype (Scala et al., 1995). Srivastava et al. (1999) showed that RI-α antisense oligonucleotide inhibited the growth of MDA-MB-231 breast cancer cells in a dose-dependent manner and induced apoptosis. Other studies evaluated the effects of blocking PKAI on MCF-10A cells treated with taxol or taxotere. Treatment with this agent was able to overcome the effect of HER-2 overexpression on MCF-10A (Ciardiello et al., 2000). Recent studies have demonstrated the utility of the combination of GEM 231 (second-generation antisense oligonucleotide targeted against RI-α subunit) and irinotecan in nude mouse with tumors derived from MCF-7 cells (Wang et al., 2002).

The transferring receptor gene (*TfR*) is the principal transport protein that mediates iron uptake into cells, and the iron is required for enzymes involved in DNA synthesis. It is a type II transmembrane protein with a molecular mass of 85 kDa. TfR interacts with two proteins, transferrin (Tf) and the hereditary hemochromatosis protein involved in the cellular transport of iron (Bennett et al., 2000). The density of transferring receptors has also been correlated with the rate of DNA synthesis and metastatic potential of tumor cells (Ryschich et al., 2004). Yang et al. (2001) used an mRNA TfR antisense oligonucleotide in breast carcinoma cell lines MCF-7, T47-D, and MDAMB- 231, finding a significant reduction in live tumor cells after exposure to antisense TfR-ON (1 umol/L for 72 h). In fact, the IC50 (50% inhibition of DNA synthesis) of TfR ON for MCF-7, T47-D, and MDAMB-231 cells was 0.5, 0.5, and 1.0 umol/L, respectively, whereas the IC50 for normal breast cells was 30 umol/L.

Integrins, a family of heterodimeric glycoproteins with α and β subunits, participate in both cell-cell adhesion and in binding to a large number of basement membrane and ECM ligands (laminin, fibronectin, collagen, vitronectin, entactin, tenascin,, and fibrinogen).

However, these molecules also play a critical role in cell signaling, cell proliferation, apoptosis, migration, invasion, cellular transformation, angiogenesis, and tumor progression (Clezardin, 1998). Townsend et al. (2000) inhibited α-V subunit synthesis in the MDA-MB231 human breast carcinoma cell line by a partially phosphorothioated antisense oligodeoxynucleotide (5543-ODN), inducing the appearance of apoptotic bodies. Currently in clinical development is LY900003 (Affinitak, ISIS-3521; Eli Lilly and Company, Indianapolis, IN), which presents an antisense oligonucleotide to specifically block PKC-α. Although its single-agent activity in breast cancer is modest, its potential role may be in concert with traditional chemotherapy.

Finally, molecules associated with cellular senescence such as Id may also serve as targets for ASO breast cancer therapy. Fong et al. (2003) showed that human metastatic breast cancer cells become significantly less invasive *in vitro* and less metastatic *in vivo* when Id-1 is downregulated by stable transduction with antisense Id-1. Compared with preclinical studies, far fewer clinical studies of oligonucleotides have been reported. Further *in vitro* and *in vivo* studies will be necessary to determine the application of an antisense system in the treatment of breast cancer.

Replacement of a Defective Tumor Suppressor Gene for Breast Cancer

Identification of the molecular basis of breast malignancies means that it may be possible to specifically correct the underlying mutations. Cancer cells are remarkably sensitive to the inhibition of activated oncogenes or replacement of lost tumor suppressor genes (TSG) function. Replacement of lost TSG function has been achieved by the use of recombinant vectors that carry an expression cassette for the corrected gene.

One of the first replacement strategies for breast cancer is the use of the *Rb* gene. This gene is a negative regulator of the cell cycle *via* its ability to bind the transcription factor E2F and repress transcription of genes required for S phase (Goodrich, 2006). Wang et al. (1993) showed that restoration of Rb expression reduced tumorigenicity in a nude mice breast cancer model. However, the most widespread studies in relation to the replacement of a defective TSG in breast cancer are related to p53 (Stoff-Khalili et al., 2006). Loss of p53, a nuclear phosphoprotein important in cell cycle regulation, DNA repair, apoptosis, and angiogenesis inhibition, accelerates the appearance of tumors in transgenic mice (Attardi and Jacks, 1999). Several laboratories demonstrated that intratumoral injection of a virus carrying the p53 gene decreased tumor size in pre-clinical and clinical studies. Initial *in vitro* and *in vivo* studies on the use of this protein showed induction of apoptosis and suppression of tumorigenicity (Nielsen and Maneval. 1998). Chen and Mixson (1998) used a tumor-bearing mouse model and intravenous delivery of liposome with p53 and observed decreased tumor growth and a bystander anti-tumor effect. This associated effect is highly desirable for a therapeutic gene, since it reduces the level of transduction efficiency required for successful gene therapy (McCormick, 2001). It was recently reported that p53 can induce the transcription of genes such as the cyclin-dependent kinases p21WAF/CIP or Bax (Ghosh et al., 2004), which are directly related to the apoptosis phenomenon. In fact, induction of the overexpression of p21WAF/CIP1 in some tumor cell lines suppresses growth (Sheikh et al., 1995). Finally, p53 augmented the cytotoxic effect of the chemotherapeutic drug paclitaxel (Nielsen et al., 1998), and it was recently demonstrated that lower concentrations of paclitaxel can activate p53 (Panno et al., 2006).

Breast Cancer Gene Therapy Based on Apoptosis

There are a multitude of critical steps during the pathogenesis of cancer in which avoidance of programmed cell death (apoptosis) assures the progression and maintenance of the malignant phenotype. The enhanced capacity of tumor cells to survive allows them to overcome the numerous challenges encountered, not only at the primary tumor site but also during their vascular distribution and at their multiple final destinations. Proapoptotic and anti-apoptotic molecules are related to some cell cycle control and DNA damage repair mechanisms that are decisive in the capacity of cancer cells to survive when attacked by the immune system or by drugs and radiotherapy. The universal dependence of tumor cells on mechanisms to avoid apoptosis suggests a 'window of homogeneity' that could be therapeutically exploited (Gómez-Navarro et al., 2000) (Figure 5).

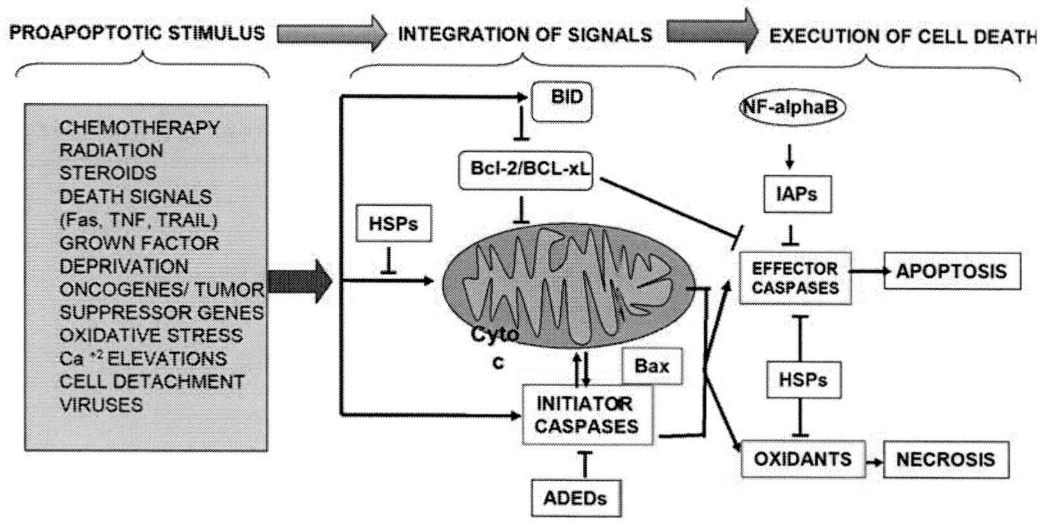

Figure 5. Apoptosis (programmed cell death). This phenomenon involves proapoptotic stimuli, a integration of signals and an execution of cell death. Execution of programmed cell death is effected by the well-defined family of caspases. Upstream, at least one family of proteins exist at each level of response to proapoptotic stimuli that is able to block a deadly signal: several members of the Bcl-2 family, heat shock proteins (HSPs), the inhibitors of apoptosis proteins (IAPs), the anti-apoptotic death effector domain proteins (ADEDs) and the nuclear factor-κB (NF-κB) family of transcription factors. Conversely, executioners of apoptosis such as Bax may be not functional, inclining the balance towards inappropriate survivalof the tumor cell. In breast cancer, many of these proteins are dysregulated.

Apoptosis and Bcl-2 Family

Beside p53, other proteins related to apoptosis include the Bcl-2 family. Thus, apoptosis id suppressed by Bcl-XL, Bcl-2, Mcl-1 and A1/Bfl-1 and induced by Bax, Bak, Bok/Mtd,

`Bad, Bik, Bid, Bim/Bod, and HrK (Gómez-Navarro et al., 2000). Overexpression of antiapoptotic Bcl-2 family members (e.g., Bcl-2 and Bcl-XL proteins) appears to play an important role in breast cancer (Lin et al., 2001). Interestingly, expression of the *Bcl-2* gene is regulated by estrogens in mammary epithelial cells and estrogen receptor (ER)-positive breast cancer cell lines (Zapata et al., 1998). This protein correlates with favorable clinicopathologic features. In fact, patients with elevated Bcl-2 levels appear to derive the greatest benefit from endocrine therapy (Hurlimann et al., 1995).

There is an inverse relationship between Bcl-2 and p53 in breast cancer. Suppression of Bcl-2 expression was observed in a p53-wild-type breast cancer cell line transfected with mutant p53. In fact, p53 can interact with Bad and Bax, inducing mitochondrial outer membrane permeabilization and apoptosis (Schuler and Green, 2005). The former, a positive regulator of cell death, is transcriptionally up-regulated by p53 and forms a Bad/p53 complex at the mitochondria to induce apoptosis (Jiang et al., 2006). The second, promotes cell death by directly binding and antagonizing prosurvival Bcl-2 and itself induces apoptosis *via* its direct channel-forming activity in mitochondria and activation of the caspase pathway (Xiang et al., 1996). Levels of Bax expression or the Bax/Bcl-2 ratio directly correlate in breast tumors with longer patient survival (Rochaix et al., 1999). In patients with metastatic breast cancer, a loss of Bax immunostaining is a prognostic indicator of a poor response to therapy and reduced survival (Krajewski et al., 1999).

Studies of human mammary tumors generated in nude mice showed that Bcl-XS induces apoptosis in tumor cells (Ealovega et al., 1996). The *in vitro* cytotoxicity of breast cancer cells via tumor-selective expression of the *Bax* gene has also been demonstrated (Tai et al., 1999). Recent studies showed that downregulation of Bik, a protein related to the development of breast and colorectal cancers, induced significant apoptosis in breast cancer cell lines *in vitro* as well as in tumor tissues in nude mice (Zou et al., 2002).

Alternative Apoptosis Strategies in Breast Cancer

In response to various stimuli, death factors bind to their respective receptors and activate the apoptotic death program in target cells (tumor necrosis factor-α tumor necrosis factor-related apoptosis-inducing ligands -TRAIL- and Fas ligand –FasL-). A cascade of specific proteases termed caspases mediates the apoptotic process. Activated caspases cleave various cellular components, a process that leads to morphological changes of cells and nuclei and degradation of chromosomal DNA. Loss-of -function mutations in the signaling molecules involved in apoptosis cause hyper-proliferation of cells in mice and humans. TRAIL has attracted considerable attention in recent years as a promising anti-cancer reagent because recombinant soluble TRAIL derivatives induce apoptosis in a broad range of tumor cells but only rarely or not at all in non-transformed cells (Schaefer et al., 2007). This signal requires activation of effector caspase-9 by the mitochondria and can be blocked by Bcl-2 and Bcl-XL (Hinz et al., 2000).

Galectin-3 (GAL3*)* is a β-galactoside-binding lectin that exhibits anti–or proapoptotic activity depending, on the cell type and the nature of the stimulus, and can confer chemoresistance to a wide variety of cancer cell types. It was recently shown that introduction of phosphorylated galectin-3 (P-GAL3) into human breast carcinoma cells promotes TRAIL-induced apoptotic cell death. The apoptosis phenomenon is mediated by the proapoptotic molecule Bad, resulting in the inhibition of mitochondrial depolarization and the release of cytochrome c. These findings suggest a possible use of P-GAL3 to enhance TRAIL sensitivity in breast cancer cells (Mazurek, et al., 2007).

The major stress-inducible Hsp70 (also known as Hsp72 or Hsp70) may be a cancer-relevant antiapoptotic protein of this type (Jaattela et al., 1999). Interestingly, Hsp70 can be induced by TNF, Bcl2 and Bcl-Xl, but not by caspases or p53 tumor suppressor protein. This induction indicates there is a point of action in the apoptosis pathway down on activation of caspases. Clinicopathological studies in breast cancer have shown that expression of Hsp70 correlates with the response to combination chemotherapy, radiotherapy, and hyperthermia (Vargas-Roig et al., 1998). Breast cancer cells depend on the constitutive high expression of Hsp70 to suppress a transformation-associated death program. Neutralization of Hsp70 may be a new way to treat cancers that have acquired resistance to therapies that induces the classical apoptosis pathway (Nylandsted et al., 2000).

IMMUNOMODULATORY GENE THERAPY

Immunotherapy strategies against breast carcinoma are an adjuvant therapy focused on stimulation of the host's immune system to detect and block tumor cells (Strong, 2000). They can be divided into two classes: passive immunotherapy, centered on administering compounds that directly affect tumor cell viability, e.g., antitumor cytokines or antibodies; and active immunotherapy, aimed at stimulating the patient's immune response by cytokines and gene vaccines (Figure 6).

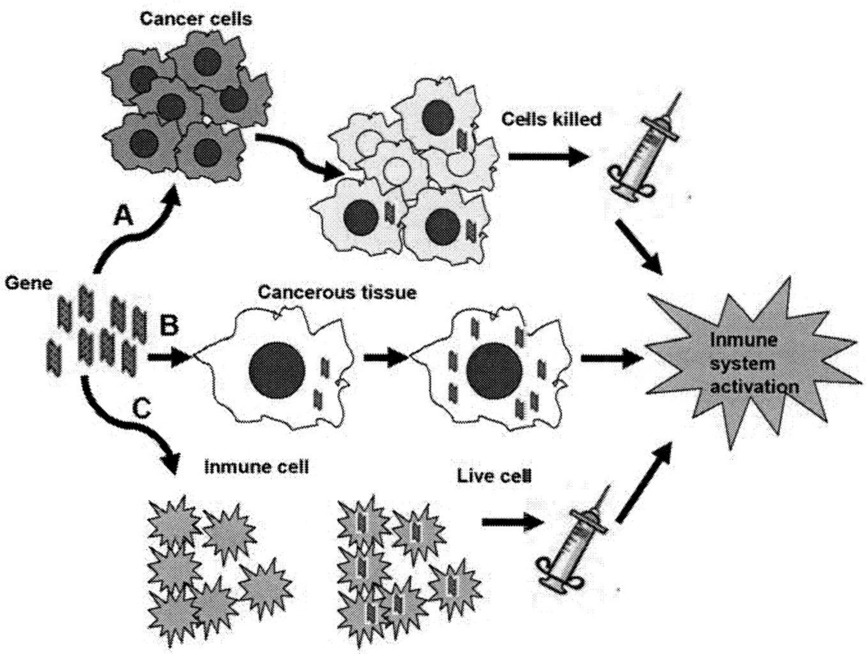

Figure 6. Immunotherapy strategies: (A) immunotherapy with altered cancer cells, (B) immunotherapy with genes *in vivo* and (C) immunotherapy using altered immune cells.

Cancer Immunotherapy Strategies

Cytokines such as interleukin-6 (IL-6), IL-10, interleukin-like IL-1, transforming growth factor-β (TGF-β), tumor necrosis factor-α (TNF-α), and chemokines have a relevant function in controlling the innate and acquired immune response (Knupfer and Preiss, 2007). In the context of cancer, cytokines are important for tumor progression because they can modulate tumor growth and immune cell activity (Nicolini et al., 2006). In fact, tumors appear to down-modulate the production of proinflammatory cytokines as one of the mechanisms to evade the immune system. Tumors also utilize chemokines to actively progress and evade immunosurveillance. These peptides play an important role in the maintenance of the immune system because they control the induction and activation of innate and adaptive immune responses (Dell'Agnola and Biragyn, 2007).

It has been shown that human breast cancer cells produces IL-1 and receptors, whose activation by autocrine or paracrine secretion could lead to the induction of protumorigenic effects such as proliferation, angiogenesis, and tumoral invasion (Pantschenko et al., 2003). In addition, IL-6, a pleiotropic cytokine, promotes human breast cancer cell line MCF-7 proliferation mediated by estrogen production (Honma et al., 2002) and increases doxorubicin resistance due to a pro-survival function via activation of several proteins (MCL-1, Bcl-Xl, and Bcl-2) that inhibit apoptosis (Brocke-Heidrich et al., 2004). For this reason, IL-6 production by some tumor cells in breast cancer patients could be employed in the prognosis of the disease, since cancer cells that produce cytokine have greater resistance to chemotherapeutic agents (Conze et al., 2001).

Type 1 IFNs exert immune stimulation, and transduction of the gene that encodes IFN-β by a defective-replicative adenovirus may block tumor formation by various tumor cell lines. This blocking appears to result from direct autocrine and paracrine rather than immunological effects of the cytokine (Qin et al., 1998), although tumorigenicity inhibition by IFN-β in bladder cancer was largely mediated by inhibition of angiogenesis and activation of host effector cells (Izawa et al., 2002).

Several *in vitro* and *in vivo* studies have focused on evaluating tumor cell vaccines generated by transfection of *IL-2* gene in irradiated primary breast tumor cells. This molecule induced a significant reduction in pulmonary metastasis, suggesting that active immunization with cytokine gene-modified tumor cells may be useful to inhibit metastases development (Coveney et al., 1996). This is a relevant issue since many patients have micrometastases at the time of diagnosis. In addition, the transference of breast cancer genomic DNA in an immunogenic cell line (e.g., fibroblasts) leads to a high immunogenic expression in breast cancer cells of antigens related to the malignancy. Co-transfection of this transfected line with *IL-2* and its subsequent injection significantly increased the survival of mice with intracerebral breast cancer, with less significant results being obtained when IL-18 rather than *IL-2* gene was used (Lichtor et al., 2005). However, transfection of *IL-18* gene directly into breast cancer cell line Bacp37 prevented tumorigenicity in injected nude mice (Han et al., 2004). The use of fibroblasts as recipient cells to augment vaccine cell numbers has been shown to be important for the development of immunotherapy protocols. Vaccines with a small number of breast cancer cells have been successfully developed in a mouse model, with the expression of tumor specific antigens leading to stimulation of CD8 T-cell mediated immunity with IL-2 adjuvant (Sung Kim and Cohen, 2005). This development is of interest because of the better prognosis of breast cancer disease at an early stage.

Target Antigens for Breast Cancer Immunotherapy

The early phase of cell-mediated immunity is stimulated when the tumor antigen is acquired by dendritic cells, the professional antigen presenting cells (Tagawa et al., 2006). The molecular mechanism permitting this acquisition may be an interaction between the Fas receptor present in dendritic cells and Fas ligand, a type II integral membrane protein of the TNF family expressed by tumoral cells (Tada et al., 2002). Hence, Fas ligand-expressing tumor cells could be used to construct specific vaccines aimed at stimulating antigen capture by antigen-presenting cells. Tumor-specific CD8+ CTLs are major components of tumor rejection reactions. The recognition and killing of a tumor cell by cytotoxic T cells is mediated by the appropriate presentation of peptides *via* MHC-I molecules. For this reason, one of the main mechanisms of tumoral immune escape is the alteration, downregulation, or loss of the peptide transporter associated with antigen processing (TAP), leading to a decrease in the presence of immunogenic peptides on the tumor cell surface with concurrent loss of HLA expression (Rees and Mian, 1999).

A prospective therapeutic protocol for the treatment of human breast cancer might be the upregulation of MHC class I molecule expression by 5-aza-2'-deoxycytidine, a histone deacetylase inhibitor that has shown antineoplastic activity that leads to demethylation of silenced MHC gene promoters (Bubenik, 2003). In fact, a promising gene therapy approach is overexpression of receptors and ligands of breast cancer cells, leading to their recognition and destruction by host immune system. The genetic recombination of B-cell and T-cell receptors might also lead to the recognition of a wide range of tumor-antigens and to the discrimination of small antigenic differences between normal and transformed cells.

A spontaneous immune response has been detected against NY-ESO-1, a strong immunogenic protein present in 30% of breast cancer cases, due to antigen processing by the tumor cells that generates an A2-restricted CTL epitope, making these cells susceptible to being killed (Chen et al., 2000). Immunization of nine cancer patients with the whole protein resulted in the induction or increase of NY-ESO-1 antibody response against 5 epitope, which was also recognized by antibodies in patients with anti-NY-ESO-1 production but without previous vaccination (Kawabata et al., 2007).

IgG antibodies against HER-2/neu were recently detected in 7% of HER-2/neu-overexpressed breast cancer patients, who appear to present a wide range of antibodies and cytotoxic T lymphocytes (CTLs) that are specific for breast tumor antigens but usually inadequate to inhibit cancer development (Zhou et al., 2004). In fact, there have been major advances in the design, selection and production of the recombinant antihuman HER-2/neu monoclonal antibody (trastuzumab) for use in breast cancer. Although, as stated above, only a small percentage of patients overexpress HER-2/neu (Ciampa et al., 2006), this gene could be introduced into tumor cells by gene therapy to induce this overexpression in a higher proportion of patients. These antibodies kill tumor cells by a conjugated cytotoxic pathway, binding natural killer cells to Fc surface receptor, or by direct lysis (Larin et al., 2004; Laheru et al., 2005).

Another molecule that is highly attractive as a vaccine target is EpCAM (epithelial cell adhesion molecule). This is a cell surface molecule that is essential for correct intercellular adhesion and is overexpressed 100- to 1000-fold in primary and metastatic breast cancers. This protein is related to cell migration and invasion of tumor cells, and siRNA studies have indicated that it may be susceptible to gene therapy (Osta et al., 2004). Thus, Braun et al. (1999) reported that use of murine monoclonal antibody 17-1A directed against EpCAM (Edrecolomab) in breast cancer patients with bone marrow micrometastases reduced or completely eliminated EpCAM+ cells tumor cells. Another protein of interest in gene therapy is MUC-1, which is overexpressed in > 90% of breast cancer in an underglycosylated form, exposing the extracellular domain of the peptide and allowing its use as a target of antibody-mediated therapy. Some progress has been reported in the development of a suitable human antibody (Singh et al., 2007) but no clinical trials have been carried out to date. Mice have been immunized with mammary tumoral cell lines transfected with plasmids encoding human MUC1 alone or in conjunction with CD80 (pCD80) or CD86 (pCD86) to generate cell-based or plasmid-based DNA vaccines. These vaccines delayed mammary tumor onset, inhibited the tumor growth rate, and prolonged the survival of mice (Vasilevko et al., 2003). Hence, the presence of CD80 or CD86 molecules is a potent costimulatory element that may improve vaccine adjuvant efficacy (Agadjanyan et al., 2003).

The BALB-neuT mouse is a good model for testing the efficacy of antitumor genetic vaccination. These mice develop breast cancer in a genetically inherited manner as the result of expression of an activated neu oncogene. Dendritic cells derived from the bone marrow of these mice were able to prevent and even delay onset of breast cancer in the animals when the cells were previously transfected with truncated neu oncoprotein by adenoviral transfection. It appears that adenovirus-activated dendritic cells can more intensively stimulate splenocytes, enhancing vaccine efficacy and immune response against tumor cells. This procedure may be beneficial to patients at risk of cancer development or metastases (Sakai et al., 2004). A recent paper described the virus-like replicon particle (VRP)-based vector, which transfects the non-mutated rat neu tumor antigen (c-erbB2 gene product) in a rat mammary tumor model with no use of adjunctive molecules. This vector system proved to be very efficacious, obtaining significant antitumor immune responses and curing of 36% of treated animals. Among other molecules used in vaccination are carcinoembryonic antigen (CEA), Fos-related antigen 1 (Fra-1), tumor cell-associated extracellular matrix metalloprotease inducer (EMMPRIN), B7-H4, hTERT and MAGE-1 (Stoff-Khalili et al., 2006). It has been proposed that the immunological response may be enhanced by strategies that target multiple tumor antigens (Laust et al., 2007).

Gene Immunotherapy Application: Clinical Trials

One aim of genetic immunotherapy is the development of clinical trials on treatments in which recombinant adenovirus or other vectors are injected to increase the expression of genes that encode cytokines in solid tumors or in which cancer vaccine immunotherapy is applied against antigens present in cancer cells.

Several cytokines have been evaluated for this purpose, and IL-2 was the first to be investigated. Stewart et al. (1999) conducted a phase I trial in 23 patients treated with subcutaneous injections of an E1-, E3-deleted adenovirus encoding IL-2, which was subcutaneously injected into melanoma deposits in 15 of these patients and into breast tumors in the other 8. Results demonstrated that the vector was non-toxic and, in 80% of patients, presence of human IL-2 mRNA from the adenoviral transfection could be detected at 7 days post-injection. The main immune response to IL-2 presence was an increase in lymphocytes infiltrates in tumors, accompanied by local inflammation and tumor necrosis.

Some recent human trials in breast cancer used recombinant adenoviruses as vectors for the overexpression of cytokine IL-2 and tumor antigen-specific MUC1, a glycoprotein found at the secretory poles of normal cells but hypoglycosylated in adenocarcinoma cells (Quinlin et al., 2007). Phase I studies with a vaccine vector based on replication-competent vaccinia virus, with sequences for both *MUC1* and *IL-2* genes, showed an enhancement of NK activity and T cell responses; in a phase II study of 31 patients, two partial responses were observed, with one of these patients developing liver metastases. Some disease stabilization was achieved in metastatic breast cancer patients but no objective clinical response was evidenced in trials of a nonpropagative recombinant vaccinia vector based on modified vaccinia Ankara with *IL-2* and *MUC1* genes (Liu et al., 2004). However, in a phase II study in 28 MUC1-positive breast cancer patients, clinical regression of axillary lymph nodes and liver metastases was obtained after repeated intramuscular administration of a replicative and attenuated recombinant vaccinia virus with *IL-2* and *MUC1* genes generated, with some patients showing partial tumor regression and others stabilization of their disease (Scholl et al., 2003).

Because breast cancer patient exhibit circulating antibodies and cytotoxic T lymphocytes that are specific for breast tumor antigens, clinical trials have been carried out using anti-HER-2/neu or anti-vascular endothelial growth factor receptor (bevacizumab), with a survival response of 23.1% with the former and 17% with the latter. An improved response was obtained when this antibody therapy was combined with chemotherapy (Burstein et al., 2003; Ferrara et al., 2004; Sawaki et al., 2004), although most patients showing an initial response with anti-HER-2/neu acquired resistance within a year. In 22 patients with advanced metastatic breast cancer and HER-2/neu overexpression, the combination of trastuzumab with metronomic cyclophosphamide was efficacious in controlling the disease and this combination appeared to delay acquired resistance to trastuzumab (Orlando et al., 2006).

Current aims in this field include improvement of the immunogenicity of tumor cells by manipulation and transfection of genes that encode mutated or hidden epitopes of tumor-specific antigens and exploration of their combination with components involved in immune rejection of foreign elements, e.g., cytokines, ligands, and costimulatory molecules. A further objective is the development of methods to more specifically direct transfected genes to target appropriate cells. Finally, prospective and randomized clinical trials are required to evaluate novel immunotherapy strategies.

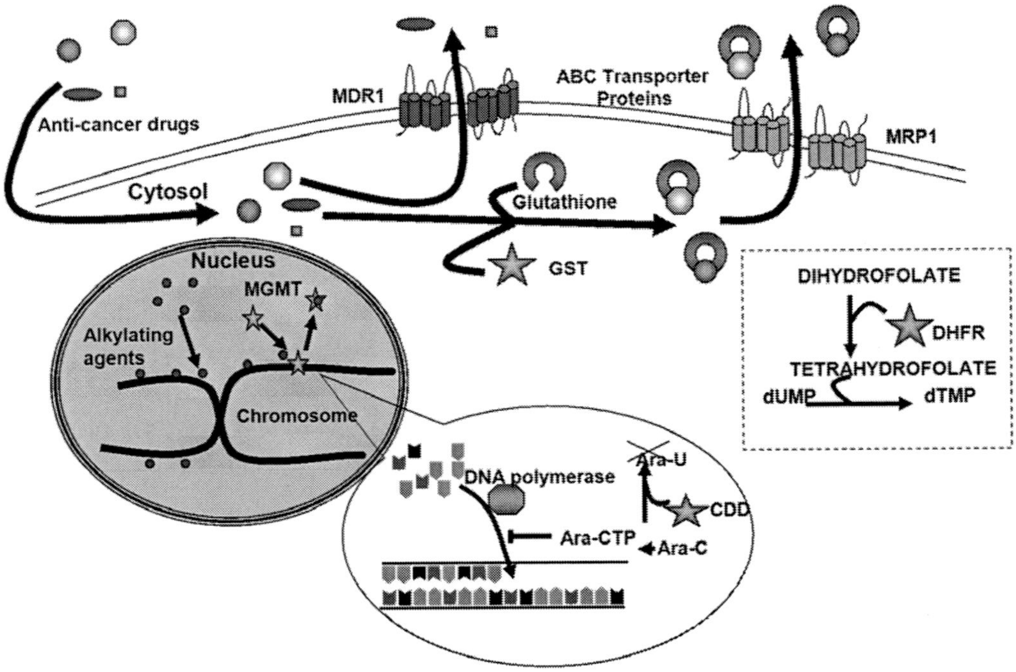

Figure 7. Drug resistance is caused by many molecular and cellular mechanisms. One prevalent mechanism is the over-expression of ATP-binding cassette (ABC) transporters, such as MDR1 (ABCB1). MDR1 gene encodes by P-glycoprotein (P-gp) which functions as a membrane pump. Activation of the P-gp by the hydrolysis of a bound ATP molecule drives a decrease in anticancer agent intracellular accumulation, resulting multidrug resistance. Methyl-guanine methyl transferase (MGMT); Glutathione S-transferase (GST); Multidrug-resistance-associated protein (MRP1); Cytidine deaminase (CDD); Dihydrofolate reductase (DHFR).

Gene Therapy for Modulation of Resistance in Breast Cancer

Although breast cancer is sensitive to chemotherapy, conventional drug doses only induce a complete response in 10-30% of patients, with duration of less than two years. Use of a high-dose chemotherapy regimen with autologous blood stem cell transplantation increases the response rate but produces inadequate bone marrow function after reconstitution. This is a major shortcoming of post-transplantation chemotherapy (Berry et al., 2002). Successful transfer of drug resistance genes into hematopoietic stem cells offers great promise as a means of protecting patients from the myelotoxicity of anticancer drugs and may permit dose intensification and better outcomes (Budak-Alpdogan et al., 2005). Numerous genes have been related to the development of drug resistance (Figure 7), the major limitation to cancer treatment with antineoplastic drugs. Although several mechanisms have been described by which tumor cells may express drug resistance (Melguizo et al., 1995), classical MDR has been associated with *MDR1* (Callaghan et al., 2006), the most widely analyzed resistance gene and the most used in cancer gene therapy. The *MDR1* gene product (Pglycoprotein, P-gp) is a 170 kDa glycoprotein consisting of two trans-membranous domains and two ATP-binding domains. In contrast to the products of other drug resistance genes, P-gp ATP-dependently excretes a broad range of hydrophobic drugs from cells, including vinca alkaloids, anthracyclines, epipodophyllotoxins, colchicine, actinomycin D, taxol and taxotere (Ambudkar et al., 2003). Moreover, besides its resistance function, the *MDR1* gene has been implicated in the differentiation of tumor cells and connected with modulation of MHC molecule expression (Prados et al., 2006).

Transfer and expression of human MDR1 in marrow cells has been used to protect hematopoietic cells against myelotoxic drugs. The first experiment was performed with docetaxel and paclitaxel, two P-gp substrates used in conventional breast cancer therapy. Using a retroviral vector, Sorrentino et al. (1992) transplanted *MDR1*-transduced bone marrow into irradiated mice, which did not develop leucopenia after paclitaxel treatment. This finding suggests that MDR1 induces chemoprotection of transduced cells. Similar results were obtained by Hanania et al. (1995) after the retroviral-mediated transfer of MDR1 gene into mouse marrow cells.

Some clinical trials have been carried out on *MDR1* gene therapy for advanced cancers. In patients with breast cancer, this gene has been transferred to hematopoietic cells using retrovirus. Thus, Cowan et al. (1999) showed that bone marrow mononuclear cells or peripheral blood stem cells transfected with *MDR1* and stimulated by IL-3 and -6 showed no enrichment of *MDR1*-transduced white blood cells. Moscow et al. (1999) reported that hematopoietic CD34+ MDR1 transfected cells were able to proliferate expressing P-gp that expelled the conventional chemotherapeutic drug. However, further investigation is necessary into the use of drug resistance genes for myeloprotection in breast cancer. Clinical trials are also required to confirm the persistence of MDR1-transduced hematopoietic cells and to explore the mutagenic risk of retroviral gene transfer (Dave et al., 2004).

Antiangiogenic Gene Therapy

Angiogenesis is a complex process of new capillary blood vessel formation from pre-existing vasculature that includes a number of overlapping steps: activation, proliferation and migration of endothelial cells (ECs), basement membranes degradation, remodeling of the extracellular matrix of tissues, formation of vascular tubes and networks, recruitment of supporting cells, including smooth muscle cells and pericytes and connection to the pre-existing vascular network (Papetti and Herman, 2002).

The angiogenic response is determined by a net balance between pro- and anti-angiogenic regulators including cytokines and mechanical forces mediated by blood flow on vascular endothelium. Cytokines include pro-angiogenic soluble growth factors, such as vascular endothelial growth factor (VEGF), basic fibroblast growth factor (bFGF), placenta-like growth factor (PIGF), transforming growth factor-ß (TGF-ß), platelet-derived growth factor (PDGF), angiopoietin 1 and 2 (Ang 1 and 2), angiogenin (An), or IL-8, but also anti-angiogenic factors including fragments of proteins (angiostatin and endostatin), thrombospondin, tissue inhibitors of metalloproteinases (TIMPs), IFN-α·and ß and many others (Liu and Deisseroth, 2006). Moreover, several disorders, such as inflammation, atherosclerosis, hemangiomas, psoriasis, restenosis rheumatoid arthritis, retinopathies and solid tumor growth and metastasis, are characterized by excessive angiogenesis (Webb and Vande Woude, 2000) (Figure 8).

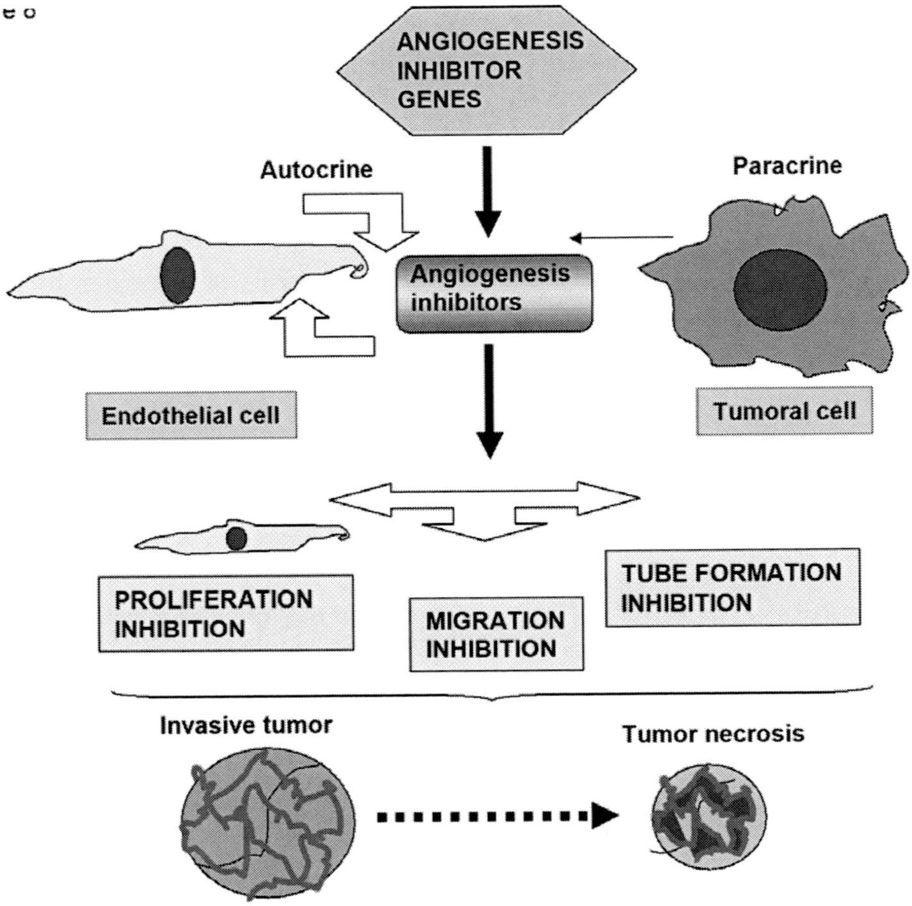

Figure 8. Therapeutic actions of anti-angiogenesis gene therapy.

Breast Cancer Angiogenesis

Continuous tumor angiogenesis is indispensable to the growth of solid tumors, because it provides the tumor with nutrients and oxygen supply and removes waste products. Initiation of tumor vessel development occurs when local environmental factors as well as genetic alterations promote conversion of tumor cells to an angiogenic phenotype (Carmeliet and Jain, 2000; Folkman, 2002). The resultant elaboration of proangiogenic cytokines by these cells permits recruitment of ECs from surrounding vessels and circulating precursors. ECs and tumor cells release angiogenesis regulators like VEGF, bFGF, PDGF, Ang 1, Ang 2 and transforming growth factor (TGF) to mediate angiogenesis (Papetti and Herman, 2002). In addition to the presence of angiogenesis factors, activation of oncogenes and loss of tumor suppressor genes are also essential for an angiogenesis phenotype that supports tumorigenicity (St Croix et al., 2000).

Tumor vessel development is generally deficient in mechanisms that induce vessel maturation and quiescence as seen in physiologic angiogenesis (Fidler and Ellis, 2004). Tumor blood vessels are immature, with a tortuous architecture, showing abnormal branching and blind endings, with dilated and irregularly shaped and a great permeability, lack functional pericytes in many areas and the loss of the basement membrane (McDonald and Baluk, 2002). Moreover, alterations in ECs are detected, with an increased proliferation and the expression of several proteins, such as integrins and receptors for angiogenic growth factors (VEGFR1 and VEGFR2). Therefore, although tumors stimulate neovessel formation, this abnormal angiogenesis results in a predominantly hypoxic and acidic intratumor microenvironment (Dickson et al., 2005) which stimulates proangiogenic factors such as VEGF via HIF-β, HIF-1α and HIF-2α factors (Pugh and Ratcliffe, 2003).

The acquisition of the angiogenic phenotype occurs early in the multistage process of breast cancer development. *In vivo* studies demonstrated that angiogenic switch occurs before that the typical morphological changes of cancer occur. In addition, increased intratumor microvessel density in primary breast cancers appears to adversely affect disease-free survival and overall survival in patients with breast cancer (Guidi et al., 2000). More recently, it has been demonstrated that the oncogene *HER-2/neu* (overexpressed approximately in 25–30% of invasive breast cancers) up-regulates cancer-cell production of angiogenic factors such as transforming growth factor (TGF)-β, Ang 1 and plasminogen-activator inhibitor-1 (PAI-1) and also VEGF (Konecny et al., 2004).

In patients, overexpression of VEGF in early stage breast cancer has been associated with increased metastatic potential and resistance to systemic adjuvant therapies (both chemotherapy and hormonal therapy) (Gasparini, 2000). Recent preclinical results have suggested that breast cancer cells may express VEGF receptors on their cell surface, and that this combination of ligand and receptor may act as an autocrine loop, paralleling the paracrine loop of breast cancer cell and ECs (Huh et al., 2005). Clinical studies showed that VEGFR-1 and VEGFR-2 were strongly expressed in endothelial cells within blood microvessels, and weakly in tumor cells. VEGFR-1 expression permits the identification of patients with poor outcome, particularly those with node negative tumors, with high risk of metastasis and relapse (Dales et al., 2003). Other endothelial growth factors may be involved in breast cancer-associated angiogenesis. The platelet derived-endothelial cell growth factor (PD-ECGF), members of FGF family, and TGF-β1 are overexpressed in human breast cancer (Relf et al., 1997).

Anti-Angiogenic Strategies

Inhibition of angiogenesis represents a promising alternative strategy to block tumor growth and metastasis. This therapy often targets EC division and migration, because these cells have low mutagenic potential. Moreover, since a single vessel can support the growth of many tumor cells, its destruction would impair the viability of many tumor cells, and, even more importantly, the same anti-angiogenic molecule could possibly be used to treat different tumors (Benouchan and Colombo, 2005). The major potential targets of antiangiogenic therapy are: (1) proliferating and migrating endothelial cells; (2) neutralization or sequestration of angiogenesis mediators and their receptors; (3) block of functions of basement membrane and extracellular matrix; (4) inhibition of endothelial cell adhesion molecules; and (5) indirect cytokines-mediated mechanisms (Morabito et al., 2004). A varietiy of compounds have been developed and are under clinical testing in advanced breast cancer. In addition, several chemotherapeutic agents routinely employed in breast cancer treatment such as bevacizumab (a humanized monoclonal antibody), have true antiangiogenic activity at clinical level (Schneider and Sledge, 2007). However, only three therapeutic strategies are capable to block tumor growth through regression of neovascularization: vascular targeting, gene therapy and direct inhibition of proliferating and migrating ECs.

Anti-Angiogenic Gene Therapy for Breast Cancer

Gene therapy strategies that result in constitutive expression of an antiangiogenic protein in ECs would be expected to be more effective than a gene therapy approach targeting a tumor cell. In these cells the mutations might quickly develop an escape mechanism of drug resistance (Tandle et al., 2004). Furthermore, antiangiogenic therapy requires prolonged administration of therapeutic proteins to maintain tumour suppression. Compared with alternative strategies requiring systemic administration of antiangiogenic recombinant proteins, monoclonal antibodies and other drugs, gene therapy theoretically allows a one-off administration of an easily produced vector, resulting in a long term expression and steady state levels of therapeutic agents (Lau and Bicknell, 1999). Moreover, this may circumvent problems associated with frequent oral or intravenous dosing of recombinant proteins, such as cost and maintenance of function during mass production of these agents. Gene therapy offers the opportunity for the patient to become his/her own source of production, an endogenous factory for antiangiogenic protein production (Feldman and Libutti, 2000). In addition, potential side effects of antiangiogenic therapy could be avoided by employing regulatable promoter systems allowing "switching on or off" transgene expression (Dickson et al, 2005). Particularly attractive features of gene transfer is the possibility of targeting gene delivery to selective tissues, thus achieving localized gene expression and high regional drug concentrations without increasing the systemic levels of the therapeutic agents, which would reduce side effects.

In breast cancer, several preclinical experiences in anti-angiogenic gene therapy have been done using viral and non-viral methods. Xu et al. (1997) found a significant reduction in intra-tumoral blood vessel count following an intravenously administered liposome:p53 complex *in vivo* which was acting through thrombospondin I (TSP-1), a protein that inhibits angiogenesis. In addition, the combination of liposomes complexed to both BAP-p53 and BAP-TSPf (a plasmid encoding an antiagiogenic fragment of TSP-I) reduced the tumor size and blood vessels density in mice implanted with two breast cancer tumor cell lines (Chen and Mixson, 1998). More recently, Hahn et al., (2004) demonstrated significant antiangiogenic effects of the N-terminal fragment of TSP-2 against a murine breast cancer cell line following intra-tumoral injection of a fibroblast cell line engineered to express this transgene.

On the other hand, liposomes complexed to plasmid containing the angiostatin or endostatin gene, two angiogenesis inhibitors, effectively restrict tumor growth of breast cancer xenografts following direct intra-tumoral or intravenous injection (Chen et al., 1999). Moreover, an inhibition of breast cancer metastatic growth has been showed by the expression of angiostatin using an adenoviral vector (Gyorffy et al., 2001). Another study, reported delivery of endostatin by adenovirus vectors in two tumor models: the syngenic MidT2-1 mammary tumor model in FVB mice and the MDA-MB-231 human breast tumor model in SCID mice. In the first case, a block in tumor growth by suppression of tumor angiogenesis *in vivo* was obtained. The second type of tumor, however, was not influenced by endostatin gene therapy, probably due to the different sensitivity of blood vessels to endostatin itself (Jin et al., 2001). Also, efficacy of endostatin gene therapy in the treatment of breast cancer using retroviral vectors has been demonstrated (Indraccolo et al., 2002)

Interferons α, β and γ regulate multiple biological activities such as cell growth and differentiation, oncogene expression, host immunity and have anti-angiogenic properties (Folkman, 2004). Moloney leukemia virus-based retroviral vectors for expression of murine *IFN-α(1)* were used to transduce human breast cancer cell lines (MCF7 and MDA-MB435). This gene induced a long-lasting inhibition of tumor growth in nude mice that was associated with reduced vascularization (Indraccolo et al., 2002). Similarly, *IFN-β* gene transduction by a replication-defective adenovirus and *in vivo* delivery into breast cancer generated high local concentrations of IFN-β, inhibited tumor growth and in many cases caused complete tumor regression (Qin et al., 1998).

The soluble, truncated form of VEGF receptor-2 (VEGFR-2), sFLK-1, is a well-known inhibitor of endothelial cells. Kou et al. (2005) showed that retroviral-mediated sFLK-1 breast gene therapy induce a reduction of microvessel density and proliferative cell nuclear antigen in animal tumor models. In other experience, authors used a replication-deficient adenoviral vector containing antisense VEGF cDNA (Ad5CMV- αVEGF) to down-regulate expression and increase the efficiency of delivery of the antisense sequence in the human breast cancer cell line MDA231-MB. The results showed that injection of the Ad5CMV-αVEGF vector into intramammary xenografts of these cells established in nude mice inhibited tumour growth and reduced the amount of VEGF protein and the density of microvessels (Im et al, 2001)

At present, new anti-angiogenic gene therapy strategies are developed. Potential use of engineered gelatin-based nanoparticulate vectors for systemic delivery of therapeutic genes to breast cancer xenografts *in vivo* has been demonstrated. Plasmid DNA encoding sFlt-1 was encapsulated in the control and polyethylene (glycol) (PEG)-modified gelatin-based nanoparticles. The *in vivo* expressed sFlt-1 was therapeutically active as shown by suppression of tumor growth and microvessel density measurements. PEG-modified gelatin-based nanovectors can serve as a safe and effective systemically administered gene delivery vehicle for solid tumor (Kommareddy and Amiji, 2007). Another strategy is the use of endothelial progenitor cells (EPCs) as angiogenesis-selective targeting vectors for the delivery of cytotoxic genes with anti-tumor effects. They can be genetically modified by being transduced *in vitro* with viral vectors and re-introduced into the systemic circulation (De Palma et al., 2003).

Although many preclinical experiences investigating a breast cancer gene therapy approach for the delivery of antiangiogenic agents give promise to its potential as an effective anticancer strategy, several challenges remain to be addressed. New studies will be required to develop effective regulatable expression systems that improve the safety of chronic delivery and tropic for tumor vasculature. Moreover, studies are necessary to examine in detail possible synergistic effects between various combinations of genes and between anti-angiogenic genes and conventional therapies. Maximal antitumor effects are achieved when antiangiogenic agents are used in combination therapy such as chemotherapy, radiotherapy and hormonal therapy (Persano et al., 2007).

SUICIDE GENE THERAPY IN BREAST CANCER

Suicide gene therapy assays in cancer test the hypothesis that tumor growth can be suppressed by delivering genes encoding a cytotoxic protein to tumor cells. Suicide gene therapy can be divided into two categories: enzyme-activating prodrug therapy, using the transfection of genes able to express enzymes that selectively activate specific prodrugs; and toxin gene therapy, which incorporates genes expressing toxic molecules that can affect cellular viability by disturbing the cell membrane.

Enzyme-Activating Prodrug Therapy

Enzyme-activating prodrug therapy relies on activation of an inactive prodrug to a cytotoxic molecule. This process involves targeted delivery of genes to cancer cells followed by administration of the prodrug, which is activated by the foreign enzyme expressed in the tumor. The most commonly used enzymes for enzyme-activating prodrug therapy in breast cancer can be divided into two types. The first consists of enzymes of non-mammalian origin, e.g., viral thymidine kinase, bacterial cytosine deaminase, carboxypeptidase G2, and nitroreductase. The second type comprises enzymes of human origin, e.g., cytochrome *P*450 isoforms (Prados et al., 2005).

Antitumor gene therapy using genetic prodrug activation therapy should, in theory, be limited to the cells that have been transduced with suicide genes. However, many researchers have reported induction of cell death in untransduced tumour cells. This phenomenon, designated *bystander effect,* can be defined as the cytotoxic effect on nontransduced cancer cells after prodrug administration, when only a fraction of the tumor mass is genetically modified to express an activating enzyme (Stribbling et al., 2000). Two major categories of bystander effect have been identified: local and immune-mediated. In the first case, the killing of neighboring cells is due to the transfer of toxic metabolic products through gap junctions, via apoptotic vesicles, our by diffusion of soluble toxic metabolites (Touraine et al., 1998). The local bystander effect can also be induced by contact with dead or dying cells due to the transfer of apoptotic factors (Greco and Dachs, 2001). In the second category, immune stimulation induces inflammatory infiltrate with tumor regression in immunocompetent animals (Stoff-Khalili et al., 2006) and can also induce regression of distant tumor deposits (Dilber and Smith, 1997).

Herpes Simplex Thymidine Kinase

The herpes simplex thymidine kinase gene is the most widely studied suicide gene therapy system. Expression of the *HSV-tk* gene confers enhanced tumor sensitivity to nucleoside analogues such as ganciclovir (GCV) and acyclovir (ACV). HSV-tk converts GCV or ACV to their non-phosphorylated forms, which are relatively non-toxic to mammalian cells, are trapped in the cytoplasm, and then become further phosphorylated to the triphosphorylated form by kinases of the host cells. Upon division of the tumor cell, the toxic triphosphorylated compounds are incorporated into the cellular DNA, thereby inhibiting DNA replication and RNA polymerase activity, eventually leading to cell death (Witlox et al., 2007). This molecular mechanism of action implies that this enzyme-prodrug system will only be effective for actively dividing cells and will not affect quiescent cells in a tumor. Nevertheless, this system may induce cell death in tissues with low mitotic indices by a p53-independent apoptosis mechanism (Vassaux and Lemoine, 2000) (Figure 9).

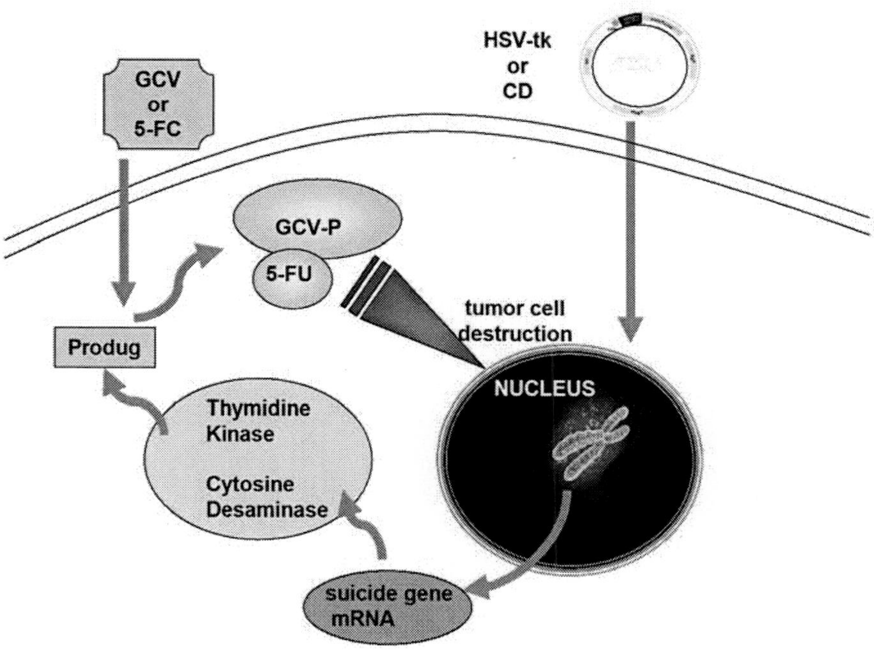

Figura 9. Sequence events in suicide gene therapy with the herpes simplex virus thymidine kinase (HSV-tk) and cytosine deaminase (CD) genes. Suicide gene is transferred to the target cells with the aid of vectors. These genes encode for an enzyme which modifies the prodrug generating a toxic drug. Ganciclovir (GCV) and 5-fluorocytosine (5-FC) are used in the HSV-tk and CD systems, respectively, generating ganciclovir triphosphate (GCV-P) and 5-fluorouracil (5-FU). These drugs inhibit DNA polymerase or RNA synthesis, leading to cell destruction.

Gadal et al. (2004) also showed *in vitro* and *in vivo* that the HSV-tk/GCV treatment system is not very efficacious in the MCF-7 breast cancer cellular line, since it significantly inhibited cell growth but did not induce early or late apoptosis. In contrast, this treatment was highly effective in a mouse breast cancer model, showing significant inhibition of tumor development during at least 60 days post-treatment. This contradiction between *in vivo* and *in vitro* results may be explained by an immune response enhancement mechanism and an endothelial cell cytotoxicity resulting in tumor ischemia (Levy et al., 2006). Other authors (Grignet-Debrus, et al., 2005) studied the Varicella zoster virus (VZV) thymidine kinase, which has very low affinity for GCV. However, both enzymes have very high affinity for pyrimidine nucleoside analogues (E)-5-(2-bromovinyl)-2`-doxyuridine (BVDU or brivudin) (Degreve et al., 1997). Studies of MCF-7, T-47D, and MDA-MB-435 breast cancer cells with VZV-TK and ACV, GCV, and BVDU showed that these compounds lacked growth-inhibitory activity on parental tumor cells, and that ACV and GCV exerted no selective toxicity on vector-expressing cells except for T47D TK^+ cells, on which GCV exhibited weak cytototoxic activity. In contrast, BVDU exerted a very strong cytotoxic effect on tumor cells expressing TK, with an IC_{50} ratio ranging from 400 to 2000. Degreve et al. (1997) tested *in vivo* the efficacy of the VZV-TK/BVDU system on MDA-MB-435-derived tumor induced in nude mice by subcutaneous injections. BVDU initially reduced the tumor growth followed by a slow growth to reach a significantly reduced tumor size in comparison with controls.

Bacterial Cytosine Deaminase

Cytosine desaminase (CD), an enzyme of bacterial or fungal origin, converts non-toxic 5-fluorocytosine (5-FC) into 5-fluorouracil (5-FU), which is extremely toxic to human cells when phosphorylated to monophosphate and triphosphate forms, which can irreversibly inhibit thymidylate-synthetase enzyme and RNA transcription (Prados et al., 2005). One of the main advantages of this system over HSV-tk/gancyclovir is a strong bystander effect that does not require cell-to-cell contact, since 5-FU can diffuse into and out of cells by non-facilitated diffusion (Seymour and Mothersill, 1999). Experiments conducted *in vitro* by exposing mixed transfected and untransfected populations to 5-FC showed that 1-30% of cells expressing CD could generate sufficient 5-FU to inhibit the growth of neighboring cells that did not express the enzyme, even when sparsely seeded (Ichikawa et al., 2000) (Figure 9).

Anderson et al. (2000) used two recombinant adenoviral vectors containing tumor targeting expression cassettes of either the ALA (human α-lactalbumin) or BLG (ovine β-lactoglobulin) promoters driving the *C. albicans* CD gene (Ad.ALA.CD and Ad.BLG.CD), finding *in vitro* growth inhibition of transduced breast cancer cells. Moreover, these cells exhibited selective sensitization to prodrug when compared with immortalized nontumorigenic breast cells or non breast cancer cells. *In vivo*, nude mice with T47D breast tumors cells showed a tumor regression profile when injected with tumor-selective adenovectors in conjunction with prodrug. Furthermore, survival was prolonged in animals treated with both vector and prodrug, showing that expression of CD is effective in tumor eradication (Anderson et al., 2000).

Bifidobacterial Selective Targeting-Cytosine Deaminase (BEST-CD) therapy has also been successfully used in breast cancer. *Bifidobacterium* selectively localizes to and proliferates in solid tumors after systemic application. Hypoxic or necrotic regions are characteristic of many murine and human solid tumors, including the majority of primary breast tumors. Therefore this system allows combination of the cytosine deaminase gene and

Bifidobacterium longum (*B. longum*), which can selectively germinate and grow in hypoxic regions of solid tumors after intravenous injection (Fujimori, 2006).

Carboxypeptidase G2

The bacterial enzyme carboxypeptidase G2 (CPG2) is able to cleave the glutamic acid moiety from the prodrug 4-[(2-chloroethyl)(2-mesyloxyethyl)amino]benzoyl-L-glutamic acid (CMDA), releasing the DNA-cross-linking mustard drug 4-[(2-chloroethyl)(2-mesyloxyethyl)amino]benzoic acid without further catalytic requirements (Niculescu-Duvaz et al., 2003; 2004). Transfection with the CPG2 gene led to production of an active enzyme that can convert CMDA into a cytotoxic agent. This enzyme produces an 11-95-fold increase in the sensitivity of CPG2-transfectant to the prodrug (Marais et al., 1996). However, the breast tumor cell line MDA MB361 showed only modest sensitivity to CMDA activated by intra-cellular expression of CPG2, mainly because the prodrug could not enter the cells (Marais et al., 1997). To overcome this problem, CPG2 was expressed tethered to the outer surface of mammalian cells, resulting in effective cell killing by CMDA *in vitro* and *in vivo* (Marais et al, 1997; Stribbling et al., 2000). Moreover, the CPG2/CMDA system has been shown to induce a robust bystander effect (Dachs et al., 2005). In nude mice, regression and cure of breast carcinoma xenografts was obtained when only 10% of the cells expressed the tethered CPG2 (Stribbling et al., 2000).

Escherichia Coli B Nitroreductase

Nitroreductase (NTR) is a monomeric enzyme that converts non-toxic monofunctional alkilating agents to their dysfunctional forms. E. Coli nitroreductase has been used to metabolize the prodrug 5-(aziridin-1-yl)-2,4-dinitrobenzamide (CB1954) to 5-(aziridin-1-yl)-4-(hydroxyamino)-2-nitrobenzamide in presence of reduced form nicotinamide adenine dinucleotide or reduced form nicotinamide adenine dinucleotide phosphate, which acts as a reductant. The metabolized prodrug is then acetylated to 5-(aziridin-1-yl)-4-(aacetylamino)-2-nitrobenzamide, which is capable of cross-linking cellular DNA, resulting in apoptosis (Vassaux and Lemoine, 2000).

In vitro studies showed that NTR expression resulted in a 2600-fold increase in sensitivity to CB1954 compared with parental lines (Weedon et al., 2000). In order to further address the efficacy of NTR-CB1954 as an anti-cancer therapeutic system *in vivo*, Cui et al. (2002) developed transgenic mice in which nitroreductase was specifically expressed in tumor cells or in *c-myc* overexpressing cells in the mammary gland. Studies with this animal model demonstrated that the NTR-CB1954 system can effectively suppress *myc*-dependent tumor formation in the mammary gland of transgenic mice.

Cytochrome P450

The enzyme cytochrome P450 (CYP) involves isozymes with different substrates, specificities and activities against cyclophosphamide (CP) and iphosphamide (IP). CYPs are present in the liver and only at low levels in other tissues or human tumors, including colon, breast, lung, liver, kidney and prostate tumors (Yu et al., 2001). Consequently, substantial increases in intratumoral production of active drug metabolites and enhanced anticancer activity may be obtained by delivery of P450 gene-activated prodrug to tumor cells (Chen and Waxman, 2002). Cyclophosphamide is commonly used in combination with other chemotherapeutic drugs in the treatment of tumors, including breast cancer (Hudis and Schmitz, 2004). Preclinical P450 gene therapy studies using (CP) have shown a substantial improvement in antitumor activity associated with a decrease in systemic toxicity compared with conventional chemotherapy. Kan et al. (2001) showed that *in vitro* transduction of T47D (human breast cancer cell line) with MetXia-P450 led to sensitization to cyclophosphamide. These observations were replicated in nude mice using HT29, MDA-MB-231 and MDA-MB-468 (human breast cancer) xenografts. Mice treated with both MetXia-P450 and cyclophosphamide showed a significant delay in tumor growth compared with those treated with cyclophosphamide alone. It was recently shown that P450 activity is dependent on electrons supplied by cytochrome P450 reductase (CPR). Since endogenous CPR activity may not be sufficient for optimal P450 activity, overexpression of CPR has been considered a valuable approach in gene-directed enzyme prodrug therapy. Lengler et al. (2006) analyzed the effects of CPR on cytochrome P450 isoform 2B1 (CYP2B1) activity in human breast tumor cell lines T47D and Hs578T. A CPR-mediated increase in CYP2B1 activity was only observed in human breast tumor cell line Hs578T, revealing an effect of CPR on CYP2B1 activity that is dependent on the cell type used. Therefore, careful evaluation is required of the therapeutic benefit of combining cytochrome P450 and CPR in each target tissue to be treated.

Clinical Trials of Enzyme-Activating Prodrug Therapy

The first clinical trial was designed to test the safety and efficacy of a tumor-specific genetic prodrug activation therapy using human erbB-2 gene promoter. This study, the first targeted gene therapy for breast cancer and the first to use the CD system in human subjects, yielded encouraging results for the development of genetic prodrug activation therapies that exploit the transcriptional profile of cancer cells. This approach was shown to be safe and resulted in targeted expression of the CD gene in 90% of cases. However, no significant tumor regression was reported (Pandha et al., 1999). Recent phase I/II clinical trials supported the clinical development of retroviral vector-based P450 gene-directed enzyme prodrug therapies to deliver P450 2B6 to advanced breast cancer patients receiving oral cyclophosphamide. Nine patients received three dose levels of MetXia-P450. One (11%) patient with breast cancer had a partial response and received 7 months of oral cyclophosphamide. Four (44%) patients had stable disease for at least 3 months and the rest had progressive disease. Gene transfer was detected at all dose levels, and these initial observations of an antitumor response indicate that MetXia-P450 should undergo further clinical assessment (Braybrooke et al., 2005).

Toxin Gene Therapy: Suicide Genes which do not Require the Use of a Prodrug

We have described above strategies based on putative killer-suicide genes that convert a nontoxic prodrug into a toxic metabolite. However, administration of prodrugs often results in the release of toxic metabolites and limited bioavailability. Thus, these limitations were detected in pre-clinical studies in an *in vivo* pancreatic cancer model (Fogar et al., 2003).

One of the most promising recently developed alternatives to these therapeutic systems has been the introduction of suicide genes that do not require the use of a prodrug to be effective in tumoral cells. These genes, which encode cytotoxic products, include fusogenic membrane proteins such as vesicular stomatitis virus (VSV) glycoprotein and gibbon ape leukemia virus (GALV) envelope protein (Diaz et al., 2000; Fielding et al., 2000). When these proteins are expressed in a target cell, they cause membrane fusions with neighboring cells, leading to the formation of large multinuclear syncytia in which cells finally die either by apoptosis or necrosis (Bateman et al., 2002).

Numerous proteins have been used for this purpose in cancer gene therapy experiments. Diphtheria toxin subunit A (DT-A) is a strong inhibitor of protein synthesis that inactivates elongation factor 2 (EF-2) (Zheng et al., 2003). The conjugate VEGF-DT385 diphtheria toxin inhibited endothelial cell proliferation, angiogenesis, and solid breast tumor growth in a xenotransplant model system (Wild et al., 2004). Other toxins with a direct cell-killing function include anthrax (*Bacillus anthracis*) toxin or cholera (*Vibrio cholerae*) toxin B (Zitzer et al., 1997; Frankel et al., 2002). It has been suggested that some bacterial or plant toxins, e.g., Pseudomonas aeruginosa exotoxin A (Yerushalmi et al., 2000), ricin (Rodriguez et al., 1998) and, more recently, saporin (SAP) (Zarovni et al., 2006), may be suitable candidates for cancer gene therapies. In contrast to suicide genes that act by disrupting DNA synthesis, these toxins are potent inhibitors of protein synthesis, which acts in a cell cycle-independent manner, killing both quiescent and rapidly dividing tumor cells. Thus, these toxins may offer effective therapy for aggressively growing tumors and other more slowly growing tumor types (Martin et al., 2000). However, validation of this new system requires analysis of its biologic effect using controlled expression systems, e.g., the well-established tetracycline (Tet)-responsive system (Tet-On, Tet-Off), the ecdysone-inducible promoter (EcP), the T7 promoter/T7 RNA polymerase system (T7P) or the glycocorticoid responsive mouse mammary tumor virus (MMTV) promoter. In general, expression of these genes can be controlled by a significant number of tumor tissue-selective promoters and enhancer elements, which have demonstrated their potential for use in gene therapy. Genes and promoters with specific actions in different cancers will need to be selected to explore the potential of this new therapeutic approach (Lo et al., 2005).

Gene Therapy with Gef Gene

The *gef* gene has been identified as a member of a gene family that encodes homologous cell-killing functions in *Escherichia coli*. It is a porin-like membrane protein of about 50 amino-acids that is anchored in the cytoplasmic membrane at the N-terminal portion and in the cytoplasm at the C-terminal portion (Gerdes et al., 1990). Mutagenesis studies with gef protein have shown that its cytoplasmic portion contains the toxic domain. The *gef* gene induces the arrest of cell respiration in *Escherichia coli*, and cells subsequently undergo morphological changes (characteristic "ghost" cells) and become non-viable (Poulsen et al., 1991). Some researchers have analyzed the effect of this gene with suicide cassettes consisting of members of the *gef* gene family in combination with inducible promoters (Molin et al., 1993).

Application of this gene in breast cancer gene therapy was recently analyzed. Using the MCF-7 breast cancer cell line, Boulaiz et al. (2003) developed a new MCF-7 cell line transfected with a mammalian expression vector containing the *gef* gene (MCF-7/TG) under control of the MMTV promoter. Induction of gef expression led to a marked decrease in the rate of cell growth, which was first observed on day 4 of induction and became significant by day 6. By days 10 and 15, growth was inhibited by 75% and 67.9%, respectively.

Although the *gef* gene has shown considerable cytotoxic effects in breast cancer cells, the mechanism is not clear. Induction of apoptosis by nonmammalian genes is a frequent mechanism of tumoral cell damage (Noteborn et al., 2004). Transcription factor E2F, diphtheria toxin A gene, and chicken anemia virus-derived protein VP3 (apoptin) induced apoptosis in melanoma, glioblastoma and osteosarcoma cell lines, respectively (Dong et al., 1999; Paulus et al., 1997; Pietersen et al., 1999). In fact, there is evidence that apoptosis inhibition may be important in tumor formation (Lauber et al., 2004). Experiments with MCF-7/TG showed that *gef* gene expression induced apoptosis at 48 h of induction (Boulaiz et al., 2003). Moreover, morphological modifications in these cells included membrane blebbing and the appearance of "craters" on the cell surface (Krueger et al., 2003). These changes are characteristic of apoptosis, as previously described by Armstrong et al. (1992) in MDA-MB-468 breast cancer cells treated with trifluorothymidine. However, the most significant finding in *gef* gene-expressing MCF-7/TG cells was the ultrastructural changes (Boulaiz et al., 2005). The presence of compaction and segregation of the chromatin at the nuclear periphery was a cytological hallmark of apoptosis. Initially, the fine structure of this chromatin was similar to that of condensed chromatin clumps in healthy cells, with the granular appearance of cross-sectioned chromatin fibers being clearly visible. At more advanced stages of apoptosis, progression of chromatin compaction was associated with redistribution of chromatin fibers, resulting in electron-dense domains of degraded chromatin with a homogeneous appearance. Another important feature was the reorganization of ribonucleoprotein-containing structures, including the nucleolus with the appearance of nucleoplasmic and presence of dilated mitochondria, demonstrated to be a critical step in several apoptotic pathways (Boya et al., 2001). These changes have also been observed in MCF-7 cells transfected with antisense Hsp70 cDNA (Nylandsted et al., 2000). However, confocal laser scanning microscopy observations revealed that gef-induced apoptosis occurred after 48 h of induction. In prokaryotic cells, death occurred at 7 h after induction (Ronchel et al., 1998), which may reflect structural and functional differences between human and bacterial cell membranes or the need for an adequate amount of gef protein in eukaryotic cells. This latter requirement has been observed in prokaryotic cells, in which a critical concentration of gef protein (unlike other killer proteins such as protein E) was required to provoke cell death (Ronchel et al., 1998).

Other changes found in induced MCF-7TG may be related to its specific mechanisms of action. For example, an aberrant cell cycle control has been demonstrated, characterized by premature progression from G_1 to S-phase and G_2 delay. These results are consistent with findings in other tumor cell lines in which apoptotic mechanisms have been induced (Wei et al., 1998). After 48 and 96h of gef expression, MCF-7 cells showed a gradual disappearance of G_1-phase cells and a corresponding accumulation of S-phase cells. Because they are unable to accomplish normal mitosis, these cells do not proliferate, and apoptotic cell death is induced. However, although numerous models of apoptosis have been described in tumor cells the pathway by which the *gef* gene acts in breast cancer cells remains under investigation.

Finally, one of the most interesting observations in breast cancer cells treated with *gef* gene therapy is the significant reduction in Ki-67 antigen expression (Boulaiz et al., 2005). This antigen is a marker of breast cancer cell proliferation with prognostic and diagnostic relevance (Aas et al., 2003; Petit et al., 2004). MCF-7TG cells showed a 30-37.86% reduction in KI-67 expression (depending on the time of induction) in comparison with the parental cells, indicating the antiproliferative effect of *gef* gene. Some authors have proposed the hypothesis that this change is related to the metastatic capacity of breast cancer cells, although this remains controversial (Bubb et al., 2002).

Experimental results obtained in breast cancer with the *gef* gene have shown that it significantly impairs proliferation in breast cancer tumor cells. The possibility of using selective transcriptional control sequences with *gef* therefore offers the gene therapist a tool of significant potential in which the use of a prodrug is not necessary.

Bacteriophage Proteins in the Treatment of Breast Cancer

The potential use of the bacteriophage Lambda encoded S105 holin protein was recently for tumoral gene therapy using MCF-7 breast cancer cells (Agu et al., 2006). The λ-holin protein has a membrane pore-forming activity that, in conjunction with an endolysin, leads to lysis of *E. coli* (Young et al., 1995). Although eukaryotic cells differ from prokaryotic cells in cellular structure, this toxic product may act in the membranes of cell organelles, because of the relationship between the eukaryotic endomembrane system and prokaryotic membrane structure (Emelyanov, 2003). In fact, some bacterial toxins, e.g., *Vibrio cholerae* cytolysin (VCC) or *Helicobacter pylori* VacA, can directly interact with the eukaryotic cytoplasm membrane, leading to osmotic swelling and cell lysis (Szabo et al., 1999; Coelho et al., 2000). It was shown that use of a Tet-inducible promoter with λ-holin significantly reduced growth rates of murine mammary adenocarcinoma cell-derived tumors in syngeneic Balb/c mice. Similar results were obtained in cervix carcinoma (HeLa) cell lines and an embryonic kidney cell line (HEK293) (Agu et al., 2006). Typically, when the λ-holin protein was expressed, breast cancer cells appeared swollen, multinucleated and in some cases extensively vacuolated, with a loss of cell viability within 48 to 96 h after induction. Although the most sensitive cell type appeared to be HEK293 (98% dead cells after 48 h), breast cancer cells also showed enhanced membrane permeability, known to be a common feature of dying cells either in late apoptosis or necrosis. Evaluation of breast tumor growth rates obtained from λ-holin protein-expressing mice revealed significantly reduced tumor growth versus controls. These results suggest that toxic proteins such as λ-holin may be used in the treatment of breast cancer. Moreover, a targeted delivery of cytoxically acting gene products appears to be feasible when constitutively active viral promoters are replaced with tissue-or tumor-specific promoters (Ozturk-Winder et al., 2002). Finally, other phage lysis genes have been analyzed as possible candidates for gene therapy. The *E gene* can induce a transmembrane tunnel structure in prokaryotic cells, formed asa result of its oligomerization. Driven by the high osmotic pressure inside the cell, the cytoplasmic content is expelled into the surrounding medium, thereby giving rise to empty bacterial cell envelopes (ghosts)

(Haidinger et al., 2003). Our group is investigating the possible application of this gene in breast cancer treatment.

Apoptin, a new Promise in Gene Therapy

Apoptin, a protein encoded by an avian virus, is able to enter the nuclei of cancerous cells and develop toxicity after phosphorylation. In contrast, this protein remains in the cytoplasm of normal cells (Rohn et al., 2005). The signaling pathways involved in apoptin-induced cell death are not well understood. Apoptin acts p53-independently and is even stimulated by the anti-apoptotic protein Bcl-2. Activation of upstream caspases is not required, whereas the activation of downstream caspases is involved in rapid apoptin-induced cell death (Teodoro et al., 2004). This protein can induce apoptosis in a great variety of human tumors including breast cancer (Noteborn, 2002). Some gene therapy experiments using MCF-7 breast cancer cells showed that apoptin is effective in this type of tumor, triggering the intrinsic/mitochondrial apoptotic-signaling cascade. At mitochondrial level, apoptin-triggered signals cause the release of various proapoptotic mitochondrial molecules that either directly propagate the apoptotic process or activate downstream molecules in the apoptotic signaling pathway (Maddika et al., 2005). Although there have been only a few *in vitro* and *in vivo* experiments with apoptin-transgenic mice, results obtained suggest that it might form the basis of a future anti-tumor therapy (Figure 10).

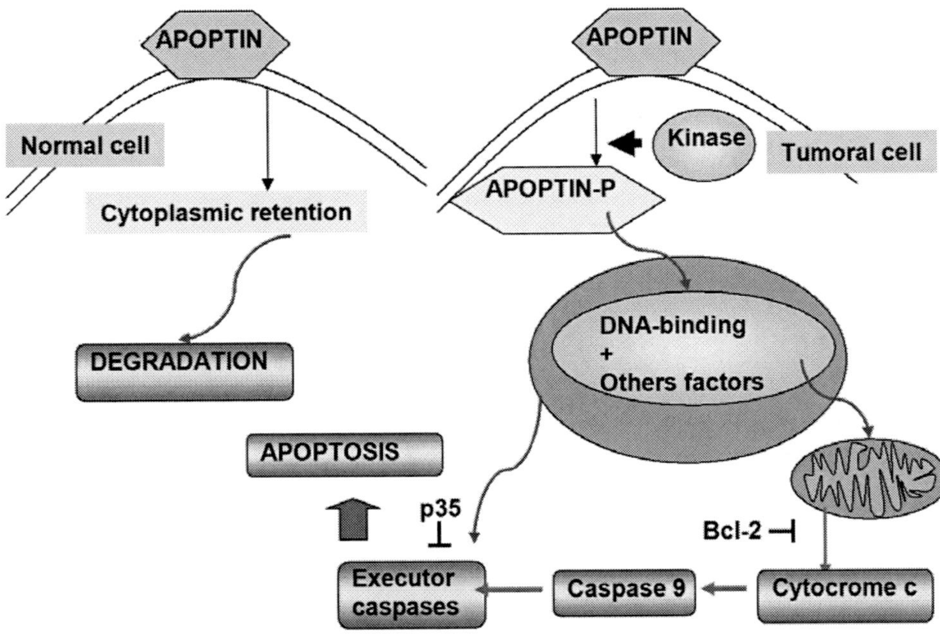

Figure 10. Apoptin mechanism of action. In normal cells, Apoptin is aggregated epitope-shielded in the cytoplasm and eventually degraded. In tumor cells, Apoptin is phosphorylated, binds to DNA and others factors triggering the apoptotic execution machinery.

Combined Gene Therapy

Conventional therapy fails in many breast cancer patients because their tumors are resistant to DNA-damaging agents, including chemotherapy and radiation therapy. Altering the genetic makeup of a cancer cell by gene transfer is a potentially powerful strategy for these cancers. However, the low efficiency of gene delivery *in vivo* and poor tumor specificity has prevented the widespread clinical implementation of this technology. One possible explanation for these unconvincing results is that first-generation viral vectors penetrate only a small portion of the tumor cells (Lumniczky and Sáfrány, 2006). Despite these obstacles, the application of combined therapy in the treatment of breast cancer is a promising new strategy (Stoff-Khalili et al., 2006).

Gene Therapy Combined with Radiation Therapy: Radiogenic Therapy

Gene therapy provides a new adjunctive approach to increase the efficacy of radiation therapy. In this combined treatment, the intratumoral introduction of genetic material results in cellular radiosensitization. A variety of strategies, e.g., gene-directed enzyme pro-drug therapy, activation of anti-tumor immune attack, application of replication-competent and oncolytic viral vectors, and hypoxia-induced gene expression are now being tested in combination with radiotherapy to modify the radiation response and overcome radiation resistance.

Radiotherapy is a well established modality for treating many forms of cancer. However, despite considerable improvements in treatment planning and delivery, the total radiation dose is often too low for tumor cure, because of the risk of normal tissue damage. Ionizing radiation exposure of mammalian cells produces a spectrum of lesions within the cell. DNA is the critical target in radiotherapy. Irradiation induces single- and double-strand DNA breaks, cell death by apoptosis or necrosis, and cell cycle checkpoint alterations (p53 and p21) (Pawlik and Keyomarsi, 2004). Radiotherapy produces various lesions in cellular macromolecules due to reactive oxygen species (Helland et al., 2006) and biological effects in non-irradiated bystander cells that have received signals from adjacent or distant irradiated cells. Several mediating mechanisms have been proposed that involve gap junction-mediated intercellular communication, secreted soluble factors, oxidative metabolism, plasma membrane-bound lipid rafts, and calcium fluxes (Hamada et al., 2007). We summarize below some different gene therapy strategies in combination with radiation therapy for breast cancer.

Combination of Radiotherapy and Suicide Gene Therapy

Gene-directed enzyme pro-drug therapy (GDEPT) is a promising tool to decrease the unfavorable side effects of radiotherapy. In GDEPT, tumor cells are transduced with suicide genes that can convert non- or mildly toxic drugs to highly toxic metabolites. This strategy can be used to improve the therapeutic ratio by reducing the dose required for an equivalent level of efficacy (Robson et al., 2005).

As noted above, the most frequently used GDEPT protocol is the thymidine kinase/GCV system. It is hypothesized that the combination of HSV-tk gene therapy and radiation may propagate DNA damage and further interferes with DNA repair mechanisms. In addition, radiation may improve adenoviral-mediated gene transfer efficiency, and radiation-induced cellular membrane damage may facilitate the transfer of cytotoxic nucleotide analogs from HSV-tk–expressing cells to neighboring nontransduced cells (Zeng et al., 1997). This combined treatment has been shown to delay local tumor growth and prolong survival in a mouse mammary tumor model (Vlachaki et al., 2001). Vlachaki et al. (2001) demonstrated that combined therapy has a considerably greater antimetastatic effect compared with HSV-tk gene therapy alone, attributing this phenomenon to the induction of a potent local and systemic immune response. The promising results of multiple courses of combined therapy also indicate that this therapy may be useful as adjuvant therapy to suppress metastasis and maintain responses in patients with disseminated disease (Vlachaki et al., 2001). More recent studies showed that when the radiation-inducible CArG promoter was used to drive HSV-*tk* expression in MCF-7 cells, a 30% higher cell kill was demonstrated compared with radiation alone (Greco et al., 2005).

Another widely investigated GDEPT strategy is the combination of cytosine deaminase (CD) with the antifungal agent 5-fluorocytosine (5-FC) (see above). Synergistic effects have been demonstrated in murine breast carcinoma cells by combining CD/5-FC GDEPT with radiation (Zhang et al., 2003). Fluorocytosine prodrug treatment also increased the therapeutic potential of radiation. Goblirsch et al. (2006) showed that cytosine deaminase enhances the effect of radiation on breast cancer in bone by reducing tumor burden, osteolysis, and skeletal fracture.

Strategies Using Apoptotic Genes Combined with Radiation Therapies

The combination of radiation and strategies to increase apoptosis is a promising therapy in cancer therapy, since apoptosis is a fundamental mechanism of cell destruction in response to ionizing radiation. Radiation and proapoptotic genes trigger apoptosis at different levels and in different pathways, suggesting that the two therapies may be synergistic or additive (Chang et al., 2006). Specific genes, e.g., *p53*, *BRCA*, and *Bcl-2* and chromosomal characteristics, e.g., telomere lengths have also been identified as playing significant roles in the radiation responsiveness of a cell (Jameela et al., 2004). p53 interacts with Bax, Bcl-XL and Bcl-2 to exert a direct apoptotic effect at mitochondria level. After radiotherapy of tumor cells, p53 promotes cell cycle arrest, initiation and transcription of DNA repair complexes, and induction of apoptosis (Fei and El-Deiry, 2003). Some preclinical studies analyzed treatment with adenoviral-mediated p53 gene transfer in conjunction with radiation therapy in non-small-cell lung cancer (NSCLC) (Szumiel, 1994). However, this combination has yet to be attempted in breast cancer (Stoff-Khalili et al., 2006). Moreover, there have been only a few reports indicating the potential value of a p53-target gene promoter, e.g., *p21* gene. Nenoi et al. (2006) showed that MCF-7 cells transfected with *p21* gene promoter were more responsive to ionizing radiation than cells transfected by electroporation.

The apoptosis-promoting gene *Bax* is downregulated in breast cancer cells and these cells are resistant to apoptosis. The pro-apoptosis protein Bax has been reported to be a possible radiation sensitizer of cancer cells. Strategies using apoptotic genes like Bax may also be beneficial if combined with radiotherapy. Interestingly, Bax itself does not cause cell death; in fact, its proapoptotic effect is exerted only after a concomitant death signal, such as deprivation of a growth factor or radiotherapy (Gómez-Navarro et al., 2000). Gene-mediated Bax-α (a splice variant of Bax) expression has been shown to increase cellular radiosensitivity in MCF-7 breast cancer cells and may potentially have a therapeutic application by enhancing radiation sensitivity in breast cancer cells (Sakakura et al., 1997).

Overexpression of cyclin D1 is often found in many different tumor cells (including breast carcinoma), which exhibit a higher induction of apoptosis. MCF7 cells containing a *cyclin D1* gene construct showed a response to ionizing radiation that was dependent on initial levels of cyclin D1. Higher levels of cyclin D1 lead to greater induction of p53 and p21. This finding suggests that breast cancer patients with wild-type p53 and pRb and an overexpression of cyclin D1 may benefit from γ-radiation treatment (Coco Martin et al., 1999).

Other promising candidates for gene replacement therapy are the melanoma differentiation associated gene-7 (*mda-7/IL-24*), tumor necrosis factor (TNF)-related apoptosis-inducing ligand (*TRAIL*), and human TESTIN (*TES*) gene. Recent studies by Chada et al. (2006) reported that animals receiving Ad-mda7 and radiotherapy underwent significant reduction in tumor growth, suggesting synergistic effects on human breast carcinoma cells. *TRAIL* is a proapoptotic gene that showed a synergistic effect on an established breast cancer xenograft (Chinnaiyan, et al., 2000) when used with radiotherapy. Finally, *TES* gene is a putative tumor suppressor gene. The mechanism of tumor suppression by TES is not fully understood. Ad-TES expression was recently shown to inhibit growth of breast and uterine cancer cells lacking TES expression *via* caspase-dependent and caspase-independent apoptosis (Sarti et al., 2005). This strategy has yet to be tested in combination with radiation but shows promise (Robson et al., 2005).

Strategies Using Hypoxia Genes Combined with Radiation Therapies

A major drawback in the radiation treatment of solid tumors is the presence of hypoxia, which can markedly reduce the effectiveness of radiotherapy. In contrast, tumor hypoxia can be exploited for gene therapy (Scott and Greco, 2004). Hypoxia is a physiological characteristic of solid tumors that induces overexpression of a number of genes. Lumniczky and Sáfrány (2006) found that gene enhancers consisting of hypoxia-responsive elements (HREs) and radiation-responsive CArG elements from the early growth response (*Egr*) 1 gene are activated by hypoxia, radiation or a combination of both stimuli. Synthetic gene promoters containing HREs from the erythropoietin (*Epo*) gene and radiation-responsive CArG elements from the Egr 1 gene have been developed to maximize targeting within the tumor. Finally, inducible nitric oxide synthase is another potent therapeutic transgene with numerous anti-cancer properties including cytotoxicity, radiosensitization, and anti-angiogenesis, making it an attractive molecule for use in cancer gene therapy (McCarthy et al., 2007).

Gene Therapy and Chemotherapy

The observation that p53 is often nonfunctional in radiotherapy- and chemotherapy-resistant tumors, the link between p53 and apoptosis, and the low toxicity of p53 in initial trials, suggest that a combination of *P53* gene therapy and other anticancer treatments may be beneficial. Tumor suppression by doxorubicin therapy with sensitization by adenovirus p53 has been demonstrated in breast cancer (Lebedeva et al., 2001). A phase II clinical trial is currently under way on the use of docetaxel and doxorubicin in combination with the local administration of Ad5CMV-*p53* (RPR/ INGN-201) in locally advanced breast cancer. Cristifanilli et al. (2006) recently reported that the combination of intratumoral administration of a nonreplicating adenoviral vector (Ad5) containing human wild-type *p53* gene (AdCMV-*p53*) with docetaxel and doxorubicin chemotherapy induces an objective clinical response and local immunomodulatory effects

Taxanes (paclitaxel and docetaxel) are antimicrotubule agents used in the treatment of breast cancer. These drugs were recently studied in combination with gene therapy using adenoviral gene type 5 *E1A*, which has been tested in multiple clinical trials for its anticancer activity (Ueno et al., 2001). This gene can downregulate HER-2/neu overexpression, thereby reversing the tumorigenic and metastatic phenotype. Association of *E1A* gene enhanced the cytoxicity of paclitaxel. A decrease in tumor growth and increase in survival rates were observed in animals treated with this combination, suggesting the need for future clinical trials on the use of E1A with chemotherapy (Liao et al., 2004).

Another area likely to be investigated in the near future is the combination of immunotherapy with established conventional tumor therapies in breast cancer. In this context, chemotherapy with taxanes has been combined with immunotherapy. Thus, Lin et al. (2003) combined *IL12* gene with paclitaxel chemotherapy in mouse mammary carcinomas and found additive responses in the decrease of tumor growth and number of lung metastases. Placlitaxel, doxorubicin, vinorelbine, gemcitabine, irinotecan and floxuridine have been combined with TRAIL gene therapy in different breast cancer cell lines, resulting in a reduction of lung metastatic nodules. These results suggest that a combination of TRAIL gene therapy and chemotherapy is effective in the treatment of breast cancer metastasis.

The use of antisense oligonucleotides and conventional chemotherapy is another example of combined therapy in breast cancer. Preclinical studies demonstrated that downregulation of specific gene products with antisense oligonucleotides sensitizes breast cancer cells to chemotherapy (gemcitabine and docetaxel), resulting in an additive or synergistic anticancer effect. In preclinical trials, these antisense targets include mouse double minutes 2 (MDM2) (Wang et al., 2001), erb-b2 (Ciardiello et al., 2001), PKC-α (Geiger et al., 1998), and Bcl-2 (Lopes de Menezes et al., 2000). In patients with solid tumors, including advanced breast cancer, a phase I trial with ISIS 2503 (antisense inhibitor of H-ras) in combination with gemcitabine and a phase I trial of a Bcl-2 antisense (G3139) with docetaxel indicated that these combined therapies were well tolerated and clinically active in heavily pretreated patients (Adjei et al., 2003).

Other combined gene therapy strategies tested for breast cancer include immunotherapy in combination with suicide gene therapy. Immunotherapy uses the transfer into tumor cells of genes of various cytokines and costimulatory molecules to stimulate an antitumoral immune response (Colombo and Forni, 1994). Direct intratumoral transfer of cytokine genes (e.g., *IL-2*, *IL-4*, IFN-γ, granulocyte colony-stimulating factor (*G-CSF*), granulocyte-macrophage-CSF (*GM-CSF*), *IL-6*, *IL-7*, and *IL-12*) has also been a strategy for augmenting tumor immunogenicity. Herpes simplex virus thymidine kinase gene therapy in combination with cytokine genes (*GM-CSF* and *IL-2*) showed beneficial effects on tumor regression and inhibition of lung metastasis in a non-immunogenic metastatic breast tumor model (Majumdar et al., 2000). Adenoviral vector-mediated strategies for breast cancer gene therapy and virotherapy also represent a promising novel therapeutic platform for breast cancer treatment. The combination of *TRAIL* gene therapy and Delta24 oncolytic adenovirus had greater antitumor activity than each used alone in both human and murine breast cancer cell lines (Guo et al., 2006).

In the immediate future, breast cancer gene therapy will probably be used as an adjuvant therapy in the local control of cancers. A multimodality approach is likely, combining surgery with concurrent or sequential gene therapy, chemotherapy, and radiotherapy.

Conclusion

Breast cancer is the most frequent cancer in females. Over the past 15 years, breast cancer mortality has been substantially reduced thanks to early detection and advances in classical breast cancer therapy (surgery, chemotherapy, radiotherapy and hormone therapy). However, new forms of therapy are urgently needed to improve the long-term survival of patients with a poor prognosis, including gene therapy. Different therapeutic strategies have been successfully used in breast cancer. Most clinical trials have focused on the intratumoral administration of an adenovirus p53 vector, although there has only been clinical evidence of tumor regression in a small minority of patients. Suicide gene therapy has been assayed in pre-clinical studies with various enzyme/prodrug systems, notably HSV-tk. The development of a new system based on toxic genes that do not need prodrugs is under investigation. In relation to immunotherapy for breast cancer, the identification of novel tumor antigens that elicit effective antitumor immune responses are likely to have a major impact on the development of genetic vaccines. siRNA and antisense technology offer a promising tool for research into future therapies and major efforts are being made in the development of clinical applications in breast cancer. MDR1-transduced hematopoietic cells have been used in advanced breast cancer patients, permitting administration of high doses of drugs such as docetaxel. Gene therapy can also be used in combination with chemotherapy and/or radiotherapy to achieve optimum outcomes with a reduction in toxic side effects. This strategy could also include suicide and immunotherapy strategies. Although many different approaches appear to be well established, there is now an urgent need for an optimal gene delivery vector. In the future, patients will probably be treated with a gene vector carrying a specific gene designed against their own specific cancer, including breast cancer.

Acknowledgments

This study was supported by the Fondo de Investigaciones Sanitarias de la Seguridad Social (FIS) through Project no. *PIO41372* headed by Prof. J. Prados. We thank Mr. Richard Davis for improving the English style of the manuscript.

References

Aas, T; Geisler, S; Eide, GE; Haugen, DF; Varhaug, JE; Bassoe, AM; et al. Predictive value of tumour cell proliferation in locally advanced breast cancer treated with neoadjuvant chemotherapy. *Eur J Cancer*, 2003, 39, 438-446.

Adjei, AA; Dy, GK; Erlichman, C; Reid, JM; Sloan, JA; Pitot, HC; et al. A phase I trial of ISIS 2503, an antisense inhibitor of H-ras, in combination with gemcitabine in patients with advanced cancer. *Clin Cancer Res*, 2003, 9, 115-123.

Agadjanyan, MG; Chattergoon, MA; Holterman, MJ; Monzavi-Karbassi, B; Kim, JJ; Dentchev, T; et al. Costimulatory molecule immune enhancement in a plasmid vaccine model is regulated in part through the Ig constant-like domain of CD80/86. *J Immunol*, 2003, 171, 4311-4319.

Agu, CA; Klein, R; Schab, S; Koning-Schuster, M; Kodajova, P; Ausserlechner, M; et al. The cytotoxic activity of the bacteriophage lambda-holin protein reduces tumour growth rates in mammary cancer cell xenograft models. *J Gene Med*, 2006, 8, 229-416.

Ahmed, M; Rahman, N. ATM and breast cancer susceptibility. *Oncogene*, 2006, 25, 5906-5911.

Ambudkar, SV; Kimchi-Sarfaty, C; Sauna, ZE; Gottesman, MM. P-glycoprotein: from genomics to mechanism. *Oncogene*, 2003, 22, 7468-7485.

Anderson, LM; Krotz, S; Weitzman, SA; Thimmapaya, B. Breast cancer-specific expression of the *Candida albicans* cytosine deaminase gene using a transcriptional targeting approach. *Cancer Gene Therapy*, 2000, 7, 845–852.

Anderson, TI; Wooster, R; Laake, K; Collins, N; Warren, W; Skrede, M; et al. Screening for ESR mutations in breast and ovarian cancer patients. *Hum Mutat*, 1997, 9, 531-536.

Armstrong, DK; Isaacs, JT; Ottaviano, YL; Davidson, NE. Programmed cell death in an estrogen-independent human breast cancer cell line MDA-MB-468. *Cancer Res*, 1992, 52, 3418-3424.

Attardi, LD; Jacks, T. The role of p53 in tumor suppression, lessons from mouse models. *Cell Mol Life Sci*, 1999, 55, 48-63.

Bateman, AR; Harrington, KJ; Kottke, T; Ahmed, A; Melcher, AA; Gough, MJ; et al. Viral fusogenic membrane glycoproteins kill solid tumor cells by nonapoptotic mechanisms that promote cross presentation of tumor antigens by dendritic cells. *Cancer Res*, 2002, 62, 6566-6578.

Bennett, MJ; Lebron, JA; Bjorkman, PJ. Crystal structure of the hereditary haemochromatosis protein HFE complexed with transferrin receptor. *Nature*, 2000, 403, 46-53.

Benouchan, M; Colombo, BM. Anti-angiogenic strategies for cancer therapy. *Int J Oncol*, 2005, 27, 563-571.

Berry, DA; Broadwater, G; Klein, JP; Antman, K; Aisner, J; Bitran, J; et al. High-dose versus standard chemotherapy in metastatic breast cancer: comparison of cancer and leukemia group B trials with data from the utologous blood and marrow transplant registry. *J Clin Oncol*, 2002, 20, 743-750.

Bjornstrom, L; Sjoberg, M. Mechanisms of estrogen receptor signaling: convergence of genomic and nongenomic actions on target genes. *Mol Endocrinol*, 2005, 19, 833-482.

Boulaiz, H; Prados, J; Marchal, JA; Concha, A; Melguizo, C; Carrillo, E; et al. Modification of Ki-67 antigen and Cell surface changes during *gef* gene induced apoptosis in human breast cancer MCF-7 cells. *Cell Mol Biol*, 2005, 51, 87-92.

Boulaiz, H; Prados, J; Melguizo, C; Garcia, A; Marchal, JA; Carrillo, E; et al. Inhibition of cell proliferation and apoptosis induction in human melanoma MCF7 cell line by gef gene. *Br J Cancer*, 2003, 89, 192-198

Boya, P; Roques, B; Kroemer, G. New EMBO members' review: viral and bacterial proteins regulating apoptosis at the mitochondrial level. *EMBO J*, 2001, 20, 4325-4331.

Braun, S; Hepp, F; Kentenich, CR; Janni, W; Pantel, K; Riethmuller, G; et al. Monoclonal antibody therapy with edrecolomab in breast cancer patients: monitoring of elimination of disseminated cytokeratin-positive tumor cells in bone marrow. *Clin Cancer Res*, 1999, 5, 3999-4004.

Braybrooke, JP; Slade, A; Deplanque, G; Harrop, R; Madhusudan, S; Foster, MD; et al. Phase I study of MetXia-P450 gene therapy and oral cyclophosphamide for patients with advanced breast cancer or melanoma. *Clin Cancer Res*, 2005, 11, 1512–1520.

Brocke-Heidrich, K; Kretzschmar, AK; Pfeifer, G; Henze, C; Loffler, D; Koczan, D; et al. Interleukin-6-dependent gene expression profiles in multiple myeloma INA-6 cells reveal a Bcl-2 family-independent survival pathway closely associated with Stat3 activation. *Blood*, 2004, 103, 242-251.

Bubb, RS; Komaki, R; Hachiya, T; Milas, I; Ro, JY; Langford, L; et al. Association of Ki-67, p53, and bcl-2 expression of the primary non-small-cell lung cancer lesion with brain metastatic lesion. *Int J Rad Oncol Biol Physics*, 2002, 53, 1216-1224.

Bubenik, J. Tumour MHC class I downregulation and immunotherapy. *Oncol Rep*, 2003, 10, 2005-2008.

Budak-Alpdogan, T; Banerjee, D; Bertino, JR. Hematopoietic stem cell gene therapy with drug resistance genes: an update. *Cancer Gene Ther*, 2005, 12, 849-863.

Burstein, HJ; Harris, LN; Marcom, PK; Lambert-Falls, R; Havlin, K; Overmoyer, B; et al. Trastuzumab and vinorelbine as first-line therapy for HER2-overexpressing metastatic breast cancer: multicenter phase II trial with clinical outcomes, analysis of serum tumor markers as predictive factors, and cardiac surveillance algorithm. *J Clin Oncol*, 2003, 21, 2889-2895.

Callaghan, R; Ford, RC; Kerr, ID. The translocation mechanism of P-glycoprotein. *FEBS Lett*, 2006, 580, 1056-1053.

Carmeliet, P; Jain, RK. Angiogenesis in cancer and other diseases. *Nature*, 2000, 407, 249-257.

Chada, S; Mhashilkar, AM; Liu, Y; Nishikawa, T; Bocangel, D; Zheng, M; et al. *mda-7* gene transfer sensities breast carcinoma cells to chemotherapy, biologic therapies and radiotherapy: correclations with expression ob bcl-2 family member. *Cancer Gene Ther*, 2006, 13, 490-502.

Chang, E; Zhu, MQ; Drezek, R; Chang, E. Novel siRNA-based molecular beacons for dual imaging and therapy. *Biotechnol J*, 2007, 4, 422-425.

Chang, JY; Zhang, X; Komaki, R; Cheung, RM; Fang, B. Tumor-specific apoptotic gene targeting overcomes radiation resistance in esophageal adenocarcinoma. *Int J Radiat Oncol Biol Phys,* 2006, 64, 1482-1494.

Chen, JL; Dunbar, PR; Gileadi, U; Jager, E; Gnjatic, S; Nagata, Y; et al. Identification of NY-ESO-1 peptide analogues capable of improved stimulation of tumor-reactive CTL. *J Immunol*, 2000, 165, 948-955.

Chen, L; Waxman, DJ. Cytochrome P450 gene-directed enzyme prodrug therapy (GDEPT) for cancer. *Curr Pharm Des*, 2002, 8, 1405-1416.

Chen, QR; Kumar, D; Stass, SA; Mixson, AJ. Liposomes complexed to plasmids encoding angiostatin and endostatin inhibit breast cancer in nude mice. *Cancer Res*, 1999, 59, 3308-3312.

Chen, QR; Mixson, JA. Systemic gene therapy with p53 inhibits breast cancer, recent advances and therapeutic implications. *Front Biosci*, 1998, 3, 997-1004.

Chi, KC; Wallis, AE; Lee, CH; De Menezes, DL; Sartor, J; Dragowska, WH; et al. Effects of bcl-2 modulation with G3139 antisense oligonucleotide on human breast cancer cells are independent of inherent bcl-2 protein expression. *Breast Cancer Res Treat*, 2000, 63, 199-212.

Chinnaiyan, AM; Prassad, U; Shankar, S; Hamstra, DA; Shanaiah, M; Chenevert, TL; et al. Combined effect of tumor necrosis factor-related apoptosis-inducing ligand and ionizing radiation in breast cancer therapy. *Proc Natl Acad Sci USA*, 2000, 97, 1754-1759.

Ciampa, A; Xu, B; Ayata, G; Baiyee, D; Wallace, J; Wertheimer, M; et al. HER-2 status in breast cancer: correlation of gene amplification by FISH with immunohistochemistry expression using advanced cellular imaging system. *Appl Immunohistochem Mol Morphol*, 2006, 14, 132-137.

Ciardiello, F; Caputo, R; Pomatico, G; De Laurentiis, M; de Placido, S; Bianco, AR; et al. Resistance to taxanes is induced by c-erbB-2 overexpression in human MCF-10A mammary epithelial cells and is blocked by combined treatment with an antisense oligonucleotide targeting type I protein kinase A. *Int J Cancer*, 2000, 85, 710-715.

Ciardiello, F; Caputo, R; Troiani, T; Borriello, G; Kandimalla, ER; Agrawal, S; et al. Antisense oligonucleotides targeting the epidermal growth factor receptor inhibit proliferation, induce apoptosis, and cooperate with cytotoxic drugs in human cancer cell lines. *Int J Cancer*, 2001, 93, 172-178.

Clezardin, P. Recent insights into the role of integrins in cancer metastasis. *Cell Mol Life Sci*, 1998, 54, 541-548.

Coco Martin, JM; Balkenende, A; Verschoor, T; Lallemand, F; Michalides, R. Cyclin D1 overexpression enhances radiation-induced apoptosis and radiosensitivity in a breast tumor cell line. *Cancer Res*, 1999, 59, 1134-1140.

Coelho, A; Andrade, JR; Vicente, AC; Dirita, VJ. Cytotoxic cell vacuolating activity from Vibrio cholerae hemolysin. *Infect Immunol*, 2000, 68, 1700-1705.

Colombo, MP; Forni, G. Cytokine gene transfer in tumor inhibition and tentative tumor therapy: where are we now? *Immunol Today*, 1994, 15, 48-51.

Conze, D; Weiss, L; Regen, PS; Bhushan, A; Weaver, D; Johnson, P; et al. Autocrine production of interleukin 6 causes multidrug resistance in breast cancer cells. *Cancer Res*, 2001, 61, 8851-8858.

Coveney, E; Clary, B; Iacobucci, M; Philip, R; Lyerly, K. Active immunotherapy with transiently transfected cytokine-secreting tumor cells inhibits breast cancer metastases in tumor-bearing animals. *Surgery*, 1996, 120, 265-272.

Cowan, KH; Moscow, JA; Huang, H; Zujewski, JA; O'Shaughnessy, J; Sorrentino, B; et al. Paclitaxel chemotherapy after autologous stem-cell transplantation and engraftment of hematopoietic cells transduced with a retrovirus containing the multidrug resistance complementary DNA (MDR1) in metastatic breast cancer patients. *Clin Cancer Res*, 1999, 5, 1619-1628.

Cristifanilli, M; Krishnamurthy, S; Guerra, L; Broglio, K; Arun, B; Booser, DJ; et al. A nonreplicating adenoviral vector that contains the wild-type p53 transgene combined with chemotherapy for primary breast cancer: safety, efficacy, and biologic activity of a novel gene-therapy approach. *Cancer*, 2006, 107, 935-944.

Cui, W; Barry, A; Gusterson, BA; Clark, AJ. Inhibition of *myc*-dependent breast tumor formation in transgenic mice. *Breast Cancer Res and Treat*, 2002, 71, 9-20.

Czauderna, F; Santel, A; Hinz, M; Fechtner, M; Durieux, B; Fisch, G; et al. Inducible shRNA expression for application in a prostate cancer mouse model. *Nucleic Acids Res*, 2003, 31, e127.

Dachs, GU; Tupper, J; Tozer, GA. From bench to bebside for gene-directed enzyme prodrug therapy of cancer. *Anti-Cancer Drug*, 2005, 16, 349-359.

Dales, JP; Garcia, S; Bonnier, P; Duffaud, F; Carpentier, S; Djemli, A; et al. Prognostic significance of VEGF receptors, VEGFR-1 (Flt-1) and VEGFR-2 (KDR/Flk-1) in breast carcinoma. *Ann Pathol*, 2003, 23, 297-305.

Dave, UP; Jenkins, NA; Copeland, NG. Gene therapy insertional mutagenesis insights. *Science*, 2004, 16, 303-333.

De Palma, M; Venneri, MA; Roca, C; Naldini, L. Targeting exogenous genes to tumor angiogenesis by transplantation of genetically modified hematopoietic stem cells. *Nat Med*, 2003, 9, 789-795.

Degreve, B; Andrei, G; Izquierdo, M; Piette, J; Morin, K; Knaus, EE; et al. Varicella-zoster virus thymidine hinase gene and antiherptic pyrimidine nucleoside analogues in a combined gene/chemotherapy treatment for cancer. *Gene Ther*, 1997, 4, 1107-1114.

Dell'Agnola, C; Biragyn, A. Clinical utilization of chemokines to combat cancer: the double-edged sword. *Expert Rev Vaccines*, 2007, 6, 267-283.

Diaz, RM; Bateman, A; Emiliusen, L; Fielding, A; Trono, D; Russell, SJ; et al. A lentiviral vector expressing a fusogenic glycoprotein for cancer gene therapy. *Gene Ther*, 2000, 7, 1656-1663.

Dickson, PV; Nathwani, AC; Davidoff, AM. Delivery of antiangiogenic agents for cancer gene therapy. *Technol Cancer Res Treat*, 2005, 4, 331-341.

Dilber, MS; Smith, CIE. Suicide genes and bystander killing: local and distant effects. *Gene Therapy*, 1997, 4, 273-274.

Dong, YB; Yang, HL; Elliot, MJ; Liu, TJ; Stilwell, A; Atienza, C; et al. Adenovirus-mediated E2F-1 gene transfer efficiently induces apoptosis in melanoma cells. *Cancer*, 1999, 86, 2021-2033.

Ealovega, MW; McGinnis, PK; Sumantran, VN; Clarke, MF; Wicha, MS. bcl-xs gene therapy induces apoptosis of human mammary tumors in nude mice. *Cancer Res*, 1996, 56, 1965-1969.

El-Deiry, WS. The role of p53 in chemosensitivity and radiosensitivity. *Oncogene*, 2003, 22, 7486-7495.

Emelyanov, VV. Mitochondrial connection to the origin of the eukaryotic cell. *Eur J Biochem*, 2003, 270, 1599-1618.

Emi, M; Kim, R; Tanabe, K; Uchida, Y; Toge, T. Targeted therapy against Bcl-2-related proteins in breast cancer cells. *Breast Cancer Res*, 2005, 7, 940-952.

Fei, P; El-Deiry WS. p53 and radiation responses. *Oncogene*, 2003, 22, 5774-5783.

Feldman, AL; Libutti, SK. Progress in antiangiogenic gene therapy of cancer. *Cancer*, 2000, 89, 1181-1194.

Ferrara, N; Hillan, KJ; Gerber, HP; Novotny, W. Discovery and development of bevacizumab, an anti-VEGF antibody for treating cancer. *Nat Rev Drug Discov*, 2004, 3, 391-400.

Fidler, IJ; Ellis, LM. Neoplastic angiogenesis - not all blood vessels are created equal. *N Engl J Med*, 2004, 351, 215-216.

Fielding, AK; Chapel-Fernandes, S; Chadwick, MP; Bullough, FJ; Cosset, FL; Russell, SJ. A hyperfusogenic gibbon ape leukemia envelope glycoprotein: targeting of a cytotoxic gene by ligand display. *Hum Gene Ther*, 2000, 11, 817-826.

Fire, A; Xu, S; Montgomery, M; Kostas, S; Driver, S; Mello, C. "Potent and specific genetic interference by double-stranded RNA in *Caenorhabditis elegans*". *Nature*, 1998, 391, 806-811.

Fogar, P; Greco, E; Basso, D; Habeler, W; Navaglia, F; Zambon, CF; et al. Suicide gene therapy with HSV-TK in pancreatic cancer has no effect in vivo in a mouse model. *Eur J Surg Oncol*, 2003, 29, 721-730.

Folkman, J. Role of angiogenesis in tumor growth and metastasis. *Semin Oncol*, 2002, 29, 15-18.

Folkman, J. Endogenous angiogenesis inhibitors. *APMIS*, 2004, 112, 496-507.

Fong, S; Itahana, Y; Sumida, T; Singh, J; Coppe, JP; Liu, Y; et al. Id-1 as a molecular target in therapy for breast cancer cell invasion and metastasis. *Proc Natl Acad Sci USA*, 2003, 100, 13543-13548.

Frankel, AE; Powell, BL; Duesbery, NS; Vande Woude, GF; Leppla, SH. Anthrax fusion protein therapy of cancer. *Curr Protein Pept Sci,* 2002, 3, 399-407.

Fujimori, M. Genetically Engineered *Bifidobacterium* as a drug delivery system for systemic therapy of metastatic breast cancer patients. *Breast Cancer*, 2006, 13, 27-31.

Gadal, F; Bastias, J; Wei, MX; Crepin, M. 'Suicide' gene therapy of breast cancer cells is only cytostatic *in vitro* but anti-tumoral *in vivo* on breast MCF7-ras tumor. *In Vivo*, 2004, 18, 813-818.

Gasparini, G. Prognostic value of vascular endothelial growth factor in breast cancer. *Oncologis*t, 2000, 5, 37-44.

Geiger, T; Muller, M; Dean, NM; Fabbro, D. Antitumor activity of a PKC-alpha antisense oligonucleotide in combination with standard chemotherapeutic agents against various human tumors transplanted into nude mice. *Anticancer Drug Des*, 1998, 13, 35-45.

Gerdes, K; Poulsen, LK; Thisted, T; Nielsen, A; Martinussen, J; Anderssen, PH. The hok killer gene family in Gram negative bacteria. *New Biologist*, 1990, 2, 964-956.

Ghosh, A; Stewart, D; Matlashewski, G. Regulation of human p53 activity and cell localization by alternative splicing. *Mol Cell Biol*, 2004, 24, 7987-7997.

Goblirsch, M; Zwolak, P; Ramnaraine, ML; Pan, W; Lynch, C; Alaei, P; et al. Novel *cytosine deaminase* fusion gene enhances the effect of radiation on breast cancer in bone by reducing tumor burden, osteolysis, and skeletal fracture. *Clin Cancer Res*, 2006, 12, 3168-3176.

Gómez-Navarro, J; Arafat, W; Xiang, J. Gene therapy for carcinoma of the breast: pro-apoptotic gene therapy. *Breast Cancer Res*, 2000, 2, 32-44.

Goodrich, DW. The retinoblastoma tumor-suppressor gene; the exception that proves the rule. *Oncogene*, 2006; 25; 5233-5243.

Greco, O; Dacha, GU. Gene directed enzyme/prodrug therapy of cancer: historical appraisal and future prospectives. *J Cell Physiol*, 2001, 187, 22-36.

Greco, O; Joiner, MC; Doleh, A; Powell, AD; Hillman, GG; Scott, SD. Hypoxia- and radiation-activated Cre/loxP 'molecular switch' vectors for gene therapy of cancer. *Gene Therapy*, 2006, 13, 206-215.

Greco, O; Powell, TM; Marples, B; Joiner, MC; Scott, SD. Gene Therapy Vectors Containing CArG Elements from the Egr1 Gene are Activated by Neutron Irradiation, Cisplatin and Doxorubicin. *Cancer Gene Ther*, 2005, 12, 655-662.

Green, KA; Streuli, CH. Apoptosis regulation in the mammary gland. *Cell Mol Life Sci*, 2004, 61, 1867-1883.

Grignet-Debrus, C; Noël, A, Foidart, JM; Calberg-Bacq, C.M. Identification of factors important for the success of suicide gene therapy after a comparative study of varicella zoster and herpes simplex viral thymidine kinases efficacy on breast cancer cells. *Cell Mol Biol*, 2005, 51, 37-48.

Grillo, M; Bott, MJ; Khandke, N; McGinnis, JP; Miranda, M; Meyyappan, M; et al. Validation of cyclin D1/CDK4 as an anticancer drug target in MCF-7 breast cancer cells: Effect of regulated overexpression of cyclin D1 and siRNA-mediated inhibition of endogenous cyclin D1 and CDK4 expression. *Breast Cancer Res Treat*, 2006, 95, 185-194.

Guidi, AJ; Berry, DA; Broadwater, G; Perloff, M; Norton, L; Barcos, MP; et al. Association of angiogenesis in lymph node metastases with outcome of breast cancer. *J Natl Cancer Inst*, 2000, 92, 486-492.

Guinee, VF. Epidemiología del cáncer de mama. La mama. *Manejo multidisciplinario de las enfermedades benignas y malignas*. 2ª ed. Buenos Aires: Editorial Médica Panamericana SA; 2000, 345-357.

Guo, W; Zhu, H; Zhang, L; Davis, J; Teraishi, F; Roth, JA; et al. Combination effect of oncolytic adenovirotherapy and TRAIL gene therapy in syngeneic murine breast cancer models. *Cancer Gen Ther*, 2006, 13, 82-90.

Gyorffy, S; Palmer, K; Gauldie, J. Adenoviral vector expressing murine angiostatin inhibits a model of breast cancer metastatic growth in the lungs of mice. *Am J Pathol*, 2001, 159, 1137-1147.

Hahn, W; Ho, SH; Jeong, JG; Hahn, EY; Kim, S; Yu, SS; et al. Viral vector mediated transduction of a modified thrombospondin-2 cDNA inhibits tumor growth and angiogenesis. *Gene Ther*, 2004, 11, 739-745.

Haidinger, W; Szostak, MP; Jechlinger, W; Lubitz, W. Online Monitoring of Escherichia coli Ghost Production. *Appl Environ Microbiol*, 2003, 69, 468-474.

Hamada, N; Matsumoto, H; Hara, T; Kobayashi, Y. Intercellular and intracellular signaling pathways mediating ionizing radiation-induced bystander effects. *J Radiat Res*, 2007, 48, 87-95.

Han, MY; Zheng, S; Yu, JM; Peng, JP; Guo, QS; Wang, JL. Study on interleukin-18 gene transfer into human breast cancer cells to prevent tumorigenicity. *J Zhejiang Univ Sci*, 2004, 5, 472-476.

Hanania, EG; Fu, S; Roninson, I; Zu, Z; Deisseroth, AB. Resistance to taxol chemotherapy produced in mouse marrow cells by safety-modified retroviruses containing a human MDR-1 transcription unit. *Gene Therapy*, 1995, 2, 279-284.

Helland, A; Johnsen, H; Froyland, C; Landmark, HB; Sætersdal, AB; Holmen, M; et al. Radiation-induced effects on gene expression: An in vivo study on breast cancer. *Radiother Oncol*, 2006, 80, 230-235.

Hinz, S; Trauzold, A; Boenicke, L; Sandberg, C; Beckmann, S; Bayer, E; et al. Bcl-XL protects pancreatic adenocarcinoma cells against CD95- and TRAIL-receptor-mediated apoptosis. *Oncogene*, 2000, 19, 5477-5486.

Hodgson, SV; Morrison, PJ; Irving, M. Breast cancer genetics: unsolved questions and open perspectives in an expanding clinical practice. *Am J Med Genet C Semin Med Genet*, 2004, 129, 56-64.

Honma, S; Shimodaira, K; Shimizu, Y; Tsuchiya, N; Saito, H; Yanaihara, T; et al. The influence of inflammatory cytokines on estrogen production and cell proliferation in human breast cancer cells. *Endocr J*, 2002, 49, 371-377.

Hu, X; Su, F; Qin, L; Jia, W; Gong, C; Yu, F; et al. Stable RNA interference of ErbB-2 gene synergistic with epirubicin suppresses breast cancer growth in vitro and in vivo. *Biochem Biophys Res Commun*, 2006, 4, 778-785.

Hudelist, G; Czerwenka, K; Kubista, E; Marton, E; Pischinger, K; Singer, CF. Expression of sex steroid receptors and their co-factors in normal and malignant breast tissue: AIB1 is a carcinoma-specific co-activator. *Breast Cancer Res Treat*, 2003, 78, 193-204.

Hudis, CA; Schmitz, N. Dose-dense chemotherapy in breast cancer and lymphoma. *Semin Oncol*, 2004, 31, 19-26.

Huh, JI; Calvo, A; Stafford, J; Cheung, M; Kumar, R; Philp, D; et al. Inhibition of VEGF receptors significantly impairs mammary cancer growth in C3(1)/Tag transgenic mice through antiangiogenic and nonantiangiogenic mechanisms. *Oncogene*, 2005, 24, 790-800.

Hurlimann, J; Larrinaga, B; Vala, DL. bcl-2 protein in invasive ductal breast carcinomas. *Virchows Arch*, 1995, 426, 163-168.

Ichikawa, T; Tamiya, T; Adachi, Y; Ono, Y; Matsumoto, K; Furuta, T; et al. In vivo efficacy and toxicity of 5-fluorocytosine/cytosine deaminase gene therapy for malignant gliomas mediated by adenovirus. *Cancer Gene Ther*, 2000, 7, 74-82.

Im, SA; Kim, JS; Gomez-Manzano, C; Fueyo, J; Liu, TJ; Cho, MS; et al. Inhibition of breast cancer growth in vivo by antiangiogenesis gene therapy with adenovirus-mediated antisense-VEGF. *Br J Cancer*, 2001, 84, 1252-1257.

Indraccolo, S; Gola, E; Rosato, A; Minuzzo, S; Habeler, W; Tisato, V; et al. Differential effects of angiostatin, endostatin and interferon-alpha(1) gene transfer on in vivo growth of human breast cancer cells. *Gene Ther*, 2002, 9, 867-878.

Izawa, JI; Sweeney, P; Perrotte, P; Kedar, D; Dong, Z; Slaton, JW; et al. Inhibition of tumorigenicity and metastasis of human bladder cancer growing in athymic mice by interferon-beta gene therapy results partially from various antiangiogenic effects including endothelial cell apoptosis. *Clin Cancer Res*, 2002, 8, 1258-1270.

Jaattela, M. Escaping cell death, survival proteimens in cancer. *Exp Cell Res*, 1999, 248, 30-43.

Jameela, JKA; Raoa, VSR; Cawkwellb, L; Drewa, PJ. Radioresistance in carcinoma of the breast. *Breast*, 2004, 13, 452-460.

Jansen, B; Wacheck, V; Heere-Ress, E; Schlagbauer-Wadl, H; Hollenstein, U; Lucas, T; et al. A phase I-II study with dacarbazine and BCL-2 antisense oligonucleotide G3139 (Genta) as a chemosensitizer in patients with advanced malignant melanoma. *Proc Am Asso Clin Oncol* 1999, 18, 2049.

Jiang, P; Du, W; Heese, K; Wu, M. The Bad guy cooperates with good cop p53, Bad is transcriptionally up-regulated by p53 and forms a Bad/p53 complex at the mitochondria to induce apoptosis. *Mol Cell Biol*, 2006, 26, 9071-9082.

Jin, X; Bookstein, R; Wills, K; Avanzini, J; Tsai, V; LaFace, D; et al. Evaluation of endostatin antiangiogenesis gene therapy in vitro and in vivo. *Cancer Gene Ther*, 2001, 8, 982-989.

Jones, KL; Buzdar, AU. A review of adjuvant hormonal therapy in breast cancer. *Endocr Relat Cancer*, 2004, 11, 391-406.

Kan, O; Griffiths, L; Baban, D; Iqball, S; Uden, M; Spearman, H; et al. Direct retroviral delivery of human cytochrome P450 2B6 for gene-directed enzyme prodrug therapy of cancer. *Cancer Gene Ther*, 2001, 8, 473-482.

Kawabata, R; Wada, H; Isobe, M; Saika, T; Sato, S; Uenaka, A; et al. Antibody response against NY-ESO-1 in CHP-NY-ESO-1 vaccinated patients. *Int J Cancer*, 2007, 120, 2178-2184.

Khanna, KK; Chenevix-Trench, G. ATM and genome maintenance: defining its role in breast cancer susceptibility. *J Mammary Gland Biol Neoplasia*, 2004, 9, 247-262.

Knupfer, H; Preiss, R. Significance of interleukin-6 (IL-6) in breast cancer. *Breast Cancer Res Treat*, 2007, 102, 129-135.

Kommareddy, S; Amiji, M. Antiangiogenic gene therapy with systemically administered sFlt-1 plasmid DNA in engineered gelatin-based nanovectors. *Cancer Gene Ther*, 2007, 14, 488-498.

Konecny, GE; Meng, YG; Untch, M; Wang, HJ; Bauerfeind, I; Epstein, M; et al. Association between HER-2/neu and vascular endothelial growth factor expression predicts clinical outcome in primary breast cancer patients. *Clin Cancer Res*, 2004, 10, 1706-1716.

Kou, B; Li, Y; Shi, Y; Xia, J; Wang, X; Wu, S. Gene therapeutic exploration: retrovirus-mediated soluble vascular endothelial growth factor receptor-2 (sFLK-1) inhibits the tumorigenicity of S180, MCF-7, and B16 cells in vivo. *Oncol Res*, 2005, 15, 239-247.

Krajewski, S; Krajewska, M; Turner, BC; Pratt, C; Howard, B; Zapata, JM; et al. Prognostic significance of apoptosis regulators in breast cancer. Endocr-Relat Cancer, 1999, 6, 29-40.

Krueger, KD; Hunter, WJ; DelCore, MG; Agrawal, DK. Calphostin C as a rapid and strong inducer of apoptosis in human coronary artery smooth muscle cells. *Int. Immunopharmacol*, 2003, 3, 1751-1759.

Kurreck, J. Antisense technologies, improvement through novel chemical modifications. *Eur J Biochemistry*, 2003, 270, 1628-1644.

Laheru, DA; Pardoll, DM; Jaffee, EM. Genes to vaccines for immunotherapy: how the molecular biology revolution has influenced cancer immunology. *Mol Cancer Ther*, 2005, 4, 1645-1652.

Lapteva, N; Yang, AG; Sanders, DE; Strube, RW; Chen, SY. CXCR4 knockdown by small interfering RNA abrogates breast tumor growth in vivo. *Cancer Gene Ther*, 2004, 12, 84-89.

Larin, SS; Georgiev, GP; Kiselev, SL. Gene transfer approaches in cancer immunotherapy. *Gene Ther*, 2004, 11, 18-25.

Lau, K; Bicknell, R. Antiangiogenic gene therapy. *Gene Ther*, 1999, 6, 1793-1795.

Lauber, K; Blumenthal, SG; Waibel, M; Wesselborg, S. Clearance of apoptotic cells: getting rid of the corpses. *Mol Cell*, 2004, 14, 277-287

Laust, AK; Sur, BW; Wang, K; Hubby, B; Smith, JF; Nelson, EL. VRP immunotherapy targeting neu: treatment efficacy and evidence for immunoediting in a stringent rat mammary tumor model. *Breast Cancer Res Treat*, 2007.

Lebedeva, S; Bagdasarova, S; Tyler, T; Mu, X; Wilson, DR; Gjerset, RA. Tumor suppression and therapy sensitization of localized and metastatic breast cancer by adenovirus p53. *Hum Gene Ther*, 2001, 12, 763-772.

Lengler, J; Omann, M; Düvier, D; Holzmüller, H; Gregor, W; Salmons, B; et al. Cytochrome P450 reductase dependent inhibition of cytochrome P450 2B1 activity: Implications for gene directed enzyme prodrug therapy. *Biochemocal Pharmacology*, 2006, 72, 893-901.

Levine, AJ; Hu, W; Feng, Z. The P53 pathway: what questions remain to be explored? *Cell Death Differ*, 2006, 13, 1027-1036.

Levy, S; Zhou, B; Ballian, N; Li, Z; Liu, SH; Feanny, N; et al. Cytotoxic gene therapy for human breast cancer in vitro. *J Surg Res*, 2006, 136,154-160.

Levy-Lahad, E; Friedman, E. Cancer risks among BRCA1 and BRCA2 mutation carriers. *Br J Cancer*, 2007, 96, 11-15.

Liang, Z; Yoon, Y; Votaw, J; Goodman, MM; Williams, L; Shim, H. Silencing of CXCR4 blocks breast cancer metastasis. *Cancer Res*, 2005, 65, 967-971.

Liao, Y; Zou, YY; Xia, WY; Hung, MC. Enhanced paclitaxel cytotoxicity and prolonged animal survival rate by a nonviral-mediated systemic delivery of E1A gene in orthotopic xenograft human breast cancer. *Cancer Gene Ther*, 2004, 11, 594-602.

Liaw, D; Marsh, DJ; Li, J; Dahia, PLM; Wang, SI; Zheng, Z; et al. Germline mutations of the PTEN gene in Cowden disease, an inherited breast and thyroid cancer syndrome. *Nature Genetics*, 1997, 16, 64-67.

Lichtor, T; Glick, RP; Lin, HI; Cohen, EP. Intratumoral injection of IL-secreting syngeneic/allogeneic fibroblasts transfected with DNA from breast cancer cells prolongs the survival of mice with intracerebral breast cancer. *Cancer Gene Ther*, 2005, 12, 708-714.

Lin, J; Page, C; Jin, X; Sethi, AO; Patel, R; Nunez, G. Suppression activity of pro-apoptotic gene products in cancer cells; a potential application for cancer gene therapy. *Anticancer Res*, 2001, 21, 831-839.

Lin, T; Zhang, L; Davis, J; Gu, J; Nishizaki, M; Ji, L; et al. Combination of TRAIL gene therapy and chemotherapy enhances antitumor and antimetastasis effects in chemosensitive and chemoresistant breast cancers. *Mol Ther*, 2003, 8, 441-448.

Liu, M; Acres, B; Balloul, JM; Bizouarne, N; Paul, S; Slos, P; et al. Gene-based vaccines and immunotherapeutics. *Proc Natl Acad Sci USA*, 2004, 101, 14567-14571.

Liu, Y; Deisseroth, A. Tumor vascular targeting therapy with viral vectors. *Blood*, 2006, 107, 3027-3033.

Lo, HW; Day, CP; Hung, MC. Cancer-specific gene therapy. *Adv Genet*, 2005, 54, 235-255.

Lopes de Menezes, DE; Hudon, N; McIntosh, N; Mayer, LD. Molecular and pharmacokinetic properties associated with the therapeutics of bcl-2 antisense oligonucleotide G3139 combined with free and liposomal doxorubicin. *Clin Cancer Res*, 2000, 6, 2891-2902.

Lumniczky, K; Sáfrány, G. Cancer gene therapy: combination with radiation therapy and the role of bystander cell killing in the anti-tumor effect. *Pathol Oncol Res*, 2006, 12, 118-124.

Lv, H; He, Z; Liu, X; Yuan, J; Yu, Y; Chen, Z. Reversal of BCRP-mediated multidrug resistance by stable expression of small interfering RNAs. *J Cell Biochem*, 2007, Mar 19, [Epub ahead of print].

Maddike, S; Booy, EP; Johar, D; Gibson, SB; Ghavami, S; Los, M. Cancer-specific toxicity of apoptin is independent of death receptors but involves the loss of mitochondrial membrane potential and the release of mitochondrial cell-death mediators by a Nur77-dependent pathway. *J Cell Sci*, 2005, 118, 4485-4493.

Majumdar, AS; Zolotorev, A; Samuel, S; Tran, K; Vertin, B; Hall-Meier, M; et al. Efficacy of herpes simplex virus thymidine kinase in combination with cytokine gene therapy in an experimental metastatic breast cancer model. *Cancer Gene Ther*, 2000, 7, 1086-1099.

Marais, R; Spooner, RA; Light, Y; Martin, J; Springer, CJ. Gene directed enzyme prodrug therapy with a mustard prodrug/carboxypeptidase G2 combination. *Cancer Res*, 1996, 56, 4735-4742.

Marais, R; Spooner, RA; Stribbling, SM; Light, Y; Martin, J; Springer, CJ. A cell surface tethered enzyme improves effciency in genedirected enzyme prodrug therapy. *Nat Biotechnol*, 1997, 15, 1373-1377.

Martin, V; Cortes, ML; De Felipe, P; Farsetti, A; Calcaterra, NB; Izquierdo, M. Cancer gene therapy by thyroid hormonemediated expression of toxin genes. *Cancer Res*, 2000, 60, 3218-3224.

Mazurek N; Sun YJ; Liu, KF; Gilcrease, MZ; Schober, W; Nangia-Makker, P; et al. Phosphorylated galectin-3 mediates tumor necrosis factor-related apoptosis-inducing ligand (TRAIL) signaling by regulating PTEN in human breast carcinoma cells. *J Biol Chem*, 2007 [Epub ahead of print].

McCarthy, HO; Worthington, J; Barrett, E; Cosimo, E; Boyd, M; Mairs, RJ; et al. *p21((WAF1))*-mediated transcriptional targeting of inducible nitric oxide synthase gene therapy sensitizes tumours to fractionated radiotherapy. *Gene Ther*, 2007, 14, 246-255.

McCormick, F. Cancer gene therapy, fringe or cutting edge? *Nat Rev Cancer*, 2001, 1, 130-141.

McDonald, DM; Baluk, P. Significance of blood vessel leakiness in cancer. *Cancer Res*, 2002, 62, 5381-5385.

Melguizo, C; Prados, J; Aránega, A. Multidrug resistance and cellular differentiation. In: Aranega A. (ed). *Muscle Cells: New Strategy in Cellular and Molecular Biology*. Granada: Editorial Universidad de Granada; 1995, 67-118.

Mendelson, J; Baselga, J. Status of epidermal growth factor receptor antagonist in biology and treatment of cancer. *J Clin Oncol*, 2003, 21, 2787-2799.

Miller, WR; Watson, DM; Jack, W; Chetty, U; Elton, RA. Tumour cyclic AMP binding proteins: an independent prognostic factor for disease recurrence and survival in breast cancer. *Breast Cancer Res Treat*, 1993, 26, 89-94.

Molin, SL; Boe, LB; Jensen, CS; Kristensen, M; Givskov, M; Ramos, JL; et al. Suicidal genetic elements and their use in biological containment of bacteria. *Annu Rev Microbiol*, 1993, 47, 139-166.

Morabito, A; Sarmiento, R; Bonginelli, P; Gasparini, G. Antiangiogenic strategies, compounds, and early clinical results in breast cancer. *Crit Rev Oncol Hematol*, 2004, 49, 91-107.

Morrison, C; Sonoda, E; Takao, N; Shinohara, A; Yamamoto, K; Takeda, S. The controlling role of ATM in homologous recombinational repair of DNA damage. *EMBO J*, 2000, 19, 463-471.

Moscow, JA; Huang, H; Carter, C; Hines, K; Zujewski, J; Cusack, G. Engraftment of MDR1 and NeoR genetransduced hematopoietic cells after breast cancer chemotherapy. *Blood*, 1999, 94, 52-61.

Mullan, PB; Quinn, JE; Harkin, DP. The role of BRCA1 in transcriptional regulation and cell cycle control. *Oncogene,* 2006, 25, 5854-5863.

Nenoi, M; Daino, K; Ichimura, S; Takahashi, SI; Akuta, T. Low-dose radiation response of the *p21WAF1/CIP1* gene promoter transduced by adeno-associated virus vector. *Exp Mol Med*, 2006, 38, 553-564.

Nicolini, A; Carpi, A; Rossi, G. Cytokines in breast cancer. *Cytokine Growth Factor Rev*, 2006, 17, 325-537.

Niculescu-Duvaz, D; Niculescu-Duvaz, I; Friedlos, F; Martin, J; Lehouritis, P. Self-immolative nitrogen mustards prodrugs cleavable by carboxypeptidase G2 showing large cytotoxicity differentials in GDEPT. *J Med Chem*, 2003, 46, 1690-1705.

Niculescu-Duvaz, I; Scanlon, I; Niculescu-Duvaz, D; Friedlos, F; Martin, J; Marais, R; et al. Significant differences in biological parameters between prodrugs cleavable by carboxypeptidase G2 that generate 3,5-difluoro-phenol and –aniline nitrogen mustards in gene-directed enzyme prodrug therapy systems. *J Med Chem*, 2004, 47, 2651-2658.

Nielsen, L; Lipari, P; Dell, J; Gurnani, M; Hajian, G. Adenovirus-mediated p53 gene therapy and paclitaxel have synergistic efficacy in models of human head and neck, ovarian, prostate, and breast cancer. *Clin Cancer Res*, 1998, 4, 835-846.

Nielsen, LL; Maneval, DC; P53 tumor suppressor gene therapy for cancer. *Cancer Gene Ther*, 1998, 5, 52-63.

Noteborn, MHM. Chicken anemia virus induced apoptosis: underlying molecular mechanisms. *Vet Microbiol*, 2004, 98, 89-94.

Noteborn, MHM. Apoptin as an anticancer therapy. In: La Thangue NB and Bandara LR. (eds.). *Targets for cancer chemotherapy; transcription factors and other nuclear proteins*. Humana Press, Totowa, USA; 2002, 275-287.

Nylandsted, J; Rohde, M; Brand, K; Bastholm, L; Elling, F; Jaattela, M. Selective depletion of heat shock protein 70 (Hsp70) activates a tumor-specific death program that is independent of caspases and bypasses Bcl-2. *Proc Natl Acad Sci USA*, 2000, 97, 7871-7876.

O'Shaughnessy, J. Extending survival with chemotherapy in metastatic breast cancer. *Oncologist*, 2005, 10, 20-29.

Orlando, L; Cardillo, A; Ghisini, R; Rocca, A; Balduzzi, A; Torrisi, R; et al. Trastuzumab in combination with metronomic cyclophosphamide and methotrexate in patients with HER-2 positive metastatic breast cancer. *BMC Cancer*, 2006, 6, 225.

Osta, WA; Chen, Y; Mikhitarian, K; Mitas, M; Salem, M; Hannun, YA; et al. EpCAM is overexpressed in breast cancer and is a potential target for breast cancer gene therapy. *Cancer Res*, 2004, 64, 5818-5824.

Ozturk-Winder, F; Renner, M; Klein, D; Muller, M; Salmons, B; Gunzburg, WH. The murine whey acidic protein promoter directs expression to human mammary tumors after retroviral transduction. *Cancer Gene Ther*, 2002, 9, 421-431.

Pandha, HS; Martin, LA; Rigg, A; Hurst, HC; Stamp, GW; Sikora, K; et al. Genetic prodrug activation therapy for breast cancer: a phase I clinical trial of erbB-2-directed suicide gene expression. *J Clin Oncol*, 1999, 17, 2180–2189.

Panno, M; Giordano, F; Mastroianni, F; Morelli, C; Brunelli, E; Palma, M; et al. Evidence that low doses of Taxol enhance the functional transactivatory properties of p53 on p21 waf promoter in MCF-7 breast cancer cells. *FEBS Let*, 2006, 580, 2371-2380.

Pantschenko, AG; Pushkar, I; Anderson, KH; Wang, Y; Miller, LJ; Kurtzman, SH; et al. The interleukin-1 family of cytokines and receptors in human breast cancer: implications for tumor progression. *Int J Oncol*, 2003, 23, 269-284.

Papetti, M; Herman, IM. Mechanisms of normal and tumor-derived angiogenesis. *Am J Physiol Cell Physiol*, 2002, 282, 947-970.

Patry, C; Bouchard, L; Labrecque, P; Gendron, D; Lemieux, B; Toutant, J; et al. Small interfering RNA-mediated reduction in heterogeneous nuclear ribonucleoparticule A1/A2 proteins induces apoptosis in human cancer cells but not in normal mortal cell lines. *Cancer Res*, 2003, 63, 7679-7688.

Paulus, W; Baur, I; Oberer, DM; Breakefield, XO; Reeves, AA. Regulated expression on the diphtheria toxin A gene in human glioma cells using prokaryotic transcriptional control elements. *J Neurosurg*, 1997, 87, 89-95.

Pawlik, T; Keyomarsi, K. Role of cell cycle mediating sensitivity to radiotherapy. *Int J Radiation Oncology Biol Phys*, 2004, 59, 928-942.

Persano, L; Crescenzi, M; Indraccolo, S. Anti-angiogenic gene therapy of cancer: current status and future prospects. *Mol Aspects Med*, 2007, 28, 87-114.

Petit, T; Wilt, M; Velten, M; Millon, R; Rodier, JF; Borel, C; et al. Comparative value of tumour grade, hormonal receptors, Ki-67, HER-2 and topoisomerase II alpha status as predictive markers in breast cancer patients treated with neoadjuvant anthracycline-based chemotherapy. *Eur J Cancer*, 2004, 40, 205-211.

Petrocelli, T; Slingerland, JM. PTEN deficiency: a role in mammary carcinogenesis. *Breast Cancer Res*, 2001, 3, 356-360.

Pietersen, AM; Van der Eb, MM; Rademaker, HJ; Van der Wollenberg, DJ; Rabelink, MJ; Kuppen, PJ; et al. Specific tumor-cell killing with adenovirus vector containing the apoptin gene. *Gene Ther*, 1999, 6, 882-892.

Poulsen, LK; Refn, A; Molin, S; Andersson, P. Topographic analysis of the toxic Gef protein from E. Coli. *Mol Microbiol*, 1991, 5, 1639-1648.

Prados, J; Melguizo, C; Boulaiz, H; Marchal, JA; Aránega, A. Cancer gene therapy:strategies and clinical trials. *Cell Mol Biol*, 2005, 51, 23-36.

Prados, J; Melguizo, C; Carrillo, E; Boulaiz, H; Marchal, JA; Vélez, C; et al. Cancer mechanism of multidrug resistance mediated by P-glycoprotein In: Marchal JA, Gaforio JA, Aránega A (eds). *Trends in basic and applied oncology*. Granada: Editorial Universidad de Granada; 2006, 266-283.

Pugh, CW; Ratcliffe, PJ. Regulation of angiogenesis by hypoxia: role of the HIF system. *Nat Med*, 2003, 9, 677-684.

Qin, XQ; Tao, N; Dergay, A; Moy, P; Fawell, S; Davis, A; et al. Interferon-beta gene therapy inhibits tumor formation and causes regression of established tumors in immune-deficient mice. *Proc Natl Acad Sci USA*, 1998, 95, 14411-14416.

Quinlin, IS; Burnside, JS; Dombrowski, KE; Phillips, CA; Dolby, N; Wright, SE. Context of MUC1 epitope: immunogenicity. *Oncol Rep*, 2007, 17, 453-456.

Rees, RC; Mian, S. Selective MHC expression in tumours modulates adaptive and innate antitumour responses. *Cancer Immunol Immunother*, 1999, 48, 374-381.

Relf, M; LeJeune, S; Scott, PA; Fox, S; Smith, K; Leek, R; et al. Expression of the angiogenic factors vascular endothelial cell growth factor, acidic and basic fibroblast growth factor, tumour growth factor beta-1, platelet-derived endothelial cell growth factor, placenta growth factor, and pleiotrophin in human primary breast cancer and its relation to angiogenesis. *Cancer Res*, 1997, 57, 963-969.

Robson, T; Worthington, J; McKeown, SR; Hirst, DG. Radiogenic therapy: Novel approaches for enhancing tumor radiosensitivity. *Technol Cancer Res Treat*, 2005, 4, 343-361.

Rochaix, P; Krajewski, S; Reed, JC; Bonnet, F; Voigt, JJ; Brousset, P. In vivo patterns of Bcl-2 family protein expression in breast carcinomas in relation to apoptosis. *J Pathol*, 1999, 187, 410-415.

Rodríguez, R; Lim, HY; Bartkowski, LM; Simona, JW. Identification of diphtheria toxin via screening as a potent cell cycle and p53-independent cytotoxin for human prostate cancer therapeutics. *Prostate*, 1998, 34, 259-269.

Roh, H; Hirose, CB; Boswell, CB; Pippin, JA; Drebin, JA. Synergistic anti-tumor effects of HER2/neu antisense oligodeoxynucleotides and conventional chemotherapeutic agents. *Surgery*, 1999, 126, 413-421.

Rohn, JL; Zhang, YH; Leliveld, SR; Danen-van Oorschot, AA; Henriquez, NV; Abrahams, JP; et al. Relevance of apoptin's integrity for its functional behavior. *J Virol*, 2005, 79, 1337-1338.

Ronchel, MC; Molina, L; Witte, A; Lutbiz, W; Molin, S; Ramos, JL; Ramos, C. Characterization of cell lysis in Pseudomonas putida induced upon expression of heterologous killing genes. *Appl Environ Microbiol*, 1998, 64, 4904-4911.

Rosen, EM; Fan, S; Ma, Y. BRCA1 regulation of transcription. *Cancer Lett*, 2006, 236, 175-185.

Rosen, EM; Fan, S; Pestell, RG; Goldberg, ID. BRCA1 gene in breast cancer. *J Cell Physiol*, 2003, 196, 19-41.

Royds, JA; Iacopetta, B. p53 and disease: when the guardian angel fails. *Cell Death Differ*, 2006, 13, 1017-1026.

Ryschich, E; Huszty, G; Knaebel, H; Hartel, M; Buchler, M; Schmidt, J. Transferrin receptor is a marker of malignant phenotype in human pancreatic cancer and in neuroendocrine carcinoma of the pancreas. *Eur J Cancer*, 2004, 40, 1418-1422.

Sakai, Y; Morrison, BJ; Burke, JD; Park, JM; Terabe, M; Janik, JE; et al. Vaccination by genetically modified dendritic cells expressing a truncated neu oncogene prevents development of breast cancer in transgenic mice. *Cancer Res*, 2004, 64, 8022-6028.

Sakakura, C; Sweeney, EA; Shirahama, T; Igarashi, Y; Hakomori, S; Tsujimoto, H; et al. Overexpression of bax enhances the radiation sensitivity in human breast cancer cells. *Surg Today*, 1997, 27, 90-93.

Sansal, I; Sellers, WR. The biology and clinical relevance of the PTEN tumor suppressor pathway. *J Clin Oncol*, 2004, 22, 2954-2963.

Sarti, M; Sevignani, C; Calin, GA; Aqeilan, R; Shimizu, M; Pentimalli, F; et al. Adenoviral Transduction of TESTIN Gene into breast and uterine cancer cell lines promotes apoptosis and tumor reduction *in vivo*. *Clin Cancer Res*, 2005, 11, 806-813.

Sawada, S; Mese, H; Sasaki, A; Yoshioka, N; Matsumura, T. Combination chemotherapy of paclitaxel and cisplatin induces apoptosis with Bcl-2 phosphorylation in a cisplatin-resistant human epidermoid carcinoma cell line. *Cancer Chemother Pharmacol*, 2003, 51, 505-511.

Sawaki, M; Ito, Y; Tada, K; Mizunuma, N; Takahashi, S; Horikoshi, N; et al. Efficacy and safety of trastuzumab as a single agent in heavily pretreated patients with HER-2/neu-overexpressing metastatic breast cancer. *Tumori*, 2004, 90, 40-43.

Scala, S; Budillon, A; Zhan, Z; Cho-Chung, YS; Jefferson, J; Tsokos, M; et al. Downregulation of mdr-1 expression by 8-Cl-cAMP in multidrug resistant MCF-7 human breast cancer cells. *J Clin Invest*, 1995, 96, 1026-1034.

Schaefer, U; Voloshanenko, O; Willen, D; Walczak, H. TRAIL, a multifunctional cytokine. *Front Biosci*, 2007, 12, 3813-3824.

Schneider, BP; Sledge, GW. Drug insight: VEGF as a therapeutic target for breast cancer. *Nat Clin Pract Oncol*, 2007, 4, 181-189.

Scholl, S; Squiban, P; Bizouarne, N; Baudin, M; Acres, B; Von Mensdorff-Pouilly, S; et al. Metastatic breast tumour regression following treatment by a gene-modified vaccinia virus expressing MUC1 and IL-2. *J Biomed Biotechnol*, 2003, 2003:194-201.

Schuler, M; Green, DR. Transcription, apoptosis and p53, catch-22. *Trends Genet*, 2005, 21, 182-187.

Scott, SD; Greco, O. Radiation and hypoxia inducible gene therapy systems. *Cancer Metastasis Rev*, 2004, 23, 269-276.

Service, RF. New role for estrogen in cancer? *Science,* 1998, 279, 1631-1633.

Seymour, C; Mothersill, C. Cell communication and the "bystander effect." *Radiat Res*, 1999, 151, 505-506.

Shafman, T; Khanna, KK; Kedar, P; Spring, K; Kozlov, S; Yen, T; et al. Interaction between ATM protein and c-Abl in response to DNA damage. *Nature*, 1997, 387, 520-523.

Shankar, P; Manjunath, N; Lieberman, J. The prospect of silencing disease using RNA interference. *JAMA*, 2005, 293, 1367-1373.

Sheikh, MS; Rochefort, H; Garcia, M. Overexpression of p21WAF1/CIP1 induces growth arrest: giant cell formation and apoptosis in human breast carcinoma cell lines. *Oncogene*, 1995, 11, 1899-1905.

Shi, Y. Mammalian RNAi for the masses. *Trends Genet*, 2003, 19, 9-12.

Shiloh, Y. ATM and related protein kinases: safeguarding genome integrity. *Nat Rev Cancer*, 2003, 3, 155-168.

Simoes-Wust, AP; Olie, RA; Gautschi, O; Leech, SH; Haner, R; Hall, J; et al. Bcl-xl antisense treatment induces apoptosis in breast carcinoma cells. *Int J Cancer* 2000, 87, 582-590.

Singh, R; Samant, U; Hyland, S; Chaudhari, PR; Wels, WS; Bandyopadhyay, D. Target-specific cytotoxic activity of recombinant immunotoxin scFv (MUC1)-ETA on breast carcinoma cells and primary breast tumors. *Mol Cancer Ther*, 2007, 6, 562-569.

Sorrentino, BP; Brandt, SJ; Bodine, D; Gottesman, M; Pastan, I; Cline, A; et al. Selection of drug-resistant bone marrow cells in vivo after retroviral transfer of human MDR1. *Science*, 1992, 257, 99-103.

Srivastava, RK; Srivastava, AR; Seth, P; Agrawal, S; Cho-Chung, YS. Growth arrest and induction of apoptosis in breast cancer cells by antisense depletion of protein kinase A-RI alpha subunit: p53-independent mechanism of action. *Mol Cell Biochem*, 1999, 195, 25-36.

St Croix, B, Rago, C; Velculescu, V; Traverso, G; Romans, KE; Montgomery E, et al. Genes expressed in human tumor endothelium. *Science*, 2000, 289, 1197-1202.

Stewart, AK; Lassam, NJ; Quirt, IC; Bailey, DJ; Rotstein, LE; Krajden, M; et al. Adenovector-mediated gene delivery of interleukin-2 in metastatic breast cancer and melanoma: results of a phase 1 clinical trial. *Gene Ther*, 1999, 6, 350-363.

Stoff-Khalili, MA; Dall, P; Curiel, DT. Gene therapy for carcinoma of the breast. *Cancer Gene Ther*, 2006, 13, 633-647.

Stribbling, SM; Friedlos, F; Martin, J; Davies, L; Spooner, RA; Marais, R; et al. Regressions of established breast carcinoma xenografts by carboxypeptidase G2 suicide gene therapy and the prodrug CMDA are due to a bystander effect. *Hum Gene Ther*, 2000, 11, 285–292.

Strong, TV. Gene therapy for carcinoma of the breast: Genetic immunotherapy. *Breast Cancer Res*, 2000, 2, 15-21.

Sung Kim, T; Cohen, EP. Immunity to breast cancer in mice immunized with fibroblasts transfected with a cDNA expression library derived from small numbers of breast cancer cells. *Cancer Gene Ther*, 2005, 12, 890-699.

Swarbrick, A; Akerfeldt, MC; Lee, CS; Sergio, CM; Caldon, CE; Hunter, LJ; et al. Regulation of cyclin expression and cell cycle progression in breast epithelial cells by the helix-loop-helix protein Id1. *Oncogene*, 2005, 24, 381-389.

Szabo, I; Brutsche, S; Tombola, F; Moschioni, M; Satin, B; Telford, JL; et al. Formation of anion-selective channels in the cell plasma membrane by the toxin VacA of Helicobacter pylori is required for its biological activity. *EMBO J*, 1999, 18, 5517-5527.

Szumiel, I. Ionizing radiation-induced cell death. Int J Radiat Biol, 1994, 66, 329-341.

Szyf, M; Pakneshan, P; Rabbani, SA. DNA methylation and breast cancer. *Biochem Pharmacol*, 2004, 68, 1187-1197.

Tada, Y; O-Wang, J; Takiguchi, Y; Tatsumi, K; Kuriyama, T; Okada, S; et al. Cutting edge: a novel role for Fas ligand in facilitating antigen acquisition by dendritic cells. *J Immunol*, 2002, 169, 2241-5224.

Tagawa, M; Kawamura, K; Shimozato, O; Ma, G; Li, Q ;Suzuki, N; et al. Virology- and immunology-based gene therapy for cancer. *Cancer Immunol Immunother*, 2006, 55, 1420-1425.

Tai, YT; Strobel, T; Kufe, D; Cannistra, SA. *In vivo* cytotoxicity of ovarian cancer cells through tumor- selective expression of the BAX gene. *Cancer Res*, 1999, 59, 2121-2126.

Tandle, A; Blazer, DG 3rd; Libutti, SK. Antiangiogenic gene therapy of cancer: recent developments. *J Transl Med*, 2004, 2, 22.

Tang, W; Li, Y; Yu, D; Thomas-Tikhonenko, A; Spiegelman, VS; Fuchs, SY. Targeting beta-transducin repeat-containing protein E3 ubiquitin ligase augments the effects of antitumor drugs on breast cancer cells. *Cancer Res*, 2005, 65, 1904-1908.

Teodoro, JG; Heilman, DW; Parker, AE; Green, MR. The viral protein Apoptin associates with the anaphase-promoting complex to induce G2/M arrest and apoptosis in the absence of p53. *Genes Dev*, 2004, 18, 1952-1957.

Tokino, T; Nakamura, Y. The role of p53-target genes in human cancer. *Crit Rev Oncol Hematol*, 2000, 33, 1-6.

Tolcher, AW. Targeting Bcl-2 protein expression in solid tumors and hematologic malignancies with antisense oligonucleotides. *Clin Adv Hematol Oncol*, 2005, 3, 635-642.

Toledo, F; Wahl, GM. Regulating the p53 pathway: in vitro hypotheses, in vivo veritas. *Nat Rev Cancer*, 2006, 6, 909-923.

Touraine, RL; Vahanian, N; Ramsey, WJ; Blaese, RM. Enhancement of the herpes simplex virus thymidine kinase ganciclovir bystander effect and its antitumor efficacy in vivo by pharmacologic manipulation of gap junctions. *Hum Gene The*, 1998, 9, 2385-2391.

Townsend, PA; Villanova, I; Uhlmann, E; Peyman, A; Knolle J; Baron R; et al. An antisense oligonucleotide targeting the αV integrin gene inhibits adhesion and induces apoptosis in breast cancer cells. *Eur J Cancer*, 2000, 36, 397-409.

Tuschl, T; Zamore, PD; Lehmann, R; Bartel, DP; Sharp, PA. Targeted mRNA degradation by double-stranded RNA in vitro. *Genes Dev*, 1999, 13, 3191-3197.

Ueno, NT; Yu, D; Hung, MC. E1A: tumor suppressor or oncogene? Preclinical and clinical investigations of E1A gene therapy. *Breast Cancer*, 2001, 8, 285-293.

Ursin, G; London, S; Stanczyk, FZ. A Pilot Study of Urinary Estrogen Metabolites (16alpha-OHE_1 and 2-OHE_1) in Postmenopausal Women with and without Breast Cancer. *Environmental Health Perspectives*, 1997, 105, 601-605.

Vargas-Roig, LM; Gago, FE; Tello, O; Aznar, JC; Ciocca, DR. Heat shock protein expression and drug resistance in breast cancer patients treated with induction chemotherapy. *Int J Cancer*, 1998, 79, 468-475.

Vasilevko, V; Ghochikyan, A; Sadzikava, N; Petrushina, I; Tran, M; Cohen, EP; et al. Immunization with a vaccine that combines the expression of MUC1 and B7 co-stimulatory molecules prolongs the survival of mice and delays the appearance of mouse mammary tumors. *Clin Exp Metastasis*, 2003, 20, 489-498.

Vassaux, G; Lemoine, NR. Gene therapy for carcinoma of the breast: genetic toxins. *Breast Cancer Res*, 2000, 2, 22-27.

Vlachaki, MT; Chhikara, M; Aguilar, L; Zhu, X; Chiu, KJ; Woo, S; et al. Enhanced therapeutic effect of multiple injections of HSVTK + GCV gene therapy in combination with ionizing radiation in a mouse mammary tumor model. *Int J Radiation Oncology Biol Phys*, 2001, 51, 1008-1017.

Vogelstein, B; Lane, D; Levine, AJ. Surfing the p53 network. *Nature*, 2000, 408, 307-310.

Vousden, KH; Lu, X. Live or let die: the cell's response to p53. *Nat Rev Cancer*, 2002, 2, 594-604.

Wang, H; Hang, J; Shi, Z; Li, M; Yu, D; Kandimalla, ER; et al. Antisense oligonucleotide targeted to RIalpha subunit of cAMP-dependent protein kinase (GEM231) enhances therapeutic effectiveness of cancer chemotherapeutic agent irinotecan in nude mice bearing human cancer xenografts: in vivo synergistic activity; pharmacokinetics and host toxicity. *Int J Oncol*, 2002, 21, 73-80.

Wang, H; Liu, YJ; Han, ZB; Liang, LH; Lv, LL; Han ZC. Effect of silencing hypoxia-inducible factor-1 alpha by RNA interference on human breast carcinoma cell line. *Zhongguo Yi Xue Ke Xue Yuan Xue Bao*. 2006, 28, 670-674.

Wang, H; Nan, L; Yu, D; Agrawal, S; Zhang, R. Antisense anti-MDM2 oligonucleotides as a novel therapeutic approach to human breast cancer: in vitro and in vivo activities and mechanisms. *Clin Cancer Res*, 2001, 7, 3613-3624.

Wang, NP; To, H; Lee, WH; Lee, EY. Tumor suppressor activity of RB and p53 genes in human breast carcinoma cells. *Oncogene*, 1993, 8, 279-288.

Wang, YH; Liu, S; Zhang, G; Zhou, CQ; Zhu, HX; Zhou, XB; et al. Knockdown of c-Myc expression by RNAi inhibits MCF-7 breast tumor cells growth in vitro and in vivo. *Breast Cancer Res*, 2005, 7, 220-228.

Webb, CP; Vande Woude, GF. Genes that regulate metastasis and angiogenesis. *J Neurooncol*, 2000, 50, 71-87.

Weedon, SJ; Green, NK; McNeish, IA; Gilligan, MG; Mautner, V; Wrighton, CJ; et al. Sensitisation of human carcinoma cells to the prodrug CB1954 by adenovirus vector-mediated expression of E. coli nitroreductase. *Int J Cancer*, 2000, 86, 848-854.

Wei, SJ; Chao, Y; Hung, YM; Lin, WC; Yang, DM; Shih, YL; et al. S-and G2-phase cell cycle arrests and apoptosis induced by ganciclovir in murine melanoma cells transduced with herpes simplex virus thymidine kinase. *Exp Cell Res*, 1998, 241, 66-75.

Wild, R; Yokoyama, Y; Dings, RPM; Ramakrishnan, S. VEGF–DT385 toxin conjugate inhibits mammary adenocarcinoma development in a transgenic mouse model of spontaneous tumorigenesis. *Breast Cancer Res Treat*, 2004, 85, 161-171.

Witlox, MA; Lamfers, ML; Wuisman, PI; Curiel, DT; Siegal, GP. Evolving gene therapy approaches for osteosarcoma using viral vectors: review. *Bone*, 2007, 40, 797-812.

Xiang, J; Chao, DT; Korsmeyer, SJ. BAX-induced cell death may not require interleukin 1 beta-converting enzyme-like proteases. *Proc Natl Acad Sci USA*, 1996, 93, 14559-14563.

Xu, M; Kumar, D; Srinivas, S; Detolla, LJ; Yu, SF; Stass, SA; et al. Parenteral gene therapy with p53 inhibits human breast tumors in vivo through a bystander mechanism without evidence of toxicity. *Hum Gene Ther*, 1997, 8, 177-185.

Yang, DC; Jiang, XP; Elliott, RL; Head, JF. Inhibition of growth of human breast carcinoma cells by an antisense oligonucleotide targeted to the transferrin receptor gene. *Anticancer Res*, 2001, 21, 1777-1787.

Yerushalmi, N; Brinkmann, U; Brinkmann, E; Pai, L; Pastan, I. Attenuating the growth of tumors by intratumoral administration of DNA encoding Pseudomonas exotoxin via cationic liposomes. *Cancer Gene Ther*, 2000, 7, 91-96.

Young, R; Bläsi, U. Holins: form and function in bacteriophage lysis. *FEMS Microbiol Rev*, 1995, 17, 191-205.

Yu, LJ; Matias, J; Scudiero, DA; Hite, KM; Monks, A; Sausville, EA; et al. P450 enzyme expression patterns in the NCI human tumor cell line panel. *Drug Metab Dispos*, 2001, 29, 304–312.

Zapata, JM; Krajewski, M; Krajewski, S; Huang, RP; Takayama, S; Wang, HG; et al. Expression of multiple apoptosis-regulatory genes in human breast cancer cell lines and primary tumors. *Breast Cancer Res Treat*, 1998, 47, 129-140.

Zarovni, N; Vago, R; Solda, T; Monaco, L; Fabbrini, MS. Saporin as a novel suicide gene in anticancer gene therapy. *Cancer Gene Ther*, 2006, 1, 1-9.

Zeng, M; Cerniglia, GJ; Eck, SL; Stevens, CW. High-efficiency stable gene transfer of adenovirus into mammalian cells using ionizing radiation. *Hum Gene Ther*, 1997, 8, 1025-1032.

Zhang, Z; Shirakawa, T; Hinata, N; Matsumoto, A; Fujisawa, M; Okada, H; et al. A. combination with CD/5-FC gene therapy enhances killing of human bladder cancer cells by radiation. *J Gene Med*, 2003, 5, 860-867.

Zheng, JY; Chen, D; Chan, J; Yu, D; Ko, E; Pang, S. Regression of prostate cancer xenografts by a lentiviral vector specifically expressing diphtheria toxin A. *Cancer Gene Ther*, 2003, 10, 764-770.

Zhou, J; Zhong, Y. Breast cancer immunotherapy. *Cell Mol Immunol*, 2004, 1, 247-255.

Zinkel, S; Gross, A; Yang, E. BCL2 family in DNA damage and cell cycle control. *Cell Death Differ*, 2006, 13, 1351-1359.

Zitzer, A; Palmer, M; Weller, U; Wassenaar, T; Biermann, C; Tranum-Jensen, J; et al. Mode of primary binding to target membranes and pore formation induced by Vibrio cholerae cytolysin (hemolysin). *Eur J Biochem*, 1997, 247, 209-216.

Zou, Y; Peng, H; Zhou, B; Wen, Y; Wang, SC; Tsai, EM; et al. Systemic tumor suppression by the proapoptotic gene bik. *Cancer Res*, 2002, 62, 8-12.

In: New Gene Therapy and Cancer Research
Editor: Wilma B. Gustafsson, pp. 67-112

ISBN: 978-1-60021-969-6

Chapter II

PULSED-HIGH INTENSITY FOCUSED ULTRASOUND EXPOSURES FOR NON-INVASIVE TARGETING OF GENE DELIVERY IN THE TREATMENT OF CANCER

Victor Frenkel
National Institutes of Health, 9000 Rockville Pike
Bethesda, Maryland 20892, USA

ABSTRACT

In this chapter the potential of using pulsed-high intensity focused ultrasound (HIFU), a type of therapeutic ultrasound, will be discussed. A short review of other physical means for enhanced gene delivery will first be presented. This will be followed by an overview of therapeutic ultrasound, including a description of the primary ultrasound mechanisms for producing bio-effects, as well as a short summary of the different therapeutic ultrasound applications, most of which deal with enhancing the delivery of drugs. Next, a more detailed description of the ultrasound mechanisms for enhancing gene delivery will be presented, followed by a review of the manner by which pulsed-HIFU exposures can be combined with various modes of administration of genes (local, intravascular, and systemic) *in vivo*. The last two short sections will deal with using pulsed-HIFU to remotely control the expression of delivered genes, and some safety considerations involved with employing these exposures.

INTRODUCTION

Since the first human gene transfer trial in 1998, over half of the more than 500 gene therapy trials tracked by the NIH Recombinant Advisory Committee have been intended for treating cancer (Gottesman, 2003); a trend that reflects the overall number of drugs presently in development (The Economist, 2005). The aim of gene therapy is to transfer genetic materials to targeted cells, where depending on the treatment the transgenes will either alter phenotypes or locally produce therapeutic agents (Wang and Yuan, 2006). Strategies for cancer gene therapy can be divided into distinct categories. The first is the use of toxic transgene products such as those from tumor suppressor genes, suicide genes (in combination with small molecular weight drugs), or those used to inhibit dominant oncogenes. Another involves immunomodulatory approaches related to correcting the immune system's failure to recognize cancer cells as being foreign, consequently allowing them to evade host immunity. Transgene products can be cytokines, such as some interleukins, which have immunostimulatory activity, or tumor specific antigens, which can then be recognized by monoclonal antibodies. Other strategies include the expression of molecules that effect cell adhesion, metastasis, and angiogenesis, or those that enhance cancer cell sensitivity to chemotherapy and radiotherapy. The use of tumor specific promoters is also being investigated to limit transgene expression to the cancer cells being targeted. Transgene expression is also being looked into for chemoprotection of stem cells in order to improve their resistance to the cytotoxicity of drugs (Seth, 2005). Designing strategies to slow or kill cancer cell growth is only one of 'three major recurring themes'described by Gottesman (2003) for the implementation of gene therapy in treating cancer. The development of safe and efficient gene transfer vectors and delivery systems is also required, as is testing the safety and efficacy of potential cancer gene therapies, through the translation of preclinical studies into clinical protocols and trials.

Despite more than a decade and a half since the first attempts were carried out at the National Cancer Institute (NIH), there are still to date no FDA approved gene therapy protocols for safe and effective cancer treatment. The number of potential targets for gene therapy in cancer continues to expand with an increase in understanding of human cancer biology and tumor-host interaction, reinforcing the rationale for gene therapy and the close tie between its potential success and that accumulation of knowledge. There is a growing consensus that the most direct and rational way to modify the function of specific genes in both the tumor and the host is through gene delivery. However the goals of safe and efficient gene transfer, and their specific actions, have shown themselves to be much more difficult than was previously anticipated (Gottesman, 2003); ultimately being the greatest hurdle for the implementation of gene therapy (Huber and Pfisterer, 2000; Ng & Liu, 2002).

In this review the manner by which pulsed-high intensity focused ultrasound (HIFU) can be used to enhance the delivery of DNA for potential use in gene therapy for treating cancer and other diseases will be discussed. These types of ultrasound exposures will be compared to those used similarly for other applications of drug and gene delivery, as well as other implementations of therapeutic ultrasound, both focused and non-focused. The ultrasound mechanisms, either thermal or non-thermal, will be reviewed that are relevant for the various delivery approaches. The manner by which the ultrasound energy interacts with the tissues, to alter permeability will also be described. These topics will then be summarized for the different gene delivery strategies. Finally, a short review will be given on the manner by which the exposures can be used for temporal and spatial control of delivered genes to further improve the safety and targeting of gene therapy. Some of the safety considerations involved with these exposures will also be discussed.

Enhancing Gene Delivery Through Physical Means

After decades of modern biomedical research the concept of gene therapy has finally become a reality. The idea that genes could be artificially constructed and delivered to targeted cells and tissues has opened up an entire new frontier for developing treatments for disease, including cancer. As a result, a large sphere of research has come into being to not only determine the different types of potential gene therapy applications, but also the manner by which to delivery genes safely and efficiently to targeted cells and tissues.

Whereas the feasibility of delivering genes to individual cells in vitro has clearly been shown (see also below for sonoporation), the challenge for gene delivery in vivo has produced a variety of physical methods that have been proposed and evaluated. Probably the most widely investigated method for viably transfecting cells with DNA has been electroporation. As the name suggests, electricity is used to create pores that enable the uptake the genetic material. The first published report on using the technique goes back more than two decades, where Neumann et al (1982) added plasmid DNA to a mouse cell suspension, followed by the application of a number of short (microsecond), high voltage electrical pulses. This simple procedure was shown to significantly enhance the uptake of the DNA by the cells. Since then, there have been hundreds of reports on how this technique can be used to increase transfection of cultured cells, and methods for this procedure in vivo have been developed for a range of animals, including mice embryos (Saito, 2006), and even sheep (Pringle et al., 2007). In the latter study, however, a surgical procedure was required for enhancing transfection of cells in the lungs with a reporter gene. Increased permeability, which is reversible, is thought to occur as a result of pores forming in the plasma membrane when a voltage across it exceeds its dielectric strength (Neuman et al., 1999).

Infrared lasers have also been used for *in vivo* gene transfection where the energy deposition is proposed to permeabilize cell membranes in a manner similar to electroporation (Zeira et al., 2003). Cell membranes may also be permeabilized by increased hydrodynamic pressure, a technique that has been called hydroporation. Zhang et al (2004) showed that rapid tail vein injections of large volumes of solutions containing plasmid DNA could produce high levels of transgene expression in the liver. These administrations produced increased venous pressure, enlargement of liver fenestrae, and increased membrane permeability of the hepatocytes, although, transient irregularity of heart function was also observed. This method of using high pressure for enhanced plasmid DNA delivery has been demonstrated in other animal models, including delivery to skeletal muscle in primates via the local vasculature (Vigen et al., 2007). Retroinfusion into the anterior cardiac vein of an adenovector in pigs also improved gene expression in the anterior descending coronary artery (Raake et al., 2004).

More 'ballistic' type methods for transfection have also been demonstrated that do not involve permeabilizing cell membranes in the presence of the DNA to be taken up. One *in vitro* technique employs the use of magnets to drive DNA incorporated in polymeric superparamagnetic nanoparticles into cultured cells (Chorny et al., 2007). A second, more popular and established, technique can be used in vivo, where DNA is coated on to metal particles (such as gold and silver), which are propelled directly into the skin using compressed air. This technique is being developed especially for the delivery of DNA vaccines, and has been used successfully for the immunization of animals, from rodents up to pigs and monkeys (Haynes et al., 1996). The technique, also known as biolistics, is also currently being used to stably transfect plants (Kikkert et al., 2005).

The methods listed above, however effective, are all associated one or more factors that are problematic for widespread implementation, which include being invasive and/or being limited to specific tissue types or regions of the body. Therapeutic ultrasound, as will be described below, can produce a variety of non-destructive effects in biological tissues, including those that can enhance the delivery of drugs and genes *in vivo* in a variety of tissues and organs. And because it can non-invasively produce these effects in deeper regions of the body, it can be used for both superficial and more internal applications.

Therapeutic Ultrasound

Using ultrasound for medical, or therapeutic, purposes dates back to more than half a decade, predating its using for diagnostic imaging (Clement, 2004). Therapeutic ultrasound can be broadly described as the use of ultrasound for applications other than imaging or diagnostics (Frenkel and Li, 2006), however, some exceptions do occur. Kost et al (2000), for example, have shown how low frequency ultrasound can be used transdermally to alter the permeability of the skin and consequently monitor glucose and other analytes. Pulsed-HIFU is also being developed for a technique known as acoustic radiation force impulse (ARFI) imaging, where short pulses of focused ultrasound are used to generate radiation forces in tissue. Displacements in the tissue are then determined through cross correlation ultrasound methods to detect lesions, whose elastic properties are different than those of the tissues from which they derive (Nightingale et al., 2006). ARFI imaging is also under development for verifying the formation of coagulative necrosis produced by HIFU ablation, where increased stiffness of the ablated tissue (due to protein denaturation) can also produce distinguishable decreases in displacement (Lizzi et al., 2003). Soo et al. (2006) has also proposed using acoustic streaming, induced by radiation forces in fluids (and detected by Doppler), to differentiate cysts from solid masses. In contrast to these applications of therapeutic ultrasound for diagnostic purposes, diagnostic ultrasound has also been used for therapeutic purposes. One example is the recent demonstration of continuous transcranial Doppler to enhance t-PA-induced arterial recanalization in acute ischemic stroke patients (Alexandrov et al., 2004).

Whereas the energy deposition in tissues with diagnostic ultrasound is meant to be minimal, and hence produce no biological effects, applications of therapeutic ultrasound are based on the deposition of ultrasonic energy to create their effects. The large range of therapeutic applications of ultrasound exposures is due the variety of ways that ultrasound energy can interact with cells and tissues (Mitragotri, 2005). The mechanisms by which these effects are produced can be divided into either thermal mechanisms or non-thermal mechanisms (e.g. acoustic cavitation). In some cases, these two mechanisms can work in harmony where the presence of cavitation bubbles may increase the attenuation of energy and hence improve the efficiency of ultrasound heating (Hynynen et al., 1991 UMB). Hemorrhage control using high intensity focused ultrasound also relies on thermal and cavitation effects for effective cauterization (Zderic and Vaezy, 2007). The following sections will cover the three most important ultrasound mechanisms for creating bio-effects as an introduction for describing the manner by which these mechanisms are involved in therapeutic ultrasound applications: heat generation, acoustic cavitation, and acoustic radiation forces. As will be described later in this chapter, the last two are important for gene delivery, whereas the first can be used for the remote control of gene activation.

Heat Generation

The thermal effects of ultrasound are probably the best known and understood. Heat generation in a medium results from the absorption of energy, with the rate of heat per unit volume produced is directly proportional to the tissue-specific absorption coefficient, the intensity and frequency of the ultrasound wave, and inversely proportional to the specific heat of the tissue (Nyborg, 2007). The total amount of heat generated, and consequent temperature elevation, will depend on the removal of heat through diffusion, which is tissue dependant, and convection by the vasculature, where perfusion itself can increase as a response to heating. Relatively greater heat will be formed at tissue to tissue interfaces. In certain cases, where the heating process produces changes in the tissues (e.g. coagulation for ultrasound ablation), the manner by which heat is generated will become even more complex, and therefore, harder to predict, even when using bioheat transfer models that account for all these dynamic processes (Rome et al., 2005).

Measuring ultrasound induced temperature elevations may be carried out in a number of ways. Thermocouple systems are known to be the most accurate, and by far the least expensive. However, this technique provides information is acquired invasively, and only at a single point, and it can often be difficult to correctly position the probes correctly in relation to the comparatively small focal zone of a focused beam (Silcox et al., 2005; Civale et al., 2006). Infra-red cameras provide spatial information, although these can be more expensive and are limited to superficial applications (Thomas et al., 2005). Magnetic resonance imaging (MRI) thermometry, using proton resonance frequency shift methods, can provide spatial information and measure temperature at any depth non-invasively (Mougenot et al., 2004). One major disadvantage of using this technique is the manner by which it is affected by movement, since measurements by MRI are based on changes in phase relative to images acquired prior to heating (Quesson et al., 2000). Another is the obvious high operating costs involved with MRI, and that the ultrasound device must be MR compatible. As will be discussed later, MR guided HIFU has many advantages for image-guided therapeutic ultrasound applications.

Acoustic Cavitation

Acoustic cavitation is defined as the growth, oscillation, and collapse of small stabilized gas bubbles subjected to a sound field in a fluid medium. It is considered the most important of all non-thermal mechanisms of ultrasound for producing effects in biological tissues

(Barnett 1994; Daniels et al. 1995). Cavitation bubbles grow by the process of rectified diffusion, where the amount of gas diffusing into a bubble during its expansion phase is greater than that diffusion out during contraction, and are typically considered to occur in two forms. Non-inertial (or stable) cavitation bubbles persist for a relatively large number of acoustic cycles, where the bubble radius varies about an equilibrium value. Inertial (or transient) cavitation bubbles oscillate unstably and expand to two to three times their resonant size, finally collapsing in a single compression half-cycle (Suslick, 1988). While it has been proposed that damage to biological tissues can occur from stable cavitation bubbles (Lewin and Bjorno, 1982), inertial cavitation is considered as the primary mechanism for structurally altering intact cells, including damage (Riesz and Kondo, 1992) and non-destructive increases in membrane permeability (Bommannan et al. 1992).

One of the most important factors affecting acoustic cavitation is the number and availability of small stabilized gas bubbles, also called cavitation nuclei (Barnett 1998; Bommannan et al. 1992). Cavitation activity will increase with the number of nuclei available (Crum 1979), which are ubiquitous in water and other liquids, but are scarce in animal tissues (Barnett 1998). Another factor determining whether cavitation will occur is the available space for bubbles to form and grow. Cavitation within intact cells and parenchyma is therefore more difficult to produce because of this and additional factors such as increased viscosity and components of the cell's infrastructure (Simonin, 1995). The vasculature, on the other hand, possesses both the necessary dimensions and cavitation nuclei for the initiation of cavitation when high enough ultrasound pressure fields are present. The pressure amplitude, especially the peak rarefractional pressure, is the most important ultrasound exposure parameter that will control the onset of cavitation activity. For a comprehensive review of the factors affecting acoustic cavitation, and its consequent biological effects, see Kimmel (2006).

A variety of phenomena occurs when bubbles collapse in an open medium. When a bubble implodes, large increases in temperature may result leading to the thermal dissociation of water molecules and the formation of hydroxyl molecules (Suslick, 1988). Observed sonochemical effects of acoustic cavitation, caused by free radical formation, include damage to DNA in aqueous solution, inactivation of certain proteins and enzymes, and lipid peroxidation. Cell membranes may also be damaged by sonochemical effects, however, these effects may be masked by mechanical effects which are predominant in cell lysis (Riesz & Kondo, 1992).

The most pronounced effects of transient cavitation damage take place in the near proximity of the rigid boundary, surrounded by a relatively large (to the bubble diameter) body of fluid (Kimmel, 2006). Because of the boundary asymmetrical collapse of the bubble occurs, where the far side of the bubble impacts and penetrates the bubble surface closest to the boundary, forming a 'wall-direct re-entrant jet'. A high pressure region is generated at the penetration interface (Zhang et al., 1993), where jet velocities can be as high as130 m/s, and the pressures as great as 10^9 Pa (Dear et al., 1988). The manner by which the jets form has been captured using high speed photography, demonstrating how they impact, compress and crack tissue surfaces, leaving them visibly damaged and pitted (Kodama and Takayama, 1998).

Various methods exist to detect both inertial and non-inertial cavitation *in vivo*. These include passive detection systems with acoustic hydrophones for sub-harmonic emissions (Hynynen, 1991) visualization of hyperechos in B-scan ultrasound images (Hwang et al., 2006). Histological analysis of treated using transmission electron microscopy (Frenkel et al., 1999) and scanning electron microscopy (Hwang et al., 2006) have also be used to detect damage induced in tissues due non-inertial bubble collapse. Typically, an increase in the cavitation threshold will occur with an increase in frequency. Predictions of the occurrence of inertial cavitation can be carried out using the Mechanical Index, which is a unit less parameter calculated using the peak rarefractional pressure and the exposure frequency (Kimmel, 2006). In addition, Church (2005) has also shown that the pulse length is an important exposure parameter for determining if cavitation will occur. Methods such as degassing the fluid medium (Levy et al., 1989) and over pressure (Khokhlova et al., 2006) have been used reduce or eliminate cavitation activity, and hence determine if it is indeed occuring during exposures.

Acoustic Radiation Forces

At relatively high amplitudes, under conditions of non-linearity, acoustic radiation forces are created in a medium exposed to ultrasound. The steady force that is created is proportional to the power (which itself is proportional to the absorption coefficient of the medium and the rate of energy being applied) and inversely proportional to the speed of sound of the absorbed ultrasound wave in the medium. If instead of absorbing, the medium behaves as a perfect reflector, then the radiation force is increased by a factor of two. The radiation pressure is simply the radiation force averaged over the area of the beam impinging normally to the medium (Nyborg, 2006). Based on this phenomenon, ultrasonic transducers may be calibrated by applying exposures onto a balance through a fluid medium, where the induce force is then translated into acoustic power (Lewin et al., 2003).

If radiation forces are great enough, tissue displacement may occur in the region of the focal zone of the HIFU beam. The most relevant tissue property determining the degree of displacement is Young's modulus, which itself is dependant on the conditions of the exposures, such as temperature, frequency and boundary conditions (Lizzi et al., 2003). By applying a HIFU pulse followed by collecting A-mode RF echo data a technique of remote elastography has been developed, also known as acoustic radiation force imaging (ARFI) (Walker et al., 2000). The application of this type of technology through a multitude of data acquisition techniques and post-processing has led to a number of proposed methods for non-invasive characterization of tissue. This includes estimation of elasticity and viscosity, based on temporal behavior and magnitude of shear strain induced by the displacements (Girnyk et al., 2006), the detection of cancerous lesions (Nightingale et al., 2002), and the monitoring of the formation of HIFU induced coagulative necrosis (Lizzi et al., 2003). The latter two applications are based on the fact that tissue displacement is inversely proportional to tissue stiffness, which is found to be elevated in both the lesions and ablated tissue.

When radiation forces are produced in a fluid medium, the consequent motion induced is in the form of a steady flow, also known as acoustic streaming (Nyborg, 2007). The velocity of the stream is proportional to the intensity of the ultrasound source, the surface area of the transducer, and the attenuation coefficient of the medium; while inversely proportional to the bulk viscosity and speed of sound of the medium (Dymling et al., 1991). Acoustic streaming has been shown to reduce heating due to ultrasound exposures through the process of increasing convective heat loss (Wu et al., 1994), as well as increase mass transport of nanoparticles for transdermal delivery (Frenkel et al., 2000b; Frenkel et al., 2001). It is also presently being used in the development of a novel technique for differentiating cysts from solid masses in indeterminate lesions, where the movement of fluid within the cysts is detected with Doppler sonography (Soo et al., 2006).

Acoustic radiation forces have also been shown to produce a number of biological phenomena. Mihran et al. (1990) demonstrated how even single HIFU pulses, at short duration and low energy, can modify the excitability of myelinated sciatic nerves in frogs *in vitro*. Experiments carried out in the heart of a frog showed how radiation forces can also reduce aortic pressure and induce premature ventricular contraction (Dalecki et al., 1997). Radiation forces, produced by relatively high frequency HIFU pulses of short duration, were also shown to be able to interrupt flow in blood vessels in the eyes of rabbits (Lizzi et al., 1981). The application of acoustic radiation forces have also been demonstrated to influence the position and velocity of flow of acoustic contrast agents in the vasculature, where the agents redistribute from the luminal space towards the vessel walls (Dayton et al., 2002). This phenomenon is presently being employed to develop a technique to facilitate receptor-ligand mediated adhesion of drug carrying nanoparticles (Borden et al., 2006). The direct effects of radiation forces in tissues for enhancing drug delivery will be discussed below.

Therapeutic Ultrasound Applications

Applications of therapeutic ultrasound can be divided into two separate categories: those that enhance the delivery of drugs, and those don't involve drugs and instead rely on the direct effects of ultrasound energy deposition.

Applications not Involving Drugs

A range of applications of therapeutic ultrasound exist and may be distinguished by the manner by which the ultrasound exposures are applied. In general, the greater the energy deposited in the tissue, especially the rate of energy deposition, the more pronounced the effects will be.

i) Healing

Ultrasound has been used in physical therapy since the late 1930's, and considered one of the best way to provide thermal treatment for soft tissue injuries, including joint and muscle sprains, tendonitis and bursitis. Exposures are typically provided with a relatively simple, non-focused, planar transducer. As a result, low level hyperthermia occurs, which induces vasodilation and improved blood flow to the treated region. The increased flow enhances the delivery of nutrients and oxygen as well as the removal of cellular wastes. This type of treatment is provided to relieve inflammation, pain and muscle spasms, as well as accelerate healing and increase range of motion (Byl, 1995). Recent studies have also shown how the exposures can facilitate the repair of fractures (Warden et al., 2006), and preclinical studies have demonstrated how they can speed up recovery of sciatic nerve injury (Mourad et al., 2001). These same exposures can also be used to enhance local transdermal delivery (described in detail below) of anti-inflammatory agents (Mitragotri, 2005), as well as accelerate to onset of cutaneous anesthesia using local anesthetics (Katz et al., 2004). Because of their low amplitudes, and low rates of energy deposition, these exposures do not typically produce any irreversible, macroscopic changes in the treated tissues. There are exceptions, however, such as the use of transient cavitation at wound surfaces, for wound cleaning, debridement of ulcers and stimulation of granulation (Uhlemann et al., 2003).

ii) Hemorrhage Control

Uncontrollable bleeding is one of the main causes of mortality after traumatic injury, and the ability to achieve haemostasis within minutes after trauma occurs is still a challenging problem (Starnes et al., 2006). High-Intensity Focused Ultrasound (HIFU) is a recently developed technology for hemorrhage control, based on the localized delivery of a high amount of acoustic energy to a site of injury, leading to its cauterization. HIFU application has been shown to be effective in hemorrhage control of injuries in the liver (Cornejo et al., 2004; Vaezy et al., 2004; Zderic et al. 2006a) , spleen (Noble et al., 2002), and blood vessels (Vaezy et al., 1998; Martin et al., 1999; Zderic et al. 2006b) in both short-term and long-term animal studies. Also, HIFU has recently been shown effective in producing hemostasis and pneumostasis of lung injuries (Vaezy et al. In Press). HIFU cauterization is achieved due to both thermal and mechanical effects of ultrasound (Vaezy and Zderic, 2007). Furthermore, HIFU treatment of bleeding injuries leads to formation of a coagulum that spreads over the injured site, and hardens to produce a seal which prevents re-bleeding (similar to tissue glue) (Vaezy et al. 2005). As compared to lasers, RF ablation and other hemostasis methods, HIFU has a unique ability of efficient application during profuse bleeding, thus allowing treatment of high-grade injuries.

The most important advantage of HIFU, as compared to all other hemorrhage control methods, is that it can be applied in a non-invasive manner in the treatment of hidden and inaccessible injuries located deep in the tissue, while sparing surrounding tissues from harmful exposure. A non-invasive treatment of hidden injuries can be achieved by the application of an ultrasound image-guided HIFU system, in which a HIFU therapy transducer is integrated with a commercially available diagnostic ultrasound imaging probe (Vaezy et al., 2001; Held at al., 2006). An important characteristic of diagnostic ultrasound is that HIFU application at the focus in the ultrasound image shows as a bright (hyperechoic) region, thus serving as targeting aid. This hyperecho can form during extremely short HIFU exposures (of 30 ms) which are not long enough to cause any significant biological changes in the tissues (Rabkin et al., 2006). Thus, hyperecho may be used to check whether HIFU focus is located at the region of interest (i.e., bleeding spot or tumor) and not in the healthy tissue, before the start of the HIFU cauterization treatment.

Ultrasound-image guided HIFU has been investigated for transcutaneous hemorrhage control of various vessel and solid organ injuries, such as the liver (Burgess et al. 2007). Hemorrhage control was achieved with HIFU in about one minute of application time; while the sham treated incisions continued to bleed for more than 7 minutes. This finding was important since currently there are no good methods for hemorrhage control in the inaccessible regions of solid organs. In another study, Color Doppler-guided HIFU was used to achieve extracorporeal hemorrhage control of injured peripheral blood vessels (Vaezy and Zderic, 2007). Puncture wounds (2-3 mm in diameter) were produced with a catheter in porcine femoral arteries in-vivo. Bleeding sites were then localized as a jet stream in Color Doppler images, and treated with HIFU for about 1 min. After the treatment, the blood loss was significantly lower in the HIFU-treatment group as compared to sham group (average loss - HIFU: 19 ml; sham: 81 ml). This study indicated that ultrasound-guided HIFU can be used for fast sealing of the peripheral vascular injuries, with the potential application outside of the hospital setting (ie, at the location of accident or in the battlefield). For a comprehensive review on the use of therapeutic ultrasound for hemorrhage control, see Vaezy and Zderic (2007).

iii) Ablation

A number of technologies are presently being used to induce local hyperthermia in the clinic, whether for tumor ablation or the treatment of cardiac arrhythmias. These techniques, which are minimally invasive, deposit energy using electrodes (for radio frequency ablation) or antennas (for microwaves). Lasers, on the other hand, are non-invasive, where levels of energy deposition can reach those required for comparable temperature elevations. The disadvantage of using lasers is that penetration of this type of optical energy is limited to just a few millimeters. In contrast, high intensity focused ultrasound can deposit energy deep inside the body to produce local hyperthermia in smaller and more defined regions (Rome et al., 2005).

Perhaps the best known application of using high intensity focused ultrasound is thermal ablation. The first demonstration of this was carried out more than 60 years ago, however, technological limited existed then to accurately control and monitor the treatments. Recent developments over the past decade in both targeting and control have enabled this procedure to become both practical and reliable. In a manner similar to light, ultrasonic waves can be focused onto very small volumes to greatly increase their intensity; hence the name high intensity focused ultrasound (HIFU). This is achieved using a spherically-curved transducer, typically in the range of frequencies from 0.5 to 10 MHz, where intensities are 10^3 to 10^4 W cm^{-2} (Clement, 2004). The vast majority of clinical applications of HIFU have been for ablating tissue, especially tumors (Kennedy, 2005). Relatively long, continuous exposures are utilized (on the order of seconds), which allows for sufficient heat to be produced to elevate temperatures for ablation (Hill and ter Haar, 1995). The focused beam passes through the skin and other intervening tissues over a wide area, where the spatial intensities are relatively low, and consequently produce no damage; however, at the focus the tissue is selectively destroyed. Irreversible cell death can occur by coagulative necrosis for exposures of only 1 sec, at temperatures of at least 56°C. Acoustic cavitation can also occur during these exposures and further contribute to tissue destruction An inflammatory response will the ensue, and then within a couple of weeks fibrous scar tissue will have replaced the necrosis in the treated region (Kennedy, 2005).

The advantages of HIFU over more invasive surgical procedures are numerous including, elimination of scar formation, limited blood loss and infection, and a reduced risk of other complications. HIFU ablations can also be provided on an outpatient basis, where cost and recovery times may be significantly reduced in comparison to existing techniques being used for tumor ablation: radio frequency ablation, cryoablation, and laser ablation (Kennedy, 2005). Today, HIFU is being employed for ablating prostate cancer (Thuroff et al., 2003) and uterine fibroids (Chan et al., 2002), and its use is currently undergoing clinical trials for ablating other types of cancer, including that of the breast (Wu et al., 2003), liver (Kennedy et al., 2004), and kidney (Wu et al., 2003), as well as for palliation in bone cancer patients (Catane et al., 2007). Pre-clinical studies have also shown how combining HIFU with the administration of chemotherapeutic agents can improve results for tumor growth inhibition and survival, when compared to either strategy on its own (Yang et al., 1992; Paparel et al., 2005). HIFU exposures can be targeted to specific tissues, organs or tumors using a number of imaging modalities (Sanghvi et al., 1996), including diagnostic (B-scan) ultrasound (Chen et al., 2004), magnetic resonance imaging (MRI) (McDannold et al., 2006), computed tomography (CT) (Wood et al., 2005), and optical 3D tracking (Vo et al., 2007).

Despite the evolution of the use of HIFU for thermal ablation of tissue in an increasingly efficient and sophisticated fashion, the creation of precise lesions is still limited by heterogeneous heating and cooling due to factors such as perfusion, tissue variability, and tissue charring. It has been proposed that non-thermal ultrasound mechanisms (i.e. cavitation) could be used to homogenize tissue in a controlled and predictable manner. Preliminary studies in the kidneys of rabbits were carried out using relatively short pulses (20 microseconds) and high intensities ($> 20 \times 10^3$ W cm^{-2}), with a pulse-repetition frequency such that low time average power was delivered. Gross and histological examination indicated that accurate and sharply demarcated regions of cellular damage could be produced with these novel exposures. Refinement of this technique for controlled tissue ablation, also call histotripsy, is currently underway (Roberts et al., 2006). For a comprehensive review on the use of HIFU for ablating tissue see Kennedy (2005).

Applications that Enhance Drug Delivery

The majority of novel applications of therapeutic ultrasound being developed today are based on enhancing the delivery of drugs and genes. These include techniques to enhance transdermal delivery (or sonophoresis), thrombolysis, blood brain barrier disruption, and the delivery of chemotherapeutic agents. Some of the techniques involve novel drug carriers in which drugs are sequestered, and consequently released at a targeted area by an extracorporeal ultrasound exposure. A short description of each application will follow, prior to concentrating on the topic of this review, which is gene delivery.

i) Sonophoresis

Investigations on enhancing drug delivery through the skin using ultrasound has been ongoing for more than half a century. Also known as sonophoresis (or phonophoresis), the advantage of the technique is to achieve need-free, drug delivery. (Mitragotri, 2005). The main transport barrier for administering drugs transdermally is the outer most layer of the skin, the stratum corneum (SC) (Lavon et al., 2007). A large body of research has produced a general agreement that acoustic cavitation is the main ultrasound mechanism for disrupting the lipid bilayers of the SC to create channels for improved transport through it. In addition to local applications of sonophoresis (mentioned above) that are already being used in the clinic, preclinical investigations have shown enhanced delivery of various large molecules such as insulin (Kost, 2002) and vaccines (Tezel et al., 2005). Similar exposures have also been used to enhance transcorneal transport of various molecules, where increased permeability of the cornea's stroma appears to occur from minor, and reversible, structural alterations produced in the epithelium. This type of direct ocular drug delivery is being developed to treat diseases such as glaucoma (Zderic et al., 2002; Zderic et al., 2004; Zderic et al., 2004). Controlled exposures at an epithelial-fluid interface using high frequency, low intensity ultrasound were shown to produce a controlled level of tissue erosion, where the rate limiting factor for its progression was found to be the diffusion rate of cavitation nuclei from the fluid through the disrupted tissue (Frenkel et al., 1999). This type of exposure was found to enhance the tissue's permeability to the inward flux of nanoparticles and may potentially be used for the relatively new field of ultrasound-mediated delivery in moist epithelial tissues (Frenkel et al., 2000b). Because this effect produces irreversible necrosis in the exposed cells, a reversal of the permeability will depend on the rate of new cell turnover. For an in-depth review on sonophoresis see Mitragotri and Kost (2004).

ii) Blood Brain Barrier Disruption

The first use ever reported using ultrasound in animals was with HIFU for producing precise focal lesions within the central nervous system. Craniotomies were required for the procedures, but the results demonstrated the potential of therapeutic ultrasound and heralded a new era in biomedical research and development (Fry, 1958). Soon afterward the procedures showed their suitability for human treatment when they were used to selectively ablate regions of the basal ganglia in patients with Parkinson's disease (Fry et al., 1958).

Recent advances in multi-element array tranducers, along with multi-modality imaging, has enabled the development of prototype devices for accurately carrying out HIFU exposures directly through the skull (Clement, 2004). Whereas the exposures on their own have demonstrated the ability to disrupt the blood brain barrier (BBB) (Mesiwala et al., 2002), the addition of ultrasound contrast agents (UCAs) during exposures has enabled more predictable cavitation activity, and consequent induction of these effects, where adding UCAs also lowers the intensity threshold for the onset of cavitation activity (McDannold et al., 2006). MRI guidance of HIFU (MRgHIFU) exposures is presently the standard for developing this type of procedure (Clement, 2004), which to date has facilitated the delivery to the brain of various marker molecules and antibodies (Kinoshita et al, 2006), and liposomal doxorubicin (Treat et al., 2004). The mechanism by which this procedure enhances delivery is not precisely known. It is thought that the stable oscillation of cavitating bubbles generate mechanical stress in the blood vessel walls, with little or no damage to brain tissue, and in that way increase their permeability. As a consequence the BBB can be reversibly disrupted to allow penetration of therapeutic agents (e.g. chemotherapeutic agents and thrombolytic agents, as well as new compounds to treat chronic brain diseases), which are normally unable to do so (Hynynen, 2007). For a comprehensive review on BBB disruption, see Hynynen (2007).

iii) Thrombolysis

Ultrasound has been used to enhance thrombolysis, both with and without the addition of thrombolytic agents (Pfaffenberger et al., 2005). A variety of ultrasound-mediated strategies exist for enhancing clot dissolution, including the use of catheter-delivered transducer devices (Atar 2001), as well as non-invasive, transcutaneous devices (Alexandrov et al., 2004). A large variety of in vitro studies have been carried out to elucidate the mechanisms by which improved thrombolytic activity is achieved. It is generally agreed that non-thermal mechanisms are primarily, if not exclusively, involved; especially acoustic cavitation. Studies in fibrin gels, and later in clots, showed ultrasound exposures to induce reversible fiber disaggregation (Braaten et al., 1997), improve fluid flow (Siddiqi et al., 1995), and enhance tissue plasminogen activator (tPA) penetration (Francis et al., 1995). In vivo studies using UCA showed the addition of these microbubbles could improve ultrasound-mediated thrombolysis, both with (Siegel et al., 2001; Datta et al., 2006) and without (Culp et al., 2003) thrombolytic agents. Novel strategies are also being developed where tPA is loaded into echogenic liposomes and released at the clots with ultrasound exposures (Tiukinhoy-Laing et al., 2007).

In addition to the previous studies, where typically low rates of ultrasound energy deposition were used, pulsed-HIFU exposures also recently demonstrated the ability to non-invasively enhance tPA-mediated thrombolysis. *In vitro* studies showed higher D-dimer levels with HIFU and tPA, compared to tPA alone, to corroborate improved thrombolytic rates (Frenkel et al., 2006 Radiology). Scanning electron micrographs and fluorescent antibody labeling of the tPA demonstrated that indeed the clots had been rendered more permeable in a non-destructive manner, and that improved of binding and penetration of the drug had occurred as a result of the exposures (Stone et al., 2005). Follow-up studies using a novel clot model in the marginal ear vein of a rabbit, showed that significantly improved thrombolysis, using the same exposures, could be reproduced in vivo. Preliminary investigations on the safety of the exposures revealed that no deleterious effects occurred in the endothelium of the treated vessels, or in the surrounding tissue (Stone et al., 2007). For an in-depth review of ultrasound-mediated thrombolysis, see Pfaffenberger et al. (2005).

iv) Controlled Release and Activation

Advances in the ability to chemically engineer a wide range of materials and drugs has opened a new field of virtually unlimited possibilities for using ultrasound to remotely deploy or activate therapeutically relevant agents. For example, studies have shown how biodegradable polymers implanted in rodent skin may be degraded by topical ultrasound exposures for controlled release of drugs incorporated within them (Kost et al., 1989). Here, a range of factors are possible for controlling release rates, including the ultrasound exposure parameters, the polymeric matrix, and the molecular weight of the incorporated drug (Lavon and Kost, 1998). More recently, preclinical studies have shown promising development of drug carriers that can be administered systemically, where extracorporeal ultrasound is used to induce reversible changes in the carriers and consequently release the incorporated drug. Examples of this type of carrier include liposomes (Schroeder et al., 2007) and polymeric micelles (Zeng and Pitt, 2006). The obvious benefit of using such a strategy is to increase local drug delivery in a targeted region for improved efficacy, while simultaneously minimizing systemic exposure to the drug and subsequent side effects associated with its use.

Whereas it has been shown that acoustic cavitation is the mechanism employed with the carriers (mentioned above) to induce reversible changes and consequent drug deployment, ultrasound induced heat generation recently been shown to work effectively with heat sensitive liposomes. Encapsulating drugs in liposomes has effectively been used to improve their delivery, compared to drug alone, by lowering systemic toxicity and improving uptake into cells (Allen, 1997). By incorporating lipid-conjugated polyethylene glycol (PEG) into their membranes, liposomes attain a smaller volume of distribution and prolonged clearance time. PEG provides a protective barrier against interactions with plasma proteins and the reticuloendothelial system; as a result, enhanced accumulation of chemotherapeutic agents into tumors occurs (Ranson et al., 1997).

Liposomes are normally stable in the physiological temperature range. However, they can be produced to undergo a phase change when heated, which renders them more permeable and consequently releases their payload (Kong and Dewhirst, 1999). Also known as thermosensitive liposomes (TSLs), they release their payload where local tissue temperatures are elevated (Gaber et al., 1996). TSLs have been combined with heat sources such as infrared laser (Salomir et al., 2005) or microwaves (Khoobehi et al., 1989) for improved local drug delivery, including cisplatin (Nishita, 1998), doxorubicin (Kong et al., 2000), and methotrexate (Weinstein et al., 1980).

To date, only a small number of preclinical studies have been reported where TSLs were combined with HIFU exposures as a source of hyperthermia. McDannold et al (2004) used TSLs loaded with a paramagnetic contrast agent, where the triggering temperature was set to thermal ablation levels. With this TSL and a HIFU system guided by MRI, the authors demonstrated the ability to non-invasively validate that indeed temperature elevations were achieved for ablating the targeted tissue. In another study Dromi et al (2007) used TSLs that trigger in the non-destructive range of 39 - 41°C. These TSLs (also known as low temperature sensitive liposomes, or LTSLs) were used with pulsed-HIFU exposures producing temperature elevations of only 4-5 °C (Frenkel et al., 2006a). The study, carried out in murine breast cancer tumors, grown subcutatneously in mice, showed that this drug/device combination was able to increase intra-tumoral levels of doxorubicin, compared to a commercial non-thermosensitive liposome. This enhanced local delivery consequently translated in to improved anti-tumor effects. More recently, Luk et al (2007) demonstrated that a split focus HIFU transducer can be employed to simultaneously treat larger regions of tissue and hence increase spatial rates of drug deposition with the LTSLs.

Table 1. Therapeutic ultrasound applications

Application	Mechanism(s)
I - Applications not involving drugs	
- Healing	Low level heat and mechanical stimulation
- Hemorrhage control	High level heat and cavitation (I)
- Ablation	High level heat and cavitation (I)
II - Applications that enhance drug delivery	
- Sonophoresis	Cavitation (NI) and acoustic streaming
- Blood brain barrier disruption	Cavitation (NI)
- Thrombolysis	Cavitation (I&NI) and radiation forces
- Controlled release and activation	Low level heat and cavitation (I&NI)
- Gene delivery	Cavitation (I) and radiation forces

N - inertial; NI - non-inertial

Ultrasound exposures can also be used to activate anti-tumor agents; a process known as sonodynamic therapy (SDT). The name is modified from photodynamic therapy (PDT), which is a previously developed technique that uses light as an activation source (Palumbo, 2007). The first studies on sonodynamic therapy used photosensitizers, and showed conclusively that combining the exposures with the agents produced synergic effects in regards to growth inhibition in targeted tumors (Yumita et al., 1990). The mechanisms of SDT for anti-tumor effects are complex and are dependant on the ultrasound mechanism of acoustic cavitation. These agents possess low toxicity, and their activation by ultrasound is thought to produce radicals that can initiate chain peroxidation of lipids in cellular membranes. The appeal of SDT over PDT is that by using focused ultrasound exposures, regions deep in the body may be treated (Rosenthal et al., 2004). Because of the limited penetration of light through tissue, PDT is restricted for the treatment of relatively small tumors on or under the skin, or with endoscopes or fiber optic catheters to reach the lining of some internal organs (Palumbo, 2007). For a complete review on SDT see Rosenthal et al. (2004).

HIFU Mechanisms for Enhanced Gene Delivery

To date, two separate techniques for using HIFU exposures to enhance gene delivery have been reported. One, sonoporation, relies on the ultrasound mechanism of inertial cavitation and acts on individual cells. The second technique, which induces more macroscopic changes to permeabilize whole tissues, has been proposed to occur from the generation of acoustic radiation forces.

Sonoporation

Inertial cavitation (i.e. collapsing bubbles) can be employed to alter permeability for improved delivery of genes and drugs at the level of individual cells. This process is known as sonoporation, since it uses sound energy, instead of electrical energy (for electroporation), to create pores to enhance permeability of plasma membranes. The fact that pores may be created in cell membranes non-lethally is not surprising since the fatty acids in the membranes tend to associate with one another and exclude water (Purves et al., 1992). The first demonstration of sonoporation was carried out by Fechheimer et al (1986), who exposed a cell suspension of live slime mold amoebae in the presence of a fluorescein-labelled dextran, which because of its size was impermeable to the cells. As a result of the ultrasound exposures, approximately 40% of the cells had taken up the fluorophore. This process was then shown to be reproducible in mammalian cells for delivering DNA (Fechheimer et al., 1987), after which it opened up an entire new field of endeavor for gene delivery using ultrasound.

Although it was always assumed, albeit correctly, that the effects of the ultrasound exposures for enabling uptake of materials into cells was the creation of pores in the plasma membranes due to bubble collapse, only recently was this shown to be conclusive. High-speed photography was used by Ohl et al (2006) to demonstrate the formation of wall-direct re-entrant jets, due to asymmetrical bubble collapse (as described above), for the delivery of molecules to cells. Frame rates higher than the ultrasonic frequency enabled visualizing the direct correlation between cell deformation and consequent cell membrane permeability, where propidium iodide served as membrane integrity probe (van Wamel et al., 2006). The formation of pores had previously been shown to occur during sonoporation, although indirectly. Deng et al (2004) developed an experimental system using a voltage clamp technique and individual Xenopus oocytes for real-time measurements of the process. Pore formation was validated by measuring increases in transmembrane current, which indicated a decrease in membrane resistance. Their study also showed that calcium ions entering the cell through US-induced pores were required for resealing of the membranes after the ultrasound exposures.

Ultrasound contrast agents (UCAs) consist of microscopic encapsulated bubbles that oscillate upon insonification (Postema et al., 2005). UCAs can penetrate into small blood capillaries because their average size is less than that of a red blood cell (Liu et al., 2006a). Although they were originally developed to enhance blood echogenicity (Miller, 2007), they have been use for a number of therapeutic ultrasound applications, for example to enhance blood brain barrier disruption (mentioned above) and sonoporation (van Wamel, 2006). Albunex® was the first UCA to be FDA approved. These of air-filled microspheres are produced from sonicated human serum albumin, with a diameter of 4 microns. The first published study using the UCAs showed they could effectively be used for as a contrast agent for myocardial echocardiography (Keller et al., 1989). Since then, applications for these UCAs have increased exponentially, for both imaging and therapeutic ultrasound, and newer generation UCAs have been developed. Optison®, for example, was the second generation UCA, where the microbubbles now contain octafluoropropane gas for improve contrast and stability. This allows for longer circulation time, and consequently longer imaging windows for echographers (Liu et al., 2006a). Since then, newer formulations for UCAs have been developed, such as Levovist® where these microbubbles are made up mostly of galactose, with some palmitic acid. For a comprehensive comparison of available UCAs see Liu et al (2006a).

A large number of studies – especially those in vitro – have demonstrated how this type of cavitation activity can been be made more efficient by the addition of ultrasound contrast agents, where the stabilized microbubbles serve as cavitation nucleation agents (van Wamel, 2006). As will be shown below, the addition of UCAs is especially crucial for in vivo applications for improving transfection efficiency, where a dearth of cavitation nucleation sites limits this process. Because of the lack of cavitation nucleation sites *in vivo*, and other physical parameters affecting cavitation activity (as described above), the difference between the *in vitro* and *in vivo* environments makes it difficult to predict the activity of inertial cavitation, and consequently sonoporation, *in vivo* based on experiments *in vitro*. *In vitro* experiments are, however, still important. For example, observations of the process of sonoporation with the addition of UCAs have shown how the gas content of these agents can be forced out of them, creating the possibility that similarly formulated agents could serve as drug carriers to be released remotely in targeted regions by ultrasound exposures (Postema et al., 2005)

Although sonoporation is a reversible process, and therefore non-destructive, cavitation activity (especially inertial cavitation) is extremely non-uniform and hard to control, and ultimately some of the cells that are exposed will undergo irreversible damage that will ultimately lead to cell death (Frenkel et al., 1999). Significant increases in tissue temperature can also occur as a result of the onset of cavitation activity during ultrasound exposures (Hynynen, 1991). And temperature elevations capable of harming cells may also occur due to viscous dissipation in the coating of UCAs (Stride and Saffari, 2004). As will be shown below, effective sonoporation has yet to be shown without the exclusion of cell destruction during the process. For a comprehensive review on sonoporation for gene delivery, see Miller (2007).

Whereas inertial cavitation is considered to be the primary type of cavitation activity for inducing damage to biological tissue, it has also been proposed that destructive effects can occur from non-inertial, or stable, cavitation activity. As a bubble located exterior to a cell membrane expands and contracts, vibrational energy is transferred to the membrane surface (Lewin and Bjorno, 1982), which can set the membrane in motion (Lewin & Bjorno, 1981; Lewin & Bjorno, 1982). Oscillatory and steady (time-independent) micro-streaming is also generated in the vicinity of the bubble (Lewin & Bjorno, 1982; Riesz & Kondo, 1992; Simonin, 1995), where rapid changes in the streaming velocity gradient, in the vicinity of the membrane, can cause considerable shear stress (Lewin & Bjorno, 1982). Cell membranes may be damaged as a result of this type of bubble activity (Lele et al., 1973; Lewin & Bjorno, 1981; Riesz & Kondo, 1992), leading to the destruction of cellular function (Lewin & Bjorno, 1981), and even the disruption of whole tissues and blood vessels (Martin et al., 1983).

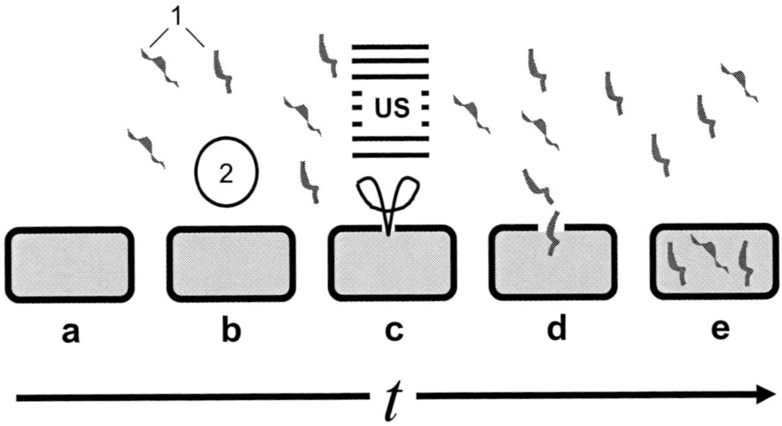

Figure 1. A schematic representation of the mechanism of sonoporation, showing a time course of a single cell. a - prior to the administration of plasmid DNA (1) and an ultrasound contrast agent (2); b - administration of plasmid DNA and ultrasound contrast agent; c - ultrasound/HIFU exposure is applied, where a wall direct re-entrant jet is formed towards the cell membrane compromising its integrity; d - plasmid enters the cytoplasm of the cell; e – membrane reseals, trapping the plasmid. Note, there is not a uniform time scale in the described process from 'a' to 'e': bubble collapse and cell membrane perforation occurs on the scale of micro-seconds; cell membranes remain open and reseal on the order of seconds.

Radiation Force Induced Displacements

Whereas pulsed-HIFU exposures are being used with UCAs to enhance blood brain barrier disruption (as described above), and can also be used with UCAs to enhance sonoporation (as will be described below), only recently have these exposures been shown to be a viable method for consistently enhancing both drug and gene delivery without the addition of UCAs. Preclinical studies in mice have shown how these exposures can enhance the delivery of high-molecular weight FITC-dextran (Yuh et al., 2005), fluorescently label polystyrene nanoparticles (Frenkel et al., 2006a), and radiolabeled monoclonal antibodies (Jang et al., 2007) in sub-cutaneous tumors, as well as fluorescein labeled lectin and fluorescently labeled polystyrene nanoparticles in murine flank muscle (Frenkel et al., 2005). The same exposures were also shown to improve binding and penetration of tPA in blood clots in vitro (Stone et al., 2005). When the exposures were evaluated in therapeutic applications similar enhancement was also observed. Improved tumor growth inhibition was found when the exposures preceded administrations of the proteasome inhibitor, Bortezomib (Velcade™), compared to the drug alone (Poff et al., 2006). And increased rates of thrombolysis were observed, both *in vitro* (Frenkel et al., 2006b) and *in vivo* (Stone et al., 2007), when the exposures were combined with tPA and compared to the administrations of the drug alone.

Mechanistic investigations of these exposures have shown that increased drug delivery occurs from both enhanced extravasation from the vasculature (Frenkel et al., 2005) and improved transport in the interstitium (Frenkel et al., 2005; Traughber et al., 2006). Whereas acoustic cavitation could potentially account for enhanced extravasation (as occurs for blood brain barrier disruption), it is highly unlikely that it is responsible for improved interstitial transport due to the physical size restrictions of intercellular spaces in the parenchyma (on the order of nanometers) and the dearth of cavitation nuclei. Indeed, real-time monitoring for cavitation *in vivo* during the exposures did not indicate the presence of cavitation activity, except for regions rich in blood vessels, where some red blood cell extravasation occurred (O'Neill et al., 2006). Further evidence that cavitation is absent during the exposures, at least inertial cavitation, is provided by histological analysis of the treated tissues where no destructive effects were observed with light microscopy (Dittmar et al., 2005; Frenkel et al., 2006; O'Neill et al., 2006; Poff et al., 2006; Jang et al., 2007) or transmission electron microscopy (Traughber et al., 2006), nor were increases found in the number of apoptotic cells (Dittmar et al., 2005; Poff et al., 2006).

In regards to a thermal mechanism, hyperthermia could similarly explain improved extravasation (Kong et al., 2000), however, it has not been shown to conclusively improve interstitial transport. Monitoring during pulsed-HIFU exposures has shown temperature elevations to occur on the order of 4 to 5 degrees celcius in tumors (Thomas et al., 2005; Frenkel et al., 2006a) and in muscle (O'Neill et al., 2007). These low temperature elevations are not surprising seeing that although ultrasound intensities are relatively high (> 1000 W cm^{-2}), duty cycles are only typically 5 to 10%, which substantially reduce time averaged energy deposition. Temperature elevations on this order have been shown to be sufficient to significantly enhance extravasation. However, hyperthermia treatments typically occur for 1 hr (Kong and Dewhirst, 1999; Kong et al., 2000), whereas pulsed-HIFU exposures at individual raster points occur for 2 min or less (Yuh et al., 2005; Frenkel et al., 2005; Frenkel et al., 2006a; Poff et al., 2006; Jang et al., 2007; Patel et al., 2007). Experiments with liposomes similar to those used by Kong et al (2000) showed that pulsed-HIFU exposures provided with the liposomes did not enhance extravasation (Dromi et al., 2007). Furthermore, recent experiments using a non-HIFU heat source was carried out, where the thermal dose was the same as the pulsed-HIFU exposures. This type of hyperthermia treatment did not produce enhanced extravasation of fluorescently labeled polystyrene nanoparticles in murine muscle compared to untreated controls; however, enhancement was observed with pulsed-HIFU (O'Neill et al., 2007).

Whereas it has been established (above) that pulsed-HIFU exposures can enhance the delivery of various agents in different tissue models, to date, conclusive evidence on the exact ultrasound mechanism(s) by which this enhancement occurs has not been provided. As stated above, all the data collected so far precludes a thermal mechanism. And regarding a non-thermal mechanism, there appears to be overwhelming evidence that cavitation alone cannot lay claim to all the effects produced. The question then arises as to what the additional mechanism is. Frenkel et al (2006 Radiology) have proposed radiation force induced displacements in the exposed tissue as the underlying mechanism for enhancing delivery when using pulsed-HIFU exposures without the addition of UCAs. Within the focal zone, displacement in the tissue is non-uniform, and further non-uniformity in displacement will occur at boundary regions between the focal zone (where displacement is highest) and tissue outside and adjacent to it (Lizzi et al., 2003). Non-uniformity in displacement between any two adjacent regions of tissue can induce shear forces, where the resulting strain will act first on the weakest structural elements in the tissue, such as junctions between individual cells (e.g. tight junctions between endothelial cells and desmosomes between cells in the parenchyma). The key to these displacements creating such alterations is thought to be the magnitude of the displacements themselves, which are typically on the order of tens of microns (Frenkel et al., 2005; Frenkel et al., 2006), or in other words, a number of times the size of individual cells.

Frenkel et al (2000a) observed non-destructive widening of intercellular spaces between epithelial cells, in response to non-focused ultrasound exposures at a fluid-tissue interface. It is hypothesized that these effects resulted from transverse waves generated at the interface, which are dampened quickly in soft tissues, thus creating a steep gradient in the shear forces that worked on the cellular junctions. As a consequence of these exposures, increased penetration of nanoparticles occurred into the tissue from the fluid medium, as well as increases in the rate of effective diffusion (Frenkel et al., 2000b). Focused ultrasound exposures have also shown the ability to induce gaps between cells (Seidl et al., 1994; Mesiwala et al., 2002 In non-cancerous tissue, possessing both normal vasculature and function lymphatics, the microvasculature pressure is greater than the interstitial fluid pressure (IFP), and hence a driving force for extravasation occurs, being also controlled by the osmotic pressure gradients across the blood vessel wall (Jain, 2005). To some degree, it is possible that creation of structural alterations (i.e. widening of intercellular gaps) that increase vascular permeability could potentially then allow for increased extravasation; especially large macromolecules and viruses, which are dependant on convection for transvascular transport. Recent studies have shown that pulsed-HIFU exposures may somehow also be lowering IFP, where levels in tumors were lower than those measured prior to exposures. Additional measurements using acoustic radiation force imaging (ARFI, described above), corroborated these results, where a reduction in elasticity of the tissue was found following the exposures. The reduced elasticity, caused by the pulsed-HIFU exposures was seen as an increase in the time required for the tissue to return back to its original position after a single radiation force induced displacement. And since these effects were produced non-destructively, these results can only be explained by a reduction in fluid pressure (O'Neill et al., unpublished data).

The idea that enhanced local drug delivery could result directly from the creation of pulsed-HIFU induced radiation forces in the issue, in the absence of contributing thermal and cavitational mechanisms, is supported by improved delivery of nanoparticles in both muscle and tumors that correlate with increased displacements generated in the exposed tissue (Frenkel et al., 2005 ISTU; Frenkel et al., 2006a). Enhanced rates of thrombolysis, which result from improved delivery of tPA (Stone et al., 2005), were also found to correlate with increases in radiation force induced displacements (Frenkel et al., 2006b). Analysis of patterns of nanoparticle delivery in the muscle at individual raster (treatment) points has also indicated extravasation to correlate positively with locally induced displacements (Frenkel et al., 2005).

A mechanism for enhanced delivery using pulsed-HIFU exposures, as described above for normal (i.e. noncancerous) tissue cannot be assumed for solid tumors. Both transvascular and interstitial transport may be irregular and insufficient for uniform and adequate delivery of therapeutic agents in tumors (Wang and Yuan, 2006). Blood vessels in tumors, compared to those in normal tissues, are leaky, possessing large gaps between endothelial cells

(McDonald and Choyke, 2003). The vasculature is also chaotic in regards to spatial distribution, diameter and microvessel length (Wang and Yuan, 2006), as well as tortuous and saccular, with haphazard interconnections, which renders them functionally abnormal (Jain, 2005). For large macromolecules and drug carriers, diffusion is not an adequate process for crossing the microvessel wall. And the hypertension (elevation of hydrostatic pressure in regions outside of blood vessels) found just past the periphery of tumors, which can be approximately the same as the microvascular pressure, will severely limit extravasation, and therefore the delivery of therapeutic agents (Boucher et al., 1990). The plasma to interstitial gradient of oncotic pressure is also generally reduced in tumors, which can further contribute to less than optimal delivery of therapeutic agents (Stohrer et al., 2000).

Additional factors in the extracellular matrix (ECM) will also limit interstitial transport and therefore further inhibit the adequate distribution of agents; especially large agents such as viral vectors (Wang and Yuan, 2006). Netti et al (2000) demonstrated the inverse relationship between tissue content of fibrillar collagen and interstitial diffusion of large macromolecules. McGuire et al (2006) also demonstrated that greater collagen content in the ECM required greater infusion pressure to initiate flow in the interstitium. The effects of collagen on limiting interstitial transport were further demonstrated, where treatment with collagenase to chemically disrupt the fibers resulted in increases in interstitial transport of antibodies (Netti et al., 2000) and oncolytic viruses (McKee et al., 2006). Collagen in the ECM acts to inhibit macromolecule transport by physically obstructing movement, where the sizes of viral vectors for example can be larger than the space between fibers (Wang and Yuan, 2006). Collagen fibers also bind and stabilize glycosaminoglycan, which can create resistance to water and solute transport (Netti et al., 2000). The manner by which size may effect drug delivery to tumors was recently demonstrated by Dreher et al (2006), where although increasing the molecular weight of macromolecules was found to increase their plasma half-life, it decreased vascular permeability for reduced extravasation, as well as penetration in to tumor tissue from the vessel wall (Dreher et al., 2006).

The mechanism (or mechanisms) linking pulsed-HIFU induced stress history to changes in fluid flow properties are not well understood. One model has been proposed that may help in explaining this link (O'Neill et al., 2005). In this purely mechanical model, the tissue is treated as a modified bi-phasic mixture of solid and fluid. The fluid phase, however, is comprised of two parts: a 'bound' fraction that moves with the tissue; and a 'free' fraction that moves through the tissue. Only the free fluid portion can contribute to the transport properties of the tissue. Thus the local hydraulic conductivity of the tissue is dependant on the free fluid volume fraction. The remaining solid and bound fluid phases act in concert as a quasi-solid whose elastic stiffness increases with bound fluid volume fraction. A transfer of fluid from the bound state to the free state therefore has a tendency to increase the local hydraulic conductivity, while simultaneously decreasing the tissue stiffness. This process is therefore driven by the decrease in strain energy. It is opposed, however, by the variety of tissue structures that prevent the free flow of fluid. These structures provide a barrier potential energy, or better yet, a barrier energy distribution, which must be overcome before bound fluid can be freed. Mechanical stimuli, such as pulsed-HIFU, might well be expected to breach some the lower energy barriers, while leaving the higher energy barriers intact. Due to the viscous nature of the tissue, this action will depend on the frequency of the stimulus as well as the power. Finally, however, the tissue is able to recover by simply rebuilding the damaged barriers.

The general model proposed above, while satisfying on a theoretical level, remains unconfirmed and lacking in substantial detail. In particular, specific 'barriers' have yet to be identified that may clearly be altered by pulsed-HIFU induced stresses. A candidate for such a barrier is the network of fibrillar collagen in the ECM, which can reduce both hydraulic conductivity (McGuire et al., 2006) and the physical passage of large macromolecules (Boucher et al., 1990 and viruses (McKee et al., 2006). Cell junctions and the dimensions of intercellular spaces can also affect hydraulic conductivity, where Darcy's law states the instantaneous discharge rate through a porous medium is proportional to the cross-sectional area to flow. It is also possible that the effect of pulsed-HIFU exposures on enhancing transport in not strictly physical, but instead results also from a biological reaction to the physical stimulus. This does not, strictly speaking, invalidate the theory outlined above, but the possibility that the cells themselves may actively participate in breaching the barriers adds a layer of complexity not envisioned in the original model. In effect, the barrier potential distribution would be determined not only by strict energy considerations, but also possibly by cell biology and physiology. It is after all, only cell biology that makes the process reversible. At this time, it is clear that significant work needs to go into measuring the barrier energy distributions of various tissues before this model can be expected to make any useful predictions, including the understanding how cell themselves might subtly contribute to the manner by which the tissue responds to pulsed-HIFU.

A number of recent investigations, however, have commenced to validate the model. The first involved pulsed-HIFU exposures in a tumor model, followed by intra-tumoral infusions of fluorescently labeled polystyrene nanoparticles. Compared to infusions alone, the exposures enabled a marked increase of nanoparticle penetration into the core of the tumors. Ultrastructural analysis of the tissue using transmission electron microscopy revealed widening of intercellular gaps (Traughber et al., 2006). These were similar to those reported by Frenkel et al (2000a; 2000b), which enabled improved nanoparticle transport in their tissue model (Frenkel et al., 2000b). In a second study, experiments in collagen type I phantoms, where concentrations of fibrillar collagen were physiologically relevant, showed the nanoparticles to penetrate the gels from an external reservoir only where the exposures were given. When the gels were observed the following day, the distribution of the nanoparticles was still restricted to regions in the gels where the pulsed-HIFU exposures were originally provided (O'Neill et al., unpublished data). It is thought that the relatively large degree of displacements produced (e.g. tens of microns) could possibly have disrupted the collagen fibers, reducing their ability to act as a functional barrier. Together these preliminary results suggest that pulsed-HIFU exposures may be improving interstitial transport by a number of mechanisms for physically enlarging pores in the ECM, as well as improving interconnectedness of the interstitium.

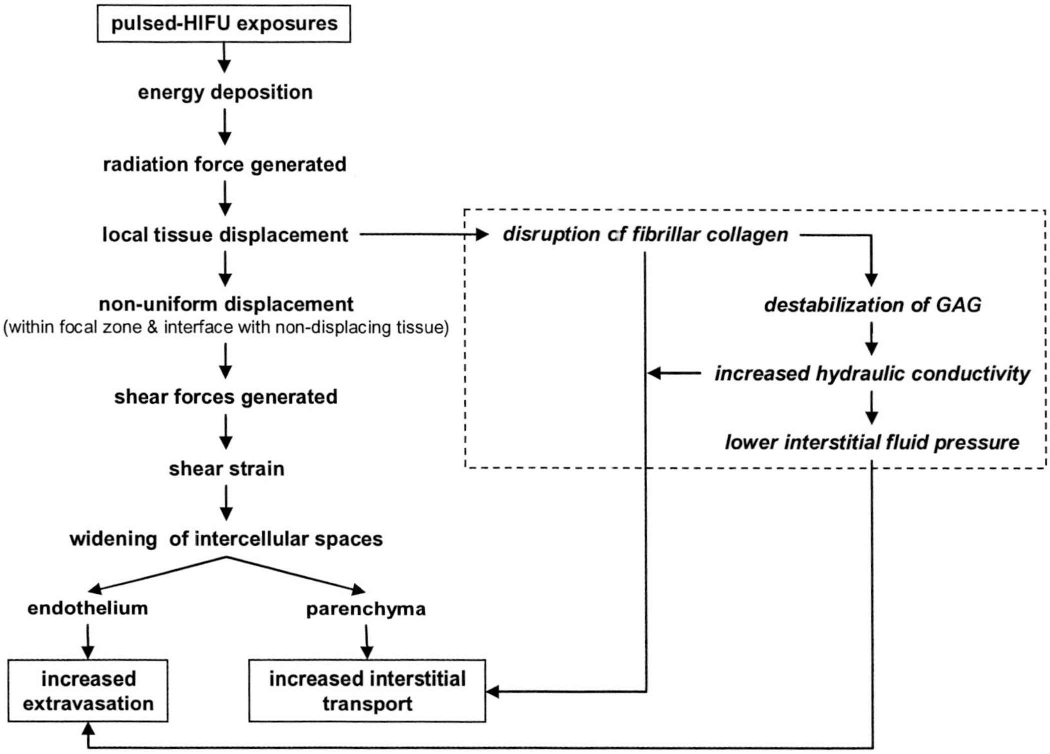

Figure 2. The proposed mechanisms by which radiation force induced displacements, generated by pulsed-HIFU exposures, create changes in the exposed tissue to enhance delivery. The flow chart on the left describes the sequence of events thought to occur in normal tissue, such as the muscle. The additional region on the right (box formed by dotted line) describes additional events that might also occur in the tumor microenvironment. (GAG = glycosaminoglycan).

Pulsed-HIFU Treatment Strategies for Enhanced Gene Delivery

So far in this chapter, clear evidence has been presented on the multitude of ways that pulsed-HIFU exposures can be used as an adjunctive modality to enhance drug delivery for various therapeutic applications. In the previous section, the two major ultrasound mechanisms for enhanced gene delivery were reviewed; sonoporation and radiation force induced displacements. In this section the manner by which these mechanisms can be employed for enhancing targeted gene delivery will reviewed. Three separate treatment strategies will be discussed, based on the manner by which the DNA, or gene carrying vectors, are administered in combination with pulsed-HIFU exposures: 1) by local injection or infusion into the targeted tissue; 2) systemically; 3) by administration into a local blood vessel associated with the targeted tissue.

Naked DNA, Viral Vectors, and Non-Viral Vectors

Although the scope of this review is not meant to include an in-depth discussion on the various systems that may be used for delivery of DNA, the following section summarizing the three different systems presently available is being provided in order to present some background for the manner by which these various systems may influence their use with pulsed-HIFU exposures. Exogenous DNA delivery to cells can presently be achieved using naked DNA, viral vectors, and non-viral vectors.

Naked DNA is the simplest non-viral gene delivery system and has been shown to produce particularly high levels of gene expression when injected directly in the muscle (Wolff et al., 1990), and to a lesser degree into the skin (Choate et al., 1997), kidneys (Kuemmerle et al., 2000, and tumors (Quijano et al., 2005). Direct injection of DNA, however, leads to lower overall levels of expression compared to viral vectors or non-viral, liposomal vectors. Because of the presence of serum nucleases, naked DNA is generally considered to be unsuitable for systemic administration (Mansouri et al., 2004). Advantages of naked DNA include ease and cost of production (Huber and Pfisterer, 2000), lack of packaging constraints, as well as low toxicity and immunogenicity (Rahim et al., 2006).

A variety of viral vectors are available for delivering genes to cells including retroviruses, herpes simplex viruses, poxviruses, lentiviruses, adenoviruses, and adeno-associated viruses (Wang and Yuan, 2006). The primary appeal to using viral vectors for gene delivery is their high transfection rates due to their natural ability to enter a cell. Among the drawbacks to using viral vectors is that large scale production is relative difficult compared to other vectors and that only relatively small sequences of DNA can be inserted into the virus genome. Toxicity, immune and inflammatory responses are also associated with viral vectors, as well as insertional mutagenesis and oncogenic effects. The development of non-viral vectors for gene delivery has in part been due to the limitations of viral vectors, especially those related to their safety (Mansouri et al., 2004).

Although various types of non-viral gene delivery vectors continue to be developed, cationic phospholipids and cationic polymers are the two most popular types presently being investigated. These systems are based electrostatic interactions between their cationic (i.e. positive) charges and the negatively charged DNA to form complexes. Advantages over viral vectors include low immunogenicity, as well as ease of preparation. The structural variability and versatility of non-viral vectors also enable the possibility of attaching ligands on their surface that can bind to receptors on targeted cells. On the other hand, these non-viral vectors have relatively low transfection efficiency compared to viral vectors (Mansouri et al., 2004). Another disadvantage is that liposome/DNA complexes have a tendency to aggregate (Wasan et al., 1996).

Local (direct) Administration

Local administration of DNA by intratumoral infusion is one of the strategies for cancer gene therapy, and presently the most common used method in clinical trials when using viral vectors (Wang et al., 2005). Not surprisingly, the majority of preclinical studies reported to date for cancer gene therapy have also involved direct (manual) injections or slow (automated) infusions into the targeted tumor tissue. Intratumoral infusion has several advantages over systemic delivery. For one, it circumvents the transvascular barrier, which is especially important for large vectors such as viruses. Secondly, interstitial transport is enhanced, where the infusions a) generate a transient pressure gradient that increases convection; and b) induce tissue deformation that can increase the connectedness and size of pores in the interstitium. Furthermore, minimal toxicity is produced in normal tissue, since systemic distribution of vectors is restricted to solid tumors (Wang and Yuan, 2006). However, recent studies have shown that under certain conditions infusion can produce dissemination of viral vectors as a result of enhanced convective transport into the leaky tumor microvasculature (Wang et al., 2005). In this section studies are discussed that employ the mechanism of sonoporation (i.e. where exposures followed injections of plasmid with UCAs) as well as other mechanical effects (where exposures preceded injections of the DNA in various systems).

Various preclinical studies have shown how pulsed-HIFU exposures can be used to improve therapeutic efficacy for treatments involving direct injections of DNA. Tumor necrosis factor alpha (TNFα) is a multifunctional cytokine that can produce cytotoxic effects against cancer epithelial cells as well as indirect effects in tumor associated vasculature (Bazzoni et al., 1996). Pulsed-HIFU exposures followed by a single intratumoral injection of TNFα was shown in one study to improve growth inhibition of a murine squamous cell carcinoma tumor model when compared to injections alone. Gross observations of the tumors indicated a larger necrotic region surrounding the needle track in the HIFU treated tumors. Histology also showed that the necrotic region extend further away, perpendicular to the needle track than for injections alone (Quijano et al., 2005). These finding are corroborated by a subsequent study using the same tumors and exposures, where a surrogate fluorophore achieved better penetration into the core of the tumors with the exposures than without (Traughber et al., 2006). In a follow up study, the same exposures and procedure were carried out in a more clinically relevant tumor/agent model. Here, infusions (i.e. slow injections) of an attenuated adenovirus were given expressing tumor necrosis factor–related apoptosis-inducing ligand (TRAIL), which induces apoptosis in cancer cells, but is not toxic in most normal host cells. The study was carried out in a human esophageal carcinoma, where the vector possessed a promoter specific to the cell line. Similar to the study using TNFα, pulsed-HIFU exposures preceding the infusions of the adenovirus produced significantly greater inhibition of tumor growth than infusions alone (Patel et al., 2007).

Local gene delivery and pulsed-HIFU exposures may also be combined with UCAs as demonstrated by Miller and Song (2003). In their study, they injected naked plasmid encoding for the bioluminescent reporter gene, luciferase, together with UCAs in murine renal carcinoma tumors, which were then followed by pulsed-HIFU. Although this treatment regimen resulted in significant increases in gene transfection compared to injections without exposures or with exposures but without UCAS, this combination treatment caused marked destructive effects evident by significantly lower growth rates of the treated tumors compared to the other two groups. Improved gene expression with the UCAs can usually be attributed to sonoporation, which as described above will enhance gene transfection. Uncontrolled destructive effects of inertial cavitation appeared to also occur as seen by the decrease in tumor growth. These conclusions are further supported by the dose dependency on the destructive effects, where increasing both pulse duration and peak rarefractional pressure amplitude (the most important exposure parameter affecting cavitation activity) caused a decrease in both tumor growth rates and expression of the reporter gene. The decrease in reporter gene activity in this case was attributed to the reduction in the overall number of viable cells and not lower transfection efficiency. Interestingly, exposures without UCAs did not significantly enhance luciferase expression compared to sham controls, where they did with the UCAs. These results are in contrast to those of Huber and Pfisterer (2000), who injected plasmid DNA encoding for beta-galactosidase into Dunning prostate tumors in rats. Pulsed-HIFU exposures, without UCAs, in their study showed a highly significant increase in the expression of the reporter gene compared to injections alone.

The ability of pulsed-HIFU exposures to enhance delivery and consequent therapeutic effects of locally infused DNA has also been demonstrated in a variety of non-cancerous tissues. In one study, the beta-galactosidase gene was injected directly into the ischemic hind limbs of rabbits and expression levels were found to increase when injections were followed by pulsed-HIFU exposures. Increased expression levels were also found when exposures were given prior to injections, however, these were relatively lower than when exposures were given afterwards. When the reporter gene was substituted with that for the vascular endothelial growth factor (VEGF), an improvement in neovascularization was acheived (Schratzberger et al., 2002). In another study, a liver specific plasmid DNA for human factor IX (for the treatment of hemophilia B) was injected directly into the liver of mice followed by pulsed-HIFU exposures. Blood samples taken showed significant increases in gene expression to occur as a result of using this procedure compared to intra-hepatic injections alone, and were further enhanced by the addition of UCAs to the injections. Varying the duration of the applied pulses was not found to strongly affect the levels of expression, though increasing the peak negative pressure did correlate positively with expression of the gene. These results correlated with expression of a fluorescent reporter seen in histological sections of the liver. Histological analysis did show damage to be produced in the liver above a pressure threshold, however, this was found to be transient, where repair was observed a few days later (Miao et al., 2005). A previous study by the group had shown that significantly higher plasma levels of factor IX could be obtained by rapid, high-volume injections of the plasmid via the tail vein (i.e. hydroporation, as described above), where injections without hydrodynamic pressure were not effective (Liu et al., 1999). Using both methods (i.e. hydroporation and the intra-hepatic injections with HIFU), plasma concentrations of factor IX approached the therapeutic range for treating hemophelia patients.

Intravenous (systemic) Administration

A second strategy for using pulsed-HIFU exposures is to administer the DNA to be delivered systemically, followed by exposures in the targeted tissue or organ. This type of procedure is thought to be especially suited for treating cardiovascular diseases, where for example transthoracic ultrasound focused on the heart could deliver genes for increasing vascularization of the myocardium in order to ameliorate congestive heart failure (Unger et al., 2001). Other targets would be skeletal muscle and blood vessels themselves. However, because of the nature of this procedure, where exposures would be targeted at regions of the vasculature contain DNA and UCAs, enhanced levels of transgene expression in solid tumors could occur similarly to the other tissues. The ability to deliver DNA by systemic administration with local enhancement being achieved using a modality such as pulsed-HIFU is attractive because of the systemic nature of cancer, itself (Zhou et al., 2005). However, this type of strategy requires both safeguards, such as tissue specific promoters, as well as vectors (e.g. liposomes) that can protect DNA in the serum from clearance and degradation, and increase circulation time. In the case where the DNA is administered prior to exposures, liposome can also protect DNA from the potential destructive effects of the exposures (e.g. cavitation) themselves (Wasan et al., 1996).

The most straightforward study to date demonstrating the feasibility of this procedure was carried out by Dittmar et al (2005). Pulsed-HIFU exposures were given in one of two bilateral, murine squamous cell carcinoma tumors grown subcutaneously in mice, followed by a tail vein injection of plasmid encoding for the reporter gene green fluorescent protein (GFP) without the addition of UCAs. Observations with fluorescent microscopy of tumor sections showed visible levels of gene expression in the exposed tumors but not in controls. Fluorescence was present almost exclusively in the first few layers of cells surrounding tumor blood vessels, however, no destructive effects were present in the exposed tissue. GFP expression was quantitatively detected in untreated tumors by western blot analysis, where nine-fold increases were found in tumors exposed to pulsed-HIFU.

One other study has reported attempts to enhance gene delivery via systemic administration using pulsed-HIFU exposures. Huber and Pfisterer (2000) injected plasmid DNA encoding for the reporter gene beta-galactosidase via the tail vein in rats with Dunning prostate tumors (as described above), with a three minute lag time before giving the exposures. Contrary to the significant enhancement they found by intratumoral injections, systemic deliveries did not result in detectable levels of the reporter gene in the tumor tissue. These results also do not support those found by Dittmar et al (2005) who admistered the DNA following exposures in mice. Comparable doses of DNA were used in each study for the relative animal models, and it is not reasonable that all the DNA had been degraded by DNases and/or scavenged by the liver in the three minute lag period between injections and exposures (Emlen and Mannik 1978). One reason perhaps that no enhancement was found in the rat study but was found with the mice, was that that ultrasound exposure intensities in the later were one order of magnitude higher. Another is perhaps because intratumoral injections can provide nucleation for cavitation to facilitate transfection (Miller and Song, 2003), whereas the occurrence in the vasculature of cavitation would be much more unlikely, since UCAs were not used. UCAs typically lower the threshold for cavitation to occur, and the introduction of nucleation sites may have made the difference at these lower intensities. This may explain why enhanced transfection occurred with direct injections into the tumors, but not by systemic administration. It is difficult, however, to speculate too far seeing the extensive differences in nearly all aspects of the two experimental systems.

Intravascular Administration

An increase in the delivery of genes can also be obtained where the DNA (usually as naked plasmid) is introduced into a large blood vessel of the targeted organ or tissue, followed by ultrasound exposures of various modalities (focused, non-focused, and intra-luminal). The advantage of such a procedure is that transfection can be restricted to a specific target tissue or organ, which is essential, for example, when using suicide genes that do not possess any targeting factors such as tissue specific promoters. A second advantage is that reduced amounts of DNA and UCAs (if being used) will be required and these agents can also concentrated for increasing transfection efficiency. The ability to combine ultrasound exposures with plasmid DNA and UCAs to enhance local gene transfection in an isolated blood vessel was demonstrated by Hashiya et al (2004). The study was carried out in a rat carotid artery model, however, a catheter based ultrasound device was used. This obvious disadvantage of such a procedure is the ultrasound device, which is inserted in the vessel, and therefore carries the risks of any endovascular procedure, especially vessel rupture (Qureshi et al., 2000).

Regarding the use of such a strategy with pulsed-HIFU, one study to date has definitively shown its feasibility. Plasmid DNA encoding for the LacZ enzyme was infused into isolated segments of the carotid artery of rabbits, which was then given a pulsed-HIFU exposures. Compared to minimal levels of expression that were detected when just administering the DNA, the exposures did significantly enhance expression. However, when UCAs were added, a further significant increase in expression did occur, indicating that sonoporation was an active mechanism for transfection. A positive correlation was found between gene expression and the ultrasound pressure amplitude, both with and without the addition of UCAs. As in other studies employing different strategies (i.e. local injection, see Miller and Song (2003)), the addition of UCAs also lowered the intensity threshold for producing damage in the treated vessels, which appeared in the form of visible hemorrhage in the vessel wall (Huber et al., 2003).

An up to date review of the literature has indicated that studies have yet to be carried out using this type of procedure for the treatment of cancer. As expected, most studies involving this type of targeting have been for vascular diseases where, for example, enhanced delivery of E2F decoy oligodeoxynucleotides improved inhibition of intimal hyperplasia following balloon injury in a carotid artery model in rats (Hashiya et al. 2004). This type of strategy, however, can be compared to other interventional oncology techniques, were vessels, limbs, or organs are isolated for an organ specific drug application to increase efficacy of anti-tumor agents in the treatment of irresectable tumors. A multitude of examples exist, such as isolated limb perfusion of melphalan for advanced stages of melanoma (Hayes et al., 2007). For such procedures, the addition of recombinant human tumor necrosis factor (rhTNF) has also been used because of its selective effect on endothelial cells in tumour angiogenic vessels. In perhaps a somewhat analogous manner to the effects of pulsed-HIFU exposures, treatment with rhTNF can result in improved penetration and efficicacy of chemotherapeutic agents, such as melphalan, by making the tumor blood vessels leakier. The mechanism of rhTNF on the vasculature is the disruption of VE-cadherin complexes at endothelial cell junctions resulting in gaps between the cells (Menon et al., 2006).

Can Pulsed-HIFU Induce longer Term Increases in Membrane Permeability?

Regarding all strategies described above, where pulsed-HIFU exposures are given prior to DNA administration, the question arises in regards to effects created at the level of individual cells, and more specifically, to their plasma membranes. Transfection efficiency is surely not on the scale of sonoporation, where cavitation is actively assisting in permeabilizing cell membranes for uptake of DNA. Since cells may be transfected by simply injecting DNA into tissue (as described above), perhaps increased gene expression could be explained in the same manner for this type of strategy (i.e. exposures prior to administration) as have been described for other non-gene based agents, where both extravasation and interstitial transport are enhanced. In the case of sonoporation, it has been shown that these effects occur on the scale of seconds (Deng et al., 2004). Could pulsed-HIFU exposures (given prior to administrations) be producing more lasting effects for increasing transfection of DNA, and in that way adding another layer of enhancing effects for gene delivery?

Table 2. Pulsed-HIFU enhanced gene delivery strategies

DNA administration	Method	References
1) Direct injection	- DNA injections follow exposures	142*, 151*, 163*, 186*
	- DNA injections precede exposures	63*, 117*, 119**, 163*
2) Systemic injection	- DNA injections follow exposures	34*
3) Intra-vascular	- DNA administered prior to exposures	64*,**

* - w/o UCAs; ** - w/ UCAs

This question does not seem that unreasonable in light of previous studies that have shown other physical stimuli to produce more enduring effects for increasing membrane permeability. In one study, for example, stress waves induced in breast cancer cell membranes using lasers were found to increase membrane permeability to the fluorophore calcein-AM for up to 80 secs after the lasers were turned off (Lee et al., 1996). Another study using aortic endothelial cells investigated the effects of physiological levels of fluid shear stress. Results of the study showed this type of stress could enhance permeability of the cells to flourescein conjugated to bovine serum albumin, up to 10-fold, where reversing this permeability to pre-treatment values occurred only after 60 mins (Jo et al., 1991). If indeed pulsed-HIFU exposures are enhancing delivery by large strains generated through local tissue displacement (where deformation of individual cells would also occur), and that these macroscopic effects are lasting up to 24 and even 48 hrs, perhaps it is not unreasonable that locally induced stresses at the level of cells is being generated for enhanced uptake of DNA. Such a hypothesis, of course, will have to be validated experimentally.

Temporal Control of Gene Expression Using Heat Shock Protein Promoters

Safe and effective gene therapy requires tight control, both spatial and temporal, of transgene expression. In the different treatment strategies discussed above, the aim of the procedures was to enhance spatial targeting and efficiency of gene delivery, however, these strategies did not include mechanisms for temporal control. Tissue specific promoters can also be employed to limit transgene expression to targeted tissues, and in that way add a layer of targeting and safety to gene therapy procedures (Greenberger et al., 2004). As described above, one such promoter for an esophageal carcinoma was recently used with pulsed-HIFU exposures with an adenovector expressing TRAIL (Patel et al., 2007). Methods have been developed to control transgene expression temporally, using gene promoters that respond to external chemical factors such as different antibiotics (Iida et al., 1996; Szulc et al., 2006), or small molecules (Clackson, 1997). One major drawback to the systemic administration of an agent, such as those listed above, is that since these agents will reach all parts of the body, expression of a transgene will occur that was not accurately delivered to the original targeted tissue (Rome et al., 2005). Even in the case of intra-tumoral infusions, conditions for the administration of the gene carriers, such as too high infusion pressure, may lead to systemic leakage from the injection site (Wang et al., 2005).

Heat shock protein (HSP) transcription in eukaryotic cells is robustly initiated within minutes of exposure to temperature elevations above those for maximum growth, and as such this heat shock response has been identified as one of the most selective and inducible ways to regulate transcription (Rome et al., 2005). Among the seven types of HSPs that respond well in terms of inducement to heat, HSP70 has demonstrated the best overall response, especially in regards to being the first to be repressed in the absence of stimulus (DiDomenico et al., 1982). Brade et al (2000), for example, demonstrated a strong thermal dose response of reporter gene expression when under the control of an HSP70B promoter. In vitro experiments carried out by Borrelli et al (2001) showed that increasing heat shock, by increasing the duration, temperature, or both, resulted in proportional increases in both temporal duration and magnitude of EGFP expression in human prostate cancer cells. A number of extremely promising pre-clinical studies to date have already been carried using HSP promoters to control transgene *in vivo* expression and consequently improve therapeutic outcomes (Rome et al., 2005).

Non-destructive HIFU exposures have demonstrated the ability to cause significant upregulation of a variety of genes including stress proteins (SP), glucose regulated proteins (GRP), and HSPs (Kramer et al., 2004). It is well know that HSP promoters, especially the HSP70 promoter, in combination with heat or other physical stimuli, can be used to selectively turn genes on remotely. Only recently, however, has the potential of HIFU exposures as a source of hyperthermia for this purpose been shown *in vivo* [Madio et al., 1998; Rome et al., 2005]. Madio et al (1998) was first to show how localized hypethermia (5 to 8 °C, for 45 min) by HIFU exposures could significantly increase levels of HSP70 mRNA in the muscle of rats. Kramer et al (2004) also found up-regulation of HSPs in tissue bordering HIFU induced thermal lesions in the prostate of patients with benign prostate hyperplasia. Interestingly, one of the proposed mechanisms for induced cellular immunity against cancer cells as a result of HIFU exposures when ablating tissue is the release of HSPs, which are known to stimulate the activity of cytotoxic T-cells (Kennedy, 2005).

A number of studies have been carried out that demonstrating the utility of HSP promoters with HIFU exposures for controlling transgene expression. Liu et al (2005) transfected tumors cells with a bioluminescent reporter gene controlled by an HSP70B promoter. In their *in vitro* experiments, they employed a strategy of using HIFU exposures to generate relatively high temperatures (60 °C) for short durations (5 sec), where the thermal dose bordered on that for inducing coagulative necrosis. These exposures were found to markedly increase gene expression, however, raising the thermal dose above this level was found to decrease the relative number of viable cells. Using the same type of exposures, the authors were then able to reproduce these results in vivo (Liu et al., 2006b). In another study, tumors that were stably transfected with a fluorescent reporter gene controlled by an HSP70 promoter were grown in rodents. Using similar HIFU exposures to those used by Madio et al (1998), marked reporter gene expression was induced, and even improved when temperatures were elevated up to 50 °C, which enabled for shorter exposures to be used (Guilhon et al., 2003). The strategy of using lower temperature elevations for longer periods has also been used to generate similar increases in transgene expression in the liver (Plathow et al., 2005) and in the prostrate (Silcox et al., 2005).

In the studies described above (Guilhon et al., 2003; Plathow et al., 2005; Silcox et al., 2005) HIFU exposures were guided by MRI, which not only enabled accurate placement of the HIFU beam, but also incorporated automated, real-time feedback control of a predefined temperature-time trajectory, which can compensate for tissue inhomogeneity and perfusion, which are known to effect heat generation. These studies indicated the clear advantage of using an MRguided HIFU system with heat shock inducible promoters, where the stimulus was delivered non-invasively in a tightly controlled manner, both spatially and temporally, and in regards to the magnitude of the stimulus. One major disadvantage, however, of this technique is that the technology is expensive and not readily available as a research resource for developing gene therapy protocols. For a comprehensive review on the use of HSP promoters for temporal and spatial control of therapeutic genes, both with and without HIFU exposures, see Rome et al (2005).

Safety Considerations for Pulsed-HIFU

Up until now, evidence has been presented on the multiple ways that pulsed-HIFU may be used to enhance the delivery therapeutic agents and in that way obtain an overall improved therapeutic efficacy. However, for any proposed treatment, it is necessary that the procedure itself does not worsen the clinical outcome (Kennedy, 2005). A fair amount of evidence has been collected regarding any destructive effects produced in the tissues by the exposures. The low level temperature elevations of 4 to 5 °C observed during a 2 min exposure with a 5 to 10% duty cycle (Thomas et al., 2005; Frenkel et al., 2006 Acad Radiol; O'Neill et al., 2007) produces a thermal dose that is far below what is required to cause coagulative necrosis as occurs with exposures for thermal ablation. Typically temperature elevations of at least 56 °C with continuous exposures for at least 1 sec are required to irreversibly cause cell death

(Kennedy, 2005). Inertial cavitation has also not been detected during real time monitoring, nor the have observations with histology shown the hemorrhage that it can typically induce. Detection of sub-harmonic generation, indicative of the presence of cavitation, as well as vessel destruction and consequent red blood cell extravasation, were indeed found when the exposures were intentionally directed at a tumor/skin interface (O'Neill et al., 2006), where under such conditions these phenomena are not unexpected.

A lack of destructive effects were similarly not found in additional tumor studies due to the exposures (Dittmar et al., 2005; Frenkel et al., 2006 Acad Radiol; Poff et al., 2006; Traughber et al., 2006; Jang et al., 2007), nor was an increase the incidence of apoptotic cells (Dittmar et al., 2005; Poff et al., 2006). Jang et al (2007) recently investigated the potential of destructive effects of the exposures on tissues adjacent to sub-cutaneous murine tumor xenografts. Damage was not found in the overlaying skin, nor in the muscle and bone behind the tumors, where both before and after the focal zone (where the beam diverges), intensities can still typically be relatively high. A similar lack of destructive effects was found in the vasculature, as reported in two rabbit studies for increased gene delivery in the carotid artery (Huber et al., 2003) and enhanced tPA-mediated thrombolysis in the marginal ear vein (Stone et al., 2007).

Further evidence is provided in regards to the non-destructive nature of these exposures, albeit this evidence is more indirect. In studies where the goal was to determine if the exposures could improve the therapeutic effect of a particular agent on slowing down the growth of tumors, the control groups that received exposures only (without the agents) had growth rates not significantly different than that of untreated controls (Quijano et al., 2005; Frenkel et al., 2006 Acad Radiol; Poff et al., 2006; Dromi et al., 2007; Patel et al., 2007). Similarly, in thrombolytic studies, the same exposures did not produce any cell lysis, when clots were observed with scanning electron microscopy (Stone et al., 2005). The exposures alone, without thrombolytics, were also not found to enhance thrombolysis both *in vitro* (Frenkel et al., 2006 Radiology) and *in vivo* (Stone et al., 2007).

Whereas pulsed-HIFU exposures may be accurately guided to targeted tissues for spatial enhancement of delivery, temporal enhancement would also seem to be a safety requirement. In one study carried out in the flank muscle of mice, fluorescently labeled polystyrene nanoparticles (100 and 200 nm in diameter) were administered systemically at various time points post-exposure. Significantly less nanoparticles were found to extravasate when administered after 24 hrs, compared to immediately after the HIFU exposures (0 hrs), and less than 5 % of the 0 hrs levels were found at 48 hrs (O'Neill et al., 2006). Although this type of study has to date been carried out in only one tissue type, the results showed that indeed the effects of the exposures on delivery enhancement can be reversible. These results are not surprising seeing that delivery enhancement is being achieved with the generation of destructive biological effects.

Perhaps the most important question regarding the safe use of pulsed-HIFU exposures in the treatment of cancer is whether or not they can enhance the dissemination of neoplastic cells. This question gains even more relevance seeing that the majority of deaths associated with cancer are by metastatic disease and not as a result of the primary tumor (Liotta and Stetler-Stevenson, 1993). Although continuous HIFU exposures for tissue ablation essentially 'fix' the tissue *in situ* by coagulative necrosis, inertial cavitation and other mechanical forces generated in the tissue could potentially increase haematogenous metastasis. However, even if an increase in disseminated cells would occur, the next question asked would then be if this would lead to increased numbers of micro-metastases, and then these to clinically relevant metasastases. In the case of HIFU for thermal ablation two studies to date have been carried out on this important issue. Regarding the question of increased dissemination, Wu et al (2004) found no detectable increase in circulating tumor cells in human patients receiving HIFU treatment. As to whether or not an increase in clinically relevant metastases occur, a study in mice with xenograft prostate tumors also found no effects of HIFU when monitoring the lungs of animals post-treatment (Oosterhof et al., 1997).

Because pulsed-HIFU work predominantly by inducing non-destructive mechanical effects, where apparent widening of intercellular spaces occurs to enhance tissue permeability, the need to determine if indeed the exposures exacerbate the metastatic process would seem even more critical. One study to date has been carried of the effects of pulsed-HIFU on metastasis, where the authors found an increase in the number of metastases in the lungs of mice in which melanoma xenograft tumors were treated (Miller and Dou, 2006). The results, however, of this study cannot be taken on face value seeing that the tumors were grown ectopically (subcutaneously) and not orthotopically by intradermal inoculation. The process of metastasis is complex, where the initial steps include separation of cells from the primary tumor, their invasion into surrounding tissues and basement membranes, and arrival into the vasculature or lymphatics (Liotta and Stetler-Stevenson, 1993; Kanna and Hunter 2005). Preference of orthotopic tumors over ectopic models for studying metastasis continues to increase as more is learned of the importance of host-tumor microenvironment interactions (Kanna and Hunter 2005). It would seem obvious that in the case of evaluating the effects of energy deposition or mechanical interventation on the metastatic process that an orthotopic model should be chosen. Recently, Shih et al (2007) used a similar human melanoma cell line (LOX) grown orthotopically in immunocompromised mice to answer the same question as to whether pulsed-HIFU exposures enhance metastasis. The cell line was stably transfected with both a fluorescent and bioluminescent report gene allowing for multi-modality, whole animal *in vivo* imaging of both primary tumor and developing metastases. Preliminary results of the study have not indicated that the exposures have any adverse effects on the metastatic process.

CONCLUSION

Since the first experiments done in with ultrasound in biological tissues, both the increase in understanding of how ultrasound energy interacts with the tissues and advances in the technology of applying this energy and guiding and monitoring it, have lead to a abounding variety of ultrasound-based diagnostic and therapeutic applications. Due to the many ways that the energy of ultrasound can produce biological effects, these therapeutic applications can range from healing tissue to ablating it in a highly controlled manner. Perhaps the largest range of applications for therapeutic ultrasound has been for enhancing the delivery of an ever increasing assortment of therapeutic agents, which themselves possess a variety of formulations and functions. These applications are presently being developed today for a host of different diseases including cancer, cardiovascular diseases, and chronic brain diseases.

More than twenty years have passed since the first demonstration of how ultrasound exposures, via acoustic cavitation, could enhance the delivery of genes to individual cells. These experiments have since lead to a profusion of investigations for developing safer and more efficient gene delivery procedures. In this chapter, the different ways that genes could be delivered using pulsed-HIFU (a type of therapeutic ultrasound) was reviewed. Various strategies were presented that combined a number of different treatment parameters: the use of plasmid DNA or viral or non-viral vectors; different modes of administration of the agents; whether or not the ultrasound exposures preceded or followed the agents' administration; and the addition or absence of UCAs. The advantages of using ultrasound were also discussed (such as being inexpensive and non-invasive), and the different ways by which the exposures can be provided and monitored with image guidance modalities (e.g. ultrasound and MRI). The manner by which the expression of delivered genes could be controlled temporally using ultrasound was also reviewed, as were some safety concerns involved with the exposures and how these are presently being addressed.

In order to effectively employ HIFU exposures in successful gene therapy protocols, and in-depth and basic understanding of the pulsed-HIFU mechanisms will be required. This will be achieved by continuing to collect experimental data and with mathematical modeling, which together will enable more efficient optimization of the exposures in regards to the multiple exposure parameters that may be selected. By having a comprehensive understanding of the manner by which the physical and acoustic characteristics of the tissues are involved, more intelligent translation of effective exposures from one tissue type to another will also be possible.

Although a wide range of gene therapy applications have been proposed and developed in preclinical studies for treating cancer and other diseases, safe and efficient gene delivery still remains the main hurdle for gene therapy to be used in the clinic. Because of the multiple ways that pulsed-HIFU can be used today for delivering genes and other therapeutic agents, it holds much promise for the future for enabling and improving the treatment of cancer and other diseases. The ability to increase the delivery of a particular therapeutic gene in a region being targeted, and consequently controlling its expression, is providing incentive for the development of new gene therapies, and will ultimately have the effect of bringing gene therapy for human treatment one step closer to being realized.

References

Alexandrov AV, Molina CA, Grotta JC, et al. Ultrasound-enhanced systemic thrombolysis for acute ischemic stroke. *N Engl J Med* 2004;351:2170-8.

Allen TM. Liposomes: opportunities in drug delivery. *Drugs* 1997; 54:8-14.

Atar S, Luo H, Birnbaum Y, et al. The use of transducer-tipped ultrasound catheter for recanalization of thrombotic arterial occlusions. *Echocardiography*. 2001;18(3):233-7.

Barnett SB, ter Haar GR, Ziskin MC et al. Current status of research on biophysical effects of ultrasound. *Ultrasound Med Biol* 1994:20(3):205-8.

Bazzoni F, Beutler B. The tumor necrosis factor ligand and receptor families. *N Engl J Med* 1996;334(26):1717-25.

Bekeredjian R, Grayburn PA, Shohet RV. Use of ultrasound contrast agents for gene or drug delivery in cardiovascular medicine. *J Am Coll Cardiol* 2005;45(3):329-35.

Boucher Y, Baxter LT, Jain RK. Interstitial pressure gradients in tissue-isolated and subcutaneous tumors: implications for therapy. *Cancer Res* 1990;50(15):4478-84.

Bommannan D, Menon GK, Okuyama H, et al. Sonophoresis: II. Examination of the mechanism(s) of ultrasound enhanced transdermal drug delivery. *Pharm Res* 1992;9(8):1043-7.

Borden MA, Sarantos MR, Stieger SM, et al. Ultrasound radiation force modulates ligand availability on targeted contrast agents. *Mol Imaging* 2006;5(3):139-47.

Borrelli MJ, Schoenherr DM, Wong A, et al. Heat-activated transgene expression from adenovirus vectors infected into human prostate cancer cells. *Cancer Res* 2001;61(3):1113-21.

Braaten JV, Gross RA, Francis CW. Ultrasound reversibly disaggregates fibrin fibres. *Thromb Haemost* 1997;78:1063-8.

Brade AM, Ngo D, Szmitko P, et al. Heat-directed gene targeting of adenoviral vectors to tumor cells. *Cancer Gene Ther* 2000;7(12):1566-74.

Burgess S, Zderic V, Vaezy S. Image-guided acoustic hemostasis for treatment of hidden liver injuries. *Ultrasound Med Biol* 2007;33:113-9.

Byl NN. The use of ultrasound as an enhancer for transcutaneous drug delivery: phonophoresis. *Phys Ther* 1995;75(6):539-53.

Catane R. Beck A, Inbar Y, et al. MR-guided focused ultrasound surgery (MRgFUS) for the palliation of pain in patients with bone metastases-preliminary clinical experience. *Ann Oncol* 2007;18(1):162-7.

Chan AH, Fujimoto VY, Moore DE, et al. An image-guided high intensity focused ultrasound device for uterine fibroids treatment. *Med Phys* 2002;29(11):2611-20.

Chen W, Carlson RF, Fedewa R, et al. The detection and exlusion of the prostate neuro-vascular bundle (NVB) in automated HIFU treatment planning using a pulsed-wave doppler ultrasound system. *Proceedings of the 4th International Symposium on Therapeutic Ultrasound*. Kyoto, Japan, 2004.

Choate KA, Khavari PA. Direct cutaneous gene delivery in a human genetic skin disease. *Hum Gene Ther* 1997;8(14):1659-65.

Chorny M, Polyak B, Alferiev IS, et al. Magnetically driven plasmid DNA delivery with biodegradable polymeric nanoparticles. *(In Press)*.

Church CC. Frequency, pulse length, and the mechanical index. *Acous Res Let Online* 2005;6(3):162-8.

Civale J, Clarke R, Rivens I, ter Haar G. The use of a segmented transducer for rib sparing in HIFU treatments. *Ultrasound Med Biol* 2006;32(11)1753-61.

Clackson T. Controlling mammalian gene expression with small molecules. *Curr Opin Chem Biol* 1997;1(2):210-8.

Clement GT. Perspectives in clinical uses of high-intensity focused ultrasound. *Ultrasonics* 2004;42(10):1087-93.

Cornejo CJ, Vaezy S, Jurkovich GJ, et al. High-intensity ultrasound treatment of blunt abdominal solid organ injury: an animal model. *J Trauma* 2004;57(1):152-6.

Culp WC, Erdem E, Roberson PK, Husain MM. Microbubble potentiated ultrasound as a method of stroke therapy in a pig model: preliminary findings. *J Vasc Interv Radiol* 2003;14(11):1433-6.

Crum L. A. Tensile strength of water. *Nature* 1979;278:148-9.

Dalecki D, Raeman CH, Child SZ, Carstensen EL. Effects of pulsed ultrasound on the frog heart: III. The radiation force mechanism. *Ultrasound Med Biol* 1997;23(2):275-85.

Daniels S, Kodama T, Price DJ. Damage to red blood cells induced by acoustic cavitation. *Ultrasound Med Biol* 1995;21(1):105-11.

Datta S, Coussios CC, McAdory LE, et al. Correlation of cavitation with ultrasound enhancement of thrombolysis. *Ultrasound Med Biol* 2006;32(8):1257-67.

Dayton PA, Allen JS, Ferrara KW. The magnitude of radiation force on ultrasound contrast agents. *J Acoust Soc Am* 2002;112(5 Pt 1):2183-92.

Dear JP, Field JE, Walton AJ. Gas compression and jet formation in cavities collapsed by a shock wave. *Nature* 1988;377:505-8.

Deng CX, Sieling F, Pan H, Cui J. Ultrasound-induced cell membrane porosity. *Ultrasound Med Biol* 2004;30(4):519-26.

DiDomenico BJ, Bugaisky GE, Lindquist S. Heat shock and recovery are mediated by different translational mechanisms. *Proc Natl Acad Sci U S A*. 1982;79(20):6181-5.

Dittmar KM, Xie J, Hunter F et al. Pulsed high-intensity focused ultrasound enhances systemic administration of naked DNA in squamous cell carcinoma model: initial experience. *Radiology* 2005;235:541-6.

Dreher MR, Liu W, Michelich CR, et al. Tumor vascular permeability, accumulation, and penetration of macromolecular drug carriers. *J Natl Cancer Inst* 2006;98(5):335-44.

Dromi S, Frenkel V, Luk A, et al. Pulsed-high intensity focused ultrasound and low temperature sensitive liposomes for enhanced targeted drug delivery and anti-tumor effect. *Clin Cancer Res* 2007;13(9):2722-7.

Du X, Qiu B, Zhan X, et al. Radiofrequency-enhanced vascular gene transduction and expression for intravascular MR imaging-guided therapy: feasibility study in pigs. *Radiology* 2005;236(3):939-944.

Dymling SO, Persson HW, Hertz TG, Lindstrom K. A new ultrasonic method for fluid property measurements. *Ultrasound Med Biol* 1991;17(5):497-500.

Emlen W, Mannik M. Kinetics and mechanisms for removal of circulating single-stranded DNA in mice. *J Exp Med* 1978;147(3):684-99.

Fechheimer M, Denny C, Murphy RF, Taylor DL. Measurement of cytoplasmic pH in Dictyostelium discoideum by using a new method for introducing macromolecules into living cells. *Eur J Cell Biol* 1986;40(2):242-7.

Fechheimer M, Boylan JF, Parker S, et al. Transfection of mammalian cells with plasmid DNA by scrape loading and sonication loading. *Proc Natl Acad Sci U S A* 1987;84(23):8463-7.

Francis CW, Blinc A, Lee S, Cox C. Ultrasound accelerates transport of recombinant tissue plasminogen activator into clots. *Ultrasound Med Biol* 1995;21:419-24.

Frenkel V, Kimmel E, Iger Y. Ultrasound-induced cavitation damage to external epithelia of fish skin. *Ultrasound Med Biol* 1999;25(8):1295-1303.

Frenkel V, Kimmel E, Iger Y. Ultrasound-induced intercellular space widening in fish epidermis. *Ultrasound Med Biol* 2000;26(3): 473-80.

Frenkel V, Kimmel E, Iger Y. Ultrasound-facilitated transport of silver chloride (AgCl) particles in fish skin. *J Control Release* 2000;68: 251-61.

Frenkel V, Deng C, O'Neill BE, et al. Pulsed-high intensity focused ultrasound (HIFU) exposures for enhanced delivery of therapeutics: mechanisms and applications. *Proceedings of the 5th International Symposium on Therapeutic Ultrasound. Boston, USA*, 2005.

Frenkel V, Etherington A, Greene M et al. Delivery of liposomal Doxorubicin (Doxil ®) in a breast cancer tumor model: investigation of potential enhancement by pulsed-high intensity focused ultrasound exposure. *Acad Radiol* 2006;13(4):469-79.

Frenkel V, Oberoi J, Stone MJ, et al. Pulsed-high intensity ultrasound (HIFU) enhances thrombolysis in and in vitro model. *Radiology* 2006;239(1):86-93.

Fry WJ. Intense ultrasound in investigations of the central nervous system. *Adv Biol Med Phys* 1958;6:281-348.

Fry FJ, Ades HW, Fry WJ. Production of reversible changes in the central nervous system by ultrasound. *Science* 1958;127(3289):83-4.

Fry FJ, Sanghvi NT, Foster RS, et al. Ultrasound and microbubbles: their generation, detection and potential utilization in tissue and organ therapy--experimental. *Ultrasound Med Biol* 1995;21(9):1227-37.

Gaber MH, Wu NZ, Hong K et al. Thermosensitive liposomes: extravasation and release of contents in tumor microvascular networks. *Int J Radiat Oncol Biol Phys* 1996;36:1177-87.

Gottesman MM. Cancer gene therapy: an awkward adolescence. *Cancer Gene Ther* 2003;10:501-8.

Greenberger S, Shaish A, Varda-Bloom N, et al. Transcription-controlled gene therapy against tumor angiogenesis. *J Clin Inv* 2004;113(7):1017-24.

Girnyk S, Barannik A, Barannik E, et al. The estimation of elasticity and viscosity of soft tissues in vitro using the data of remote acoustic palpation. *Ultrasound Med Biol* 2006;32(2):211-9.

Guilhon E, Voisin P, de Zwart JA, et al. Spatial and temporal control of transgene expression in vivo using a heat-sensitive promoter and MRI-guided focused ultrasound. *J Gene Med* 2003;5(4):333-42.

Hashiya N, Aoki M, Tachibana K et al.: Local delivery of E2F decoy oligodeoxynucleotides using ultrasound with microbubble agent (Optison) inhibits intimal hyperplasia after balloon injury in rat carotid artery model. *Biochem Biophys Res Commun* 2004;317(2):508-4.

Hayes AJ, Neuhaus SJ, Clark MA, Thomas JM. Isolated limb perfusion with melphalan and tumor necrosis factor alpha for advanced melanoma and soft-tissue sarcoma. *Ann Surg Oncol* 2007;14(1):230-8.

aynes JR, McCabe DE, Swain WF, Particle-mediated nucleic acid immunization. *J Biotechnol.* 1996;44(1-3):37-42.

Held RT, Zderic V, Nguyen TN, Vaezy S. Annular phased array high intensity focused ultrasound device for image-guided therapy. *IEEE Trans Ultrason Ferroelectr Freq Control* 2006;53:335-48.

Herweijer H, Wolff JA. Progress and prospects: naked DNA gene transfer and therapy. *Gene Ther* 2003;10:453-8.

Hill CR, ter Haar GR. High intensity focused ultrasound - potential for cancer treatment. *Br J Radiol* 1995;68(816);1296-303.

Huber PE, Pfisterer P. In vitro and in vivo transfection of plasmid DNA in the Dunning prostate tumor R3327-AT1 is enhanced by focused ultrasound. *Gene Ther* 2000;7(17):1516-25.

Huber PE, Mann MJ, Melo LG, et al. Focused ultrasound (HIFU) induces localized enhancement of reporter gene expression in rabbit carotid. *Gene Ther* 2003;10:1600-7.

Hwang JH, Tu J, Brayman AA, Matula TJ, Crum LA. Correlation between inertial cavitation dose and endothelial cell damage in vivo. *Ultrasound Med Biol* 2006;32(10):1611-9.

Hynynen K. The threshold for thermally significant cavitation in dog's thigh muscle in vivo. *Ultrasound Med Biol* 1991;17(2):157-69.

Hynynen K, Colucci V, Chung A, Jolesz F. Noninvasive arterial occlusion using MRI-guided focused ultrasound. *Ultrasound Med Biol* 1996;22(8):001-7.

Hynynen K, McDannold N, Sheikov NA, et al. Local and reversible blood-brain barrier disruption by noninvasive focused ultrasound at frequencies suitable for trans-skull sonications. *Neuroimage* 2005;24(1):12-20.

Hynynen K. Focused ultrasound for blood-brain disruption and delivery of therapeutic molecules into the brain. *Expert Opin Drug Deliv* 2007;4(1):27-35.

Iida A, Chen ST, Friedmann T, Yee JK. Inducible gene expression by retrovirus-mediated transfer of a modified tetracycline-regulated system. *J Virol* 1996;70(9):6054-9.

Jain RK. Normalization of tumor vasculature: An emerging concept in antiangiogenic therapy. *Science* 2005;307:58-62.

Jang BS, Khaibullina A, Sun H, et al. Pulsed high intensity focused ultrasound (HIFU) enhances delivery of radiolabeled monoclonal antibody b3 to a431 tumor in nude mice. *Proceedings of the 54th Annual Meeting of the Society of Nuclear Medicine*. Washington, DC, 2007.

Jo H, Dull RO, Hollis TM et al. Endothelial albumin permeability is shear dependant, time dependant, and reversible. *Am J Physiol* 1991;260 (6/2):1992-6.

Kanna C and Hunter K. Modeling metastasis *in vivo*. *Carcinogenesis* 2005;26(3):513-23.

Katz NP, Shapiro DE, Herrmann TE, et al. Rapid onset of cutaneous anesthesia with EMLA cream after pretreatment with a new ultrasound-emitting device. *Anesth Analg* 2004;98(2):371-6.

Keller MW, Glasheen W, Kaul S. Albunex: a safe and effective commercially produced agent for myocardial contrast echocardiography. *J Am Soc Echocardiogr* 1989;2(1):48-52.

Kennedy JE, Wu F, ter Haar GR et al. High-intensity focused ultrasound for the treatment of liver tumors. *Ultrasonics* 2004;42(1-9):931-5.

Kennedy JE. High-intensity focused ultrasound in the treatment of solid tumors. *Nat Rev Cancer* 2005;5:321-7

Khokhlova VA, Bailey MR, Reed JA, et al. Effects of nonlinear propagation, cavitation, and boiling in lesion formation by high intensity focused ultrasound in a gel phantom. *J Acoust Soc Am* 2006;119(3):1834-48.

Kikkert JR, Vidal JR, Reisch BI. Stable transformation of plant cells by particle bombardment/biolistics. *Methods Mol Biol* 2005;286:61-78.

Kimmel E. Cavitation bioeffects. *Crit Rev Biomed Eng* 2006;34(2):105-61.

Kinoshita M, McDannold N, Jolesz FA, Hynynen K. Noninvasive localized delivery of Herceptin to the mouse brain by MRI-guided focused ultrasound-induced blood-brain barrier disruption. *Proc Natl Acad Sci USA*. 2006;103(31):11719-23.

Kong G, Dewhirst MW. Hyperthermia and Liposomes. Intl J Hyperthermia 1999;15:345-70.

Kong G, Anyarambhatla G, Petros WP, et al. Efficacy of liposomes and hyperthermia in a human tumor xenograft model: importance of triggered drug release. *Cancer Res* 2000;60:6950-7.

Khoobehi B, Peyman GA, Niesman MR, Oncel M. Hyperthermia and temperature-sensitive liposomes: selective delivery of drugs into the eye. *Jpn J Ophthalmol* 1989;33:405-12.

Kodama T, Takayama K. Dynamic behavior of bubbles during extracorporeal shock-wave lithotripsy. *Ultrasound Med Biol* 1998;24(5):723-8.

Kost J, Leong K, Langer R. Ultrasound-enhanced polymer degradation and release of incorporated substances. *Proc Natl Acad Sci* 1989;86(20):7663-6.

Kost J, Mitragotri S, Gabbay RA, et al. Transdermal monitoring of glucose and other analytes using ultrasound. *Nat Med* 2000;6(3):347-50.

Kost J. Ultrasound-assisted insulin delivery and noninvasive glucose sensing. *Diabetes Technol Ther* 2002;4(4):489-97.

Kramer G, Steiner GE, Grobl M, et al. Response to sublethal heat treatment of prostatic tumor cells and of prostatic tumor infiltrating T-cells. *Prostate* 2004;58(2):109-20.

Kuemmerle NB, Lin PS, Krieg RJ Jr, et al. Gene expression after intrarenal injection of plasmid DNA in the rat. *Pediatr Nephrol* 2000;14(2):152-7.

Larson TR, Bostwick DG, Corica A. Temperature-correlated histopathologic changes following microwave thermoablation of obstructive tissue in patients with benign prostatic hyperplasia. *Urology* 1996;47(4):463-9.

Lavon I, Kost J. Mass transport enhancement by ultrasound in non-degradable polymeric controlled release systems. *J Control Release* 1998;54(1):1-7.

Lavon I, Grossman N, Kost J, Kimmel E, Enden G. Bubble growth within the skin by rectified diffusion might play a significant role in sonophoresis. *J Control Release* 2007;12;117(2):246-55.

Lee S, Anderson T, Zhang H, et al. Alteration of cell membrane by stress waves in vitro. *Ultrasound Med Biol* 1996; 22(9):1285-93.

Levy D, Kost J, Meshulam Y, Langer R. Effect of ultrasound on transdermal drug delivery to rats and guinea pigs. *J Clin Invest* 1989;83(6):2074-8.

Lewin PA, Bjorno L. Acoustically induced shear stresses in the vicinity of microbubbles in tissue. *J Acoust Soc Am* 1982;1(3):728-34.

Lewin PA, Barrie-Smith N, Ide M, et al. Interlaboratory acoustic power measurement. *J Ultrasound Med* 2003;22(2):207-13.

Liotta LA, Stetler-Stevenson WG. Principles of molecular cell biology of cancer: Cancer metastasis. In DeVita SHV, Rosenberg Sa (Eds): *Cancer Principles & Practice of Oncology*, 4th edition. J.B. Lippincott, Philadelphia, 1993.

Liu F, Song Y, Liu D. Hydrodynamics-based transfection in animals by systemic administration of plasmid DNA. *Gene Ther* 1999;6(7):1258-66.

Liu Y, Kon T, Li C, Zhong P. High intensity focused ultrasound-induced gene activation in sublethally injured tumor cells in vitro. *J Acoust Soc Am* 2005;118(5):3328-36.

Liu Y, Miyoshi H, Nakamura M. Encapsulated ultrasound microbubbles: therapeutic application in drug/gene delivery. *J Control Release* 2006;114(1):89-99.

Liu Y, Kon T, Li C, Zhong P. High intensity focused ultrasound-induced gene activation in solid tumors. *J Acoust Soc Am* 2006;120(1):492-501.

Lizzi FL, Coleman DJ, Driller J, et al. Effects of pulsed ultrasound on ocular tissue. *Ultrasound Med Biol* 1981;7(3):245-52.

Lizzi FL, Muratore R, Deng CX et al. Radiation-force technique to monitor lesions during ultrasonic therapy. *Ultrasound Med Biol* 2003;29(11):1593-605.

Luk A, Patel P, Durrani AK, et al. Enhanced throughput of pulsed-high intensity focused ultrasound (HIFU) exposures using split focus transducer. *Proceedings of IEEE Ultrasonics*. New York, 2007

Madio DP, van Gelderen P, DesPres D, et al. On the feasibility of MRI-guided focused ultrasound for local induction of gene expression. *J Magn Reson Img* 1998;8(1):101-4.

Mansouri S, Lavigne P, Corsi K, et al. Chitosan-DNA nanoparticles as non-viral vectors in gene therapy: strategies to improve transfection efficacy. *Eur J Pharm Biopharm* 2004;57(1):1-8.

Martin RW, Vaezy S, Kaczkowski P, et al. Hemostasis of punctured vessels using Doppler-guided high-intensity ultrasound. *Ultrasound Med Biol* 1999;25(6):985-90.

McDonald DM, Choyke PL. Imaging of angiogenesis: from microscopic to clinic. *Nat Med* 2003;9(6):713-25.

McDannold N Fossheim SL, Rasmussen H, et al. Heat-activated liposomal MR contrast agent: initial in vivo results in rabbit liver and kidney. *Radiology* 2004;230:743-52.

McDannold N, Hynynen K. Quality assurance and system stability of a clinical MRI-guided focused ultrasound system: four-year experience. *Med Phys* 2006;33(11):4307-13.

McDannold N, Vykhodtseva N, Hynynen K. Targeted disruption of the blood-brain barrier with focused ultrasound: association with cavitation activity. *Phys Med Biol* 2006;51(4):793-807.

McKee TD, Grandi P, Mok W, et al. Degradation of fibrillar collagen in a human melanoma xenograft improves the efficacy of an oncolytic herpes simplex virus vector. *Cancer Res* 2006;66(5):2509-13.

Menon C, Ghartey A, Canter R, et al. Tumor necrosis factor-alpha damages tumor blood vessel integrity by targeting VE-cadherin. *Ann Surg* 2006;244(5):781-91.

Mesiwala AH, Farrell L, Wenzel HJ et al. High-intensity focused ultrasound selectively disrupts the blood brain barrier in vivo. *Ultrasound Med Biol* 2002;28(3):389-400.

Miao CH, Brayman AA, Loeb KR et al. Ultrasound enhances gene delivery of human factor IX plasmid. *Hum Gene Ther* 2005;16:893-905.

Mihran RT, Barnes FS, Wachtel H. Temporally-specific modification of myelinated axon excitability in vitro following a single ultrasound pulse. *Ultrasound Med Biol* 1990;16(3):297-309.

Miller DL, Song J. Tumor growth reduction and DNA transfer by cavitation-enhanced high-intensity focused ultrasound in vivo. *Ultrasound Med Biol* 2003;29(6):887-93.

Miller DL, Dou C. The potential for enhancement of mouse melanoma metastasis by diagnostic and high-amplitude ultrasound. *Ultrasound Med Biol* 2006;32(7):1097-101.

Miller DL. Ultrasound-mediated gene therapy. In *Emerging Therapeutic Ultrasound.* Eds. Wu J, Nyborg WL. World Scientific Publishing Co. New Jersey, 2006.

Mitragotri S, Kost J. Low-frequency sonophoresis: a review. *Adv Drug Deliv Rev* 2004;56(5):589-601.

Mitragotri S. Healing sound: the use of ultrasound in drug delivery and other therapeutic applications. *Nat Rev Drug Discov* 2005;4(3):255-60.

Mourad PD, Lazar DA, Curra FP, et al. Ultrasound accelerates functional recovery after peripheral nerve damage. *Neurosurgery* 2001;48(5):1136-40.

Mougenot C, Salomir R, Palussiere J, et al. Automatic spatial and temporal temperature control for MR-guided focused ultrasound using fast 3D MR thermometry and multispiral trajectory of the focal point. *Magn Reson Med* 2004;52(5):1005-15.

Netti PA, Berk DA, Swartz MA, et al. Role of extracellular matrix assembly in interstitial transport in solid tumors. *Cancer Res* 2000;60:2497-503.

Neumann E, Schaefer-Ridder M, Wang Y, Hofschneider PH. Gene transfer into mouse lyoma cells by electroporation in high electric fields. *MBO J* 1982;1(7):841-5.

Neumann E, Kakorin S, Toensing K. Fundamentals of electroporative delivery of drugs and genes. *Bioelectrochem Bioenerg* 1999;48(1):3-16.

Ng K, Liu Y: Therapeutic ultrasound: its application in drug delivery. *Med Res Rev* 2002;22(2):204-23.

Nightingale K, Soo MS, Nightingale R, Trahey G. Acoustic radiation force impulse imaging: in vivo demonstration of clinical feasibility. *Ultrasound Med Biol* 2002;28:227-35.

Nishita T. Heat-sensitive liposomes containing cisplatin and localized hyperthermia in treatment of murine tumor. *Osaka City Med J* 1998;44:73-83.

Noble ML, Vaezy S, Keshavarzi A, et al. Spleen hemostasis using high-intensity ultrasound: survival and healing. *J Trauma* 2002;53(6):1115-20.

Nyborg WL. Mechanisms for bioeffects of ultrasound relevant to therapeutic applications. In *Emerging Therapeutic Ultrasound.* Eds. Wu J, Nyborg WL. World Scientific Publishing Co. New Jersey, 2006.

Ohl CD, Arora M, Ikink R, Sonoporation from jetting cavitation bubbles. *Biophys J.* 2006;91(11):4285-95.

O'Neill BE, Quinn TP, Frenkel V, Li KCP. A multi-phasic continuum damage mechanics model of mechanically induced increased permeability in tissues. *Proceedings of the Materials Research Society*, Boston, 2005.

O'Neill BE, Frenkel V, Li KCP, Quinn TP. Pulsed HIFU for enhanced drug delivery: a study of possible mechanisms. *Proceedings of the 6th International Symposium on Therapeutic Ultrasound.* Oxford, 2006.

O'Neill BE, Vo H, Angstadt M, et al. Investigations into the potential contribution of a thermal mechanism for pulsed-high intensity focused ultrasound mediated delivery. *Proceedings of IEEE Ultrasonics*. New York, Oct. 28-31, 2007

Oosterhof GO, Cornel EB, Smits GA, et al. Influence of high-intensity focused ultrasound on the development of metastases. *Eur Urol* 1997;32(1):91-5.

Palumbo G. Photodynamic therapy and cancer: a brief sightseeing tour. *Expert Opin Drug Deliv*. 2007;4(2):131-48.

Pan H, Zhou Y, Izadnegahdar O, et al. Study of sonoporation dynamics affected by ultrasound duty cycle. *Ultrasound Med Biol* 2005;31(6):849-56.

Paparel P, Curiel L, Chesnais S, et al. Synergistic inhibitory effect of high-intensity focused ultrasound combined with chemotherapy on Dunning adenocarcinoma. *Brit J Ultrasound* 2005; 95(6):881-5.

Patel P, Shah S, Sekhar KP, et al. Enhancement of AdVgTRAIL Gene Therapy using Pulsed-High Intensity Focused Ultrasound (HIFU) in a Human Esophageal Carcinoma Model in Mice. *Proceedings of the Meeting of the Radiological Society*, Chicago, 2007.

Pfaffenberger S, Devcic-Kuhar B, Kastl SP, et al. *Ultrasound thrombolysis. Tromb Haemost* 2005;94:26-36.

Plathow C, Lohr F, Divkovic G, et al. Focal gene induction in the liver of rats by a heat-inducible promoter using focused ultrasound hyperthermia: preliminary results. *Invest Radiol* 2005;40(11):729-35.

Poff J, Traughber BJ, Allen C, et al. Pulsed-high intensity focused ultrasound enhances tumor growth inhibition by bortezomib in a murine squamous cell carcinoma model. *Proceedings of the 6th International Symposium on Therapeutic Ultrasound.* Oxford, 2006.

Postema M, van Wamel A, ten Cate FJ, de Jong N. High-speed photography during ultrasound illustrates potential therapeutic applications of microbubbles. *Med Phys* 2005;32(12):3707-11.

Pringle IA, McLachlan G, Collie DD, et al. Electroporation enhances reporter gene expression following delivery of naked plasmid DNA to the lung. *J Gene Med* 2007;9(5):369-80.

Purves WK, Orians GH, Heller HG. *Life: The Science of Biology*, 3rd edition. W. H. Freeman and Co., Salt Lake City, 1992.

Qureshi AI, Luft AR, Sharma M, et al. Prevention and treatment of thromboembolic and ischemic complications associated with endovascular procedures: part I – pathophysiological and pharmacological features. *Neurosurgery* 2000;46:1344-59.

Quesson B, de Zwart JA, Moonen CT. Magnetic resonance temperature imaging for guidance of thermotherapy. *J Magn Reson Imaging* 2000;12(4):525-33.

Quijano J, Colunga A, Xie J, et al. Enhanced Regression in a Squamous Cell Carcinoma Murine Tumor Model Using Pulsed-High Intensity Focused Ultrasound (HIFU) and Naked TNF-a Plasmid. *Proceedings of the 4th annual meeting of the Society for Molecular Imaging*, Cologne, Germany, 2005.

Raake P, von Degenfeld G, Hinkel R, et al. Myocardial gene transfer by selective pressure-regulated retroinfusion of coronary veins: comparison with surgical and percutaneous intramyocardial gene delivery. *J Am Coll Cardiol*. 2004;44(5):1124-9.

Rabkin BA, Zderic V, Crum LA, Vaezy S. Biological and physical mechanisms of HIFU-induced hyperecho in ultrasound images. *Ultrasound Med Biol* 2006;32:1721-9.

Rahim AA, Taylor SL, Bush NL, et al. Spatial and acoustic pressure dependence of microbubble-mediated gene delivery targeted using focused ultrasound. *J Gene Med* 2006;8(11):1347-57.

Ranson MR, Carmichael J, O'Byrne K, et al. Treatment of advanced breast cancer with sterically stabilized liposomal doxorubicin: results of a multicenter phase II trial. *J Clin Oncol* 1997;15:3185-91.

Rome C, Couillaud F, Moonen CT. Spatial and temporal control of expression of therapeutic genes using heat shock protein promoters. *Methods* 2005;35(2):188-98.

Riesz P, Kondo T. Free radical formation induced by ultrasound and its biological implications. *Free Radic Biol Med* 1992;13:247-70.

Roberts WW, Hall TL, Ives K, et al. Pulsed cavitational ultrasound: a noninvasive technology for controlled tissue ablation (histotripsy) in the rabbit kidney. *J Urol* 2006;175(2):734-8.

Rosenthal I, Sostaric JZ, Riesz P. Sonodynamic therapy - a review of the synergistic effects of drugs and ultrasound. *Ultrason Sonochem* 2004;11(6):349-63.

Saito T. In vivo electroporation in the embryonic mouse central nervous system. *Nat Protoc* 2006;1(3):1552-8.

Salomir R, Palussiere J, Fossheim SL, et al. Local delivery of magnetic resonance (MR) contrast agent in kidney using thermosensitive liposomes and MR imaging-guided local hyperthermia: a feasibility study in vivo. *J Magn Reson Imaging* 2005;22:534-40.

Sanghvi NT, Hynynen K, Lizzi FL. New Developments in Therapeutic Ultrasound. *Proceedings of IEEE Engineering in Medicine and Biology*, Amsterdam, Holland, 1996.

Schratzberger P, Krainin JG, Schratzberger G et al. Transcutaneous ultrasound augments naked DNA transfection of skeletal muscle. *Mol Ther* 2002;6(5):576-83.

Schroeder A, Avnir Y, Weisman S, et al. Controlling liposomal drug release with low frequency ultrasound: mechanism and feasibility. *Langmuir* 2007;23(7):4019-25.

Seidl M, Steinbach P, Wörle K et al. Induction of stress fibres and intercellular gaps in human vascular endothelium by shock-waves. *Ultrasonics* 1994;32(5):397-400.

Seth P: Vector-mediated cancer gene therapy. *Cancer Biol Ther* 2005;4(5): 512-7.

Sheikov N, McDannold N, Vykhodtseva N, et al. Cellular mechanisms of the blood-brain barrier opening induced by ultrasound in presence of microbubbles. *Ultrasound Med Biol* 2004;30(7):979-89.

Shih J, Pollock C, Angstadt M, et al. The Effects of Pulsed High-Intensity Focused Ultrasound Exposures on Metastases. *Proceedings of the World Conference on Interventional Oncology*. Washington, DC, 2007.

Siddiqi F, Blinc A, Braaten JV, Francis CW. Ultraound increases flow through fibrin gels. *Thromb Haemost* 1995;73:495-8.

Siegel RJ, Atar S, Fishbein MC, et al. Noninvasive transcutaneous low frequency ultrasound enhances thrombolysis in peripheral and coronary arteries. *Echocardiography* 2001;18(3):247-57

Silcox CE, Smith RC, King R, et al. MRI-guided ultrasonic heating allows spatial control of exogenous luciferase in canine prostate. *Ultrasound Med Biol* 2005;31(7):965-70.

Simonin JP. On the mechanisms of in vitro and in vivo phonophoresis. *J Control Release* 1995;33:125-41.

Soo MS, Ghate SV, Baker JA, et al. Streaming detection for evaluation of indeterminate sonographic breast masses: a pilot study. *Am J Roentgenol* 2006;186(5):1335-41.

Starnes BW, Beekley AC, Sebesta JA, et al. Extremity vascular injuries on the battlefield: tips for surgeons deploying to war. *J Trauma* 2006;60:432-42.

Stohrer M, Boucher Y, Stangassinger M, Jain RK. Oncotic pressure in solid tumors is elevated. *Cancer Res* 2000;60(15):4251-5.

Stone MJ, Frenkel V, Oberoi J, et al. Pulsed-High Intensity Focused Ultrasound (HIFU)-enhanced Thrombolysis in Vitro: Proof of Concept and Investigation of Mechanism. *Proceedings of the 91st annual meeting of the Radiological Society of North America.* Chicago, 2005.

Stone MJ, Frenkel V, Dromi S, et al. Pulsed-high intensity focused ultrasound enhanced t-PA mediated thrombolysis in a novel in vivo clot model, a pilot study. *Thrombosis Research* (In Press).

Stride E, Saffari N. The potential for thermal damage posed by microbubble ultrasound contrast agents. *Ultrasonics* 2004;42:907-13.

Survey: The pharmaceutical industry. "Prescription for change". *The Economist* June 18, 2005.

Suslick KS. Homogenous sonochemistry. In: Suslick KS, ed. *Ultrasound: It's Chemical, Physical and Biological Effects*. New York VCH Publishers Inc, 1988.

Szulc J, Wiznerowics M, Sauvain MO, et al. A versatile tool for conditional gene expression and knockdown. *Nat Methods* 2006;3(2):109-16.

Tezel A, Paliwal S, Shen Z, Mitragotri S. Low-frequency ultrasound as a transcutaneous immunization adjuvant. *Vaccine* 2005;23(29):3800-7.

Thomas P, Stone MJ, Durrani A, et al. Infrared imaging for monitoring pulsed-high intensity focused ultrasound (HIFU) induced temperature elevations in a tissue mimicking phantom. *Proceedings of Inframation – Infrared Camera Applications Conference*. Las Vegas, USA, 2005.

Thuroff S, Chaussy C, Vallancien G, et al. High-intensity focused ultrasound and localized prostate cancer: efficacy results from the European multicentric study. *J Endourol* 2003;17(8):673-7.

Tiukinhoy-Laing SD, Huang S, Klegerman M, et al. Ultrasound-facilitated thrombolysis using tissue-plasminogen activator-loaded echogenic liposomes. *Thromb Res* 2007;119(6):777-84.

Traughber B, Frenkel V, Xie J, et al. Pulsed-high intensity focused ultrasound (HIFU) exposures combined with intratumoral injection of TNF-a plasmid enhance growth inhibition in a murine squamous cell carcinoma model. *Proceedings of the 6th International Symposium on Therapeutic Ultrasound*. Oxford, 2006.

Treat LH, McDannold N, Vykhodtseva N, Hynynen K. Transcranial MRI-guided focused ultrasound-induced blood-brain barrier opening in rats. *IEEE Ultrasonics Symposium*, Montreal, 2004.

Uhlemann C, Heinig B, Wollina U. Therapeutic ultrasound in lower extremity wound management. *Int J Low Extrem Wounds* 2003;2(3):152-7.

Vaezy S, Martin R, Yaziji H, et al. Hemostasis of punctured blood vessels using high-intensity focused ultrasound. *Ultrasound Med Biol* 1998;24(6):903-10.

Vaezy S, Shi X, Martin RW, et al. Real-time visualization of high-intensity focused ultrasound treatment using ultrasound imaging. *Ultrasound Med Biol* 2001;27(1):33-42.

Vaezy S, Noble ML, Keshavarzi A, Paun M, et al. Liver hemostasis with high-intensity ultrasound: repair and healing. *J Ultrasound Med* 2004;23(2):217-25.

Vaezy S, Vaezy S, Starr F, et al. Intra-operative acoustic hemostasis of liver: production of a homogenate for effective treatment. *Ultrasonics* 2005;43(4):265-9.

Vaezy S, Zderic V, Karmy-Jones R, et al. Hemostasis and Sealing of Air Leaks in Lung using High-Intensity Focused Ultrasound. *J Trauma (In Press).*

van Wamel A, Kooiman K, Harteveld M. Vibrating microbubbles poking individual cells: drug transfer into cells via sonoporation. *J Control Release* 2006;112(2):149-55.

Vigen KK, Hegge JO, Zhang G, et al. Magnetic resonance imaging-monitored plasmid DNA delivery in primate limb muscle. *Hum Gene Ther*. 2007;18(3):257-68.

Vo H, Patriciu A, Luk A, et al. CT-guided high intensity focused ultrasound ablation with optical 3D tracking. *Proceedings of IEEE Ultrasonics*. New York, 2007.

Walker WF, Fernandez FJ, Negron LA. A method of imaging viscoelastic parameters with acoustic radiation force. *Phys Med Biol* 2000;45(6):1437-47.

Wang Y, Yang Z, Liu S, et al. Characterisation of systemic dissemination of nonreplicating adenoviral vectors from tumours in local gene delivery. *Br J Cancer* 2005;92(8):1414-20.

Wang Y, Yuan F. Delivery of viral vectors to tumor cells: extracellular transport, systemic distribution, and strategies for improvement. *Ann Biomed Eng* 2006;34(1):114-27.

Warden SJ, Fuchs RK, Kessler CK, et al. Ultrasound produced by a conventional therapeutic ultrasound unit accelerates fracture repair. *Phys Ther* 2006; 86(8):1118-27.

Wasan EK, Reimer DL, Bally MB. Plasmid DNA is protected against ultrasonic cavitation-induced damage when complexed to cationic liposomes. *J Pharm Sci* 1996;85(4):427-33.

Wells DJ. Gene therapy progress and prospects: electroporation and other physical methods. *Gene Ther* 2005;11:1363-9.

Weinstein JN, Magin RL, Cysk RL, Zaharko DS. Treatment of solid L1210 murine tumors with local hyperthermia and temperature-sensitive liposomes containing methotrexate. *Cancer Res* 1980;40:1388-95.

Wolff JA, Malone RW, Williams P, et al. Direct gene transfer into mouse muscle in vivo. *Science* 1990;247(4949 Pt 1):1465-8.

Wood BJ, Yanof J, Frenkel V et al. CT and Ultrasound Guided Stereotactic High Intensity Focused Ultrasound (HIFU). P*roceedings of the 5th International Symposium on Therapeutic Ultrasound*. Boston, 2005.

Wu F, Wang ZB, Jin CB, et al. Circulating tumor cells in patients with solid malignancy treated by high-intensity focused ultrasound. *Ultrasound Med Biol* 2004;30(4):511-7.

Wu F, Wang ZB, Cao YD et al. A randomised clinical trial of high-intensity focused ultrasound ablation for the treatment of patients with localised breast cancer. *Br J Cancer* 2003;89(12):2227-33.

Wu F, Wang ZB, Chen WZ, et al. Preliminary experience using high intensity focused ultrasound for the treatment of patients with advanced stage renal malignancy. *J Urol* 2003;170(6 Pt 1):2237-40.

Wu J, Winkler AJ, O'Neill TP. Effect of acoustic streaming on ultrasonic heating. *Ultrasound Med Biol* 1994;20(2):195-201.

Wu J, Chappelow J, Yang J, Weimann L. Defects generated in human stratum corneum specimens by ultrasound. *Ultrasound Med Biol* 1998;24(5):705-10.

Xu Z, Fowlkes JB, Rothman ED, et al. Controlled ultrasound tissue erosion: the role of dynamic interaction between insonation and microbubble activity. *J Acoust Soc Am* 2005;117(1):424-35.

Yang R, Reilly CR, Rescorla FJ, et al. Effects of high intensity focused ultrasound in the treatment of experimental neuroblastoma. *J Pediatr Surg* 1992;27(2):246-50.

Yuh EL, Shulman SG, Mehta SA, et al. Delivery of systemic chemotherapeutic agent to tumors by using focused ultrasound: study in a murine model. *Radiology* 2005;234:431-437.

Yumita N, Nishigaki R, Umemura K, Umemura S. Synergistic effect of ultrasound and hematoporphyrin on sarcoma 180. *Jpn J Cancer Res* 1990;81(3):304-8.

Zderic V, Vaezy S, Martin RW, Clark JI. Ocular drug delivery using 20-kHz ultrasound. *Ultrasound Med Biol* 2002;28(6):823-9.

Zderic V, Clark JI, Martin RW, Vaezy S. Ultrasound-enhanced transcorneal drug delivery. *Cornea* 2004;23(8):804-11.

Zderic V, Clark JI, Vaezy S. Drug delivery into the eye with the use of ultrasound. *J Ultrasound Med* 2004;23(10):1349-59.

Zderic V, Keshavarzi A, Noble ML, et al. Hemorrhage Control in Arteries Using High-Intensity Focused Ultrasound: A Survival Study. *Ultrasonics* 2006:44:46-53.

Zderic V, Brayman AA, Sharar SR, et al. Microbubble-Enhanced Hemorrhage Control Using High Intensity Focused Ultrasound. *Ultrasonics* 2006;40:113-20.

Zderic V, Vaezy S. Hemorrhage control using high intensity focused ultrasound. *Int J Hyperthermia* 2007;23(2):1-9.

Zeira E, Manevitch A, Khatchatouriants A, et al. Femtosecond infrared laser-an efficient and safe in vivo gene delivery system for prolonged expression. *Mol Ther*. 2003;8(2):342-50.

Zeng Y, Pitt WG. A polymeric micelle system with a hydrolysable segment for drug delivery. *J Biomater Sci Polym Ed* 2006;17(5):591-604.

Zhang G, Gao X, Song YK, et al. Hydroporation as the mechanism of hydrodynamic delivery. *Gene Ther* 2004;11(8):675-82.

Zhang S, Duncan JH, Chamine GL. The final stage of collapse of a cavitation bubble near a rigid wall. *J Fluid Mech*1993;257:147-81.

Zhou QH, Miller DL, Carlisle RC, et al. Ultrasound-enhanced transfection activity of HPMA-stabilized DNA polyplexes with prolonged plasma circulation. *J Control Release* 2005;106(3):416-27.

In: New Gene Therapy and Cancer Research
Editor: Wilma B. Gustafsson, pp. 113-143
ISBN: 978-1-60021-969-6

Chapter III

CANCER THERAPY BY ANGIOGENESIS INHIBITION: CURRENT STATUS AND FUTURE PROSPECTS

Elena Favaro[1], Alberto Amadori[1] and Stefano Indraccolo[2,*]
[1]Department of Oncology and Surgical Sciences, Oncology Section, University of Padova, Italy;
[2]Istituto Oncologico Veneto - IRCCS, Padova, Italy

ABSTRACT

Discovery of the pathways involved in the molecular regulation of angiogenesis has made it possible to test the hypothesis that blocking the angiogenic switch may keep tumor growth in check, and has added a new investigational arm to the field of cancer therapy. Angiogenesis inhibitors are heterogeneous in origin and potency; pre-clinical studies have clearly indicated that these factors are essentially cytostatic and need long-term administration in order to obtain prolonged anti-tumor effects. The experimental approaches attempted to date with endogenous factors, reviewed herein, indicate overall that delivery of anti-angiogenic factors or their cDNA by gene therapy approaches is mainly effective in the preventive setting. Meanwhile, anti-angiogenic drugs have entered the clinical arena, usually in combination with chemotherapy, to treat patients with advanced solid tumors with encouraging results in terms of survival. On the other hand, resistance to angiogenesis inhibitors has rapidly emerged and the current hypothesis formulated to explain this clinically relevant phenomenon will also be presented in this chapter. Decoding the biological mechanisms underlying resistance to angiogenesis inhibition, along with the identification of useful biomarkers of response and the design of appropriate combined treatments, will eventually allow for the achievement of durable control of advanced tumors.

* Correspondence concerning this article should be addressed to: Stefano Indraccolo, M.D., Istituto Oncologico Veneto - IRCCS, via Gattamelata, 64 - 35128 Padua – Italy. Phone ++39 049 8215875 ; fax ++39 049 8072854 ; e-mail : stefano.indraccolo@unipd.it.

INTRODUCTION

A prerequisite for tumour development, local invasion and metastatic dissemination, *angiogenesis*, the multistep process of new blood vessel formation, includes the activation, proliferation and migration of endothelial cells (EC), disruption of vascular basement membranes, remodelling of the extracellular matrix of tissues, formation of vascular tubes and networks, recruitment of supporting cells, including smooth muscle cells and pericytes, and connection to the pre-existing vascular network (Folkman, 1995).

Most physiological angiogenesis occurs in the embryo. In adults the endothelium is in a quiescent state with only 0.01% of the EC undergoing cell division (Hobson & Denekamp, 1984); normal angiogenesis occurs only during the ovarian cycle, pregnancy, physiologic repair processes such as wound healing and endometrial regrowth (Folkman, 1995), or in response to pathological insults, including inflammation and hypoxic related conditions i.e. to stroke and tumors (Chen, Zhang, Gasper, & Mixson, 2001). Angiogenesis also underlies other pathological conditions such as rheumatoid arthritis, macular degeneration, psoriasis, atherosclerosis, restenosis, and diabetic retinopathy (Folkman, 2007).

Table I. Endogenous stimulators and inhibitors of angiogenesis

Angiogenesis Stimulators	**Inhibitors**
Vascular endothelial growth factor (VEGF)	Angiostatin
Basic fibroblast growth factor (bFGF)	Endostatin
Hepatocyte growth factor (HGF)	Vasostatin
Platelet-derived endothelial cell growth factor (PDGF)	Canstatin
Transforming growth factor-β (TGF-β)	Tumstatin
Placenta growth factor (PIGF)	Soluble VEGF receptors
Interleukin-8	Matrix metalloproteinase inhibitors
Angiogenin	16-kDa prolactin fragment
Angiopoietin	Interferons (IFN-α, IFN-β, IFN-γ)
Leptin	Interleukins (IL-4, IL-12, IL-18)
Granulocyte colony-stimulating factor (G-CSF)	Arrestin
Folistatin	Platelet factor-4
Tumor necrosis factor-α (TNF-α)	Restin
Pleiotrophin	Maspin
	Pigment epithelium-derived factor (PEDF)

Under normal circumstances, angiogenesis is a highly ordered process under tight regulation by endogenous angiogenesis-inducing and angiogenesis-inhibiting factors (Table I). These factors include soluble growth factors, such as vascular endothelial growth factor (VEGF), angiopoietins (Ang), basic fibroblast growth factor (bFGF), platelet-derived growth factor (PDGF), transforming growth factor-β (TGF-β), metalloproteinases (MMPs), and other membrane-associated molecules, such as integrins and cadherins (Liu & Deisseroth, 2006). Some chemokines, such as interleukin-8 (IL-8), have a less established role in normal angiogenesis but are nevertheless important in tumor angiogenesis (Yuan et al., 2000). In addition to these molecules, mechanical forces mediated by blood flow on vascular endothelium contribute to the angiogenesis process: in fact, vessels that are not perfused generally undergo regression (Papetti & Herman, 2002).

In 1971 Judah Folkman was the first to suggest that tumor growth is dependent on new blood vessel formation. Meanwhile, it is widely recognized that angiogenesis is a critical process required by solid tumors to support their growth. In fact, approximately 95% of human carcinomas originate as *in situ* lesions in an avascular epithelial layer clearly separated from the vasculature: these microscopic tumors are able to grow only after vascularization of tissues surrounding the nodule (Folkman, 1971). Within a given microenvironment, the angiogenic response results from a balance between pro- and anti-angiogenic factors, secreted both by tumour cells and components of the stroma; the prevalence of the former determines the "*angiogenic switch*" (Hanahan & Folkman, 1996), resulting in the activation of angiogenesis followed by tumor outgrowth. Several mechanisms can contribute to the angiogenic switch (Figure 1). Initially, many tumors profit from cooption of the existing vasculature. However, tumor growth around blood vessels is generally followed by EC apoptosis and loosening of vessel integrity mediated by the up-regulation of Ang2. At that point, almost invariably, the tumor induces neovascular sprouts from neighbouring vessels (Holash, Wiegand, & Yancopoulos, 1999). This process is generally driven by various pro-angiogenic proteins (such as VEGF, bFGF, PDGF and Ang2), released by the tumor cells and acting on resident EC. In some circumstances, however, circulating haematopoietic precursors may contribute to the regulation of angiogenesis (Asahara et al., 1997). In fact, functional vascular endothelial growth factor receptors (VEGFR-1 and VEGFR-2) are expressed by both haematopoietic stem cells and endothelial progenitor cells. These rare cell subsets are mobilized by tumor-released cytokines/chemokines, such as VEGF or SDF-1α into the circulation and can be recruited into the vascular bed of certain tumor types (Lyden et al., 2001). Finally, many tumors establish a sort of cross-talk with the bone-marrow through the secretion of chemokines capable of attracting differentiated haematopoietic cells, including mast cells, monocytes, macrophages, and inflammatory cells (Coussens et al., 1999). These cells can then foster tumor angiogenesis by releasing proangiogenic molecules, or metallo-proteases that permit an enhanced EC' motility (Bergers et al., 2000; Scott, Holdsworth, Balkwill, & Dias, 2000) (Figure 1).

In general, most experimental attempts to interfere with the angiogenic switch have focused on reducing activation and recruitment of intratumoral EC, either by increasing the production of anti-angiogenic factors which affect the response of EC to pro-angiogenic molecules or by neutralizing biologically active pro-angiogenic factors. Some recent strategies, however, aim to contrast recruitment of circulating precursor cells or to exploit the selective activation of angiogenesis-inducible promoters to express therapeutic factors into the tumor microenvironment, as will be illustrated below.

This chapter aims at achieving two objectives. The first is to provide up-dated information on the results of tumor angiogenesis inhibition in pre-clinical models, with special emphasis on gene therapy-based strategies, and discuss some successful examples of pharmacologic inhibition of angiogenesis in the clinical setting. The second objective is to delineate some mechanisms of resistance to anti-angiogenic drugs, a clinically-relevant phenomenon, and to underline the importance of developing new surrogate markers of angiogenesis in order to monitor the outcome of therapy or the onset of resistance in a timely, non-invasive manner.

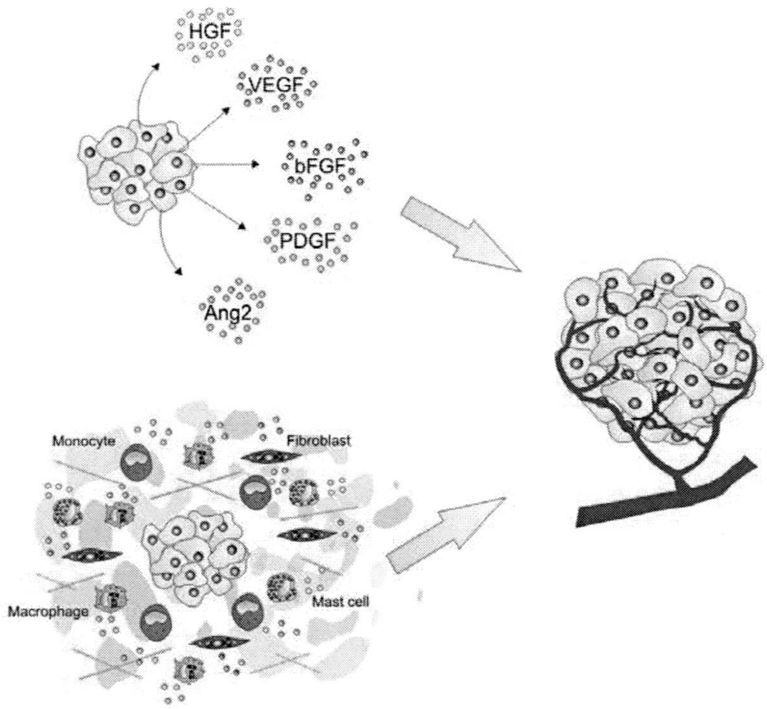

Figure 1. Cells that can contribute to the angiogenic switch. Angiogenic tumors generally induce neovascular sprouts from neighbouring vessels. This process is driven by various pro-angiogenic proteins (such as VEGF, bFGF, PDGF, HGF and Ang2), released by the tumor cells and acting on resident EC (top illustration). In some circumstances, however, tumor cells are themselves poorly angiogenic and the angiogenic switch is triggered by stromal cells including fibroblasts, monocyte/macrophages, mast cells and several types of hematopoietic progenitor cells (bottom illustration).

Anti-Angiogenesis Gene Therapy Approaches: Potential Advantages

Gene therapy based strategies of angiogenesis inhibition have attracted interest due to their potential advantages compared to conventional modalities of administration of anti-angiogenic drugs (Indraccolo, 2004). First of all, since effective suppression of pathological angiogenesis requires chronic treatment, gene delivery could be useful in prolonging expression of the therapeutic agents (Scappaticci, 2002). Moreover, gene therapy represents a method for circumventing the production problems of many recombinant proteins including their stability and solubility. Adequate production of anti-angiogenic factors by recombinant engineering methods has sometimes been problematic and may limit their clinical application; gene transfer usage, however, allows the correct folding of proteic agents and their stability *in vivo* since they are assembled in their physiologic environment (Sedlacek, 2001; Tanaka, Cao, Folkman, & Fine, 1998). A particularly attractive feature of gene transfer is the possibility of delivering genes to selective tissues, thus achieving localized gene expression and high regional drug concentrations without increasing the systemic levels of the therapeutic agents. Although this approach is valuable only for treatment of relatively localized tumors, such as SNC tumors and ovarian cancer, the confinement of the anti-angiogenic effects may avoid undesirable suppression of essential physiologic functions (Kong & Crystal, 1998) and thus reduce side effects.

Delivery of Angiogenesis Inhibitors by Gene Therapy

Extensive research has led to the identification of several negative regulators of angiogenesis (Table I), which may act either directly to inhibit cellular functions required for the angiogenic process, including EC proliferation or migration, or, alternatively, behave as indirect inhibitors through suppression of the production of angiogenic factors by tumor cells (Indraccolo, 2004).

Naturally-occurring inhibitors of angiogenesis have been known for quite a while (Zetter, 1998), their prototypes being angiostatin (O'Reilly et al., 1994) and endostatin (O'Reilly et al., 1997) which are proteolytic fragments of plasminogen and collagen type XVIII, respectively, exerting pivotal regulatory activities in tumor angiogenesis. In general, these proteins are good candidates for gene delivery, since they are produced physiologically, probably being not immunogenic, and are effective extracellularly. A second interesting group of endogenous inhibitors of angiogenesis is represented by certain cytokines and chemokines which, in addition to their effects on cells of the immune system, regulate some critical EC functions. We will comment in detail only the results obtained with representative inhibitors of the proteolytic group, including angiostatin and endostatin, and of the cytokine/chemokine group. For detailed information on other factors refer to recent reviews covering angiogenesis inhibitors (Folkman, 2006; Indraccolo, 2004; Scappaticci, 2002).

Angiostatin

Angiostatin, a 38 kDa kringle-containing internal fragment of plasminogen, belongs to a class of "cryptic" endogenous angiogenesis inhibitors which are not active until released from their parental protein by enzymatic cleavage. It is one of the most potent inhibitors of angiogenesis, and a selective inhibitor of EC proliferation and migration *in vitro*; furthermore, angiostatin has been shown to suppress tumour growth and metastases in tumour models (O'Reilly, Holmgren, Chen, & Folkman, 1996; O'Reilly et al., 1994). Angiostatin inhibits EC migration and proliferation most likely through its ability to bind a cell surface ATP synthase, which may act as a receptor (Moser et al., 1999). Moreover, by inhibiting extracellular matrix (ECM)-stimulated plasminogen activation, it determines a decrease in endothelial cell invasion (Stack, Gately, Bafetti, Enghild, & Soff, 1999). Other studies have revealed that angiostatin may induce apoptosis in EC, albeit at relatively high concentrations (Claesson-Welsh et al., 1998; Lucas et al., 1998).

Several approaches have been developed to translate the basic science behind angiostatin into therapeutic efficacy. Initial efforts aimed at the generation of recombinant angiostatin using the Pichia pastoris expression system (Sim et al., 1997), but concerns regarding the biological activity of the recombinant protein were soon raised. Moreover, production of large amounts of active angiostatin turned out to be expensive and technical problems were frequently encountered.

An attractive alternative has been represented by gene delivery. Expression of angiostatin has been obtained in tumor models both by transfecting angiostatin-expression plasmids (Fukumori et al., 2002; Matsumoto, Ohmi, & Shindo, 2001; Uesato et al., 2004), or by recombinant adenoviral (Griscelli et al., 1998; Schmitz et al., 2004; Soff, 2000; Tanaka et al., 1998; Xu et al., 2003), retroviral (Scappaticci et al., 2001) and adeno-associated viral vectors (Ma et al., 2002) that carry the angiostatin open-reading-frame. All these studies report significant inhibition of tumor growth and microvessel density in various tumor models, as discussed in detail elsewhere (Dell'Eva, Pfeffer, Indraccolo, Albini, & Noonan, 2002). However, in some other cases no delay in tumor growth was measured, even if angiostatin was found to be expressed at high levels in the circulation or in the tumor (Indraccolo, Gola et al., 2002; Joseph et al., 2003). These data may underscore that angiostatin could show efficacy as monotherapy only on certain tumor types, although factors which could predict therapeutic response remain unknown.

Endostatin

Endostatin is an endogenous angiogenesis inhibitor identified as a 20 kDa C-terminal fragment of collagen XVIII, and isolated from conditioned media of cultured hemangioendothelioma cells; for endostatin a functional receptor on vascular endothelium is integrin $\alpha_5\beta_1$ (Sudhakar et al., 2003). Endostatin seems to inhibit EC functions by several means, including its binding to $\alpha_5\beta_1$ integrins (O'Reilly et al., 1997), attenuation of VEGF receptor signalling (Kim et al., 2002) and inhibition of cyclin D1 (Hanai et al., 2002). Endostatin is picked-up from plasma and stored in platelets, and it can be released at the tumor site or by adding COX-2 inhibitors (Folkman, 2003). Presently, phase I clinical trials of endostatin as a fusion protein infusion for various cancers are underway. A comprehensive description of the results of endostatin therapy was recently published by Folkman (Folkman, 2006).

In pre-clinical tumor models, endostatin has generally been capable of preventing tumor growth and occasionally to regress established masses, with some exceptions. In example, one study (Jin et al., 2001) reported delivery of endostatin by adenovirus vectors in 2 tumor models: the syngenic MidT2-1 mammary tumor model in FVB mice and the MDA-MB-231 human breast tumor model in SCID mice. In the first case, a block in tumor growth by suppression of tumor angiogenesis *in vivo* was obtained. The second type of tumor, however, was not influenced by endostatin gene therapy, hypothetically due to the different sensitivity of blood vessels to endostatin itself or other unknown reasons.

Our group investigated the efficacy of endostatin gene therapy in the treatment of breast cancer using retroviral vectors (Indraccolo, Gola et al., 2002). Again, heterogeneous therapeutic effects were noticed; a possible explanation for these findings was that endostatin levels achieved were not enough to starve rapidly growing tumors. In fact, it has been shown that more rapidly growing tumors can require higher doses of anti-angiogenic therapy than slowly growing tumors (Beecken et al., 2001), that hints at optimization of anti-angiogenic therapy as a very important issue to be worked out before definitive conclusions about efficacy can be drawn.

A second series of studies analyzed the combined effect of angiostatin and endostatin and found a strong synergism in terms of both anti-proliferative effects on EC *in vitro* and anti-tumor effects in ovarian cancer models (Isayeva, Ren, & Ponnazhagan, 2005; Ponnazhagan et al., 2004). Raikwar and colleagues (Raikwar et al., 2005) developed an adenoviral vector Ad-hEndo-angio, expressing a unique chimeric human endostatin-angiostatin fusion protein and studied its therapeutic potential following intra-tumoral injection. Treatment resulted in enhanced inhibition and complete regression of both the treated and untreated tumors on the other flank of the mice in a vast majority of animals. Although these studies suggest that long-term expression of both inhibitors may be effective as a preventive approach against recurrent and metastasis cancer, regression of established tumors even by the combined treatment remains elusive.

Anti-Angiogenic Cytokines

Although the most popular explanation of the anti-tumor activity of cytokine gene transfer in pre-clinical models has been induction of systemic immunity, it rather quickly emerged that the mechanisms involved may be more complex. In fact, it was realized that certain cytokines, including IFNs, IL-4, IL-12 and TNF-α, are endowed with dramatic anti-angiogenic or vasculotoxic effects. Initial evidence for vascular effects of type I IFNs - the prototype of anti-angiogenic cytokines - stems from observations in immunocompetent DBA/2 mice bearing IFN-resistant erythroleukemia, or ESb lymphoma cells. Results indicated that IFN-α/β exerted an anti-tumor effect by damaging tumor blood vessels, causing disruption of tumor blood flow, which led to ischemic tumor necrosis (Dvorak & Gresser, 1989). In the same years it was suggested that IFNs may modulate the signal for angiogenesis produced by the tumor cells (Sidky & Borden, 1987). Later on, experiments of IFN-α gene transfer by various delivery systems in immunodeficient mice confirmed and extended these findings (Hottiger, Dam, Nickoloff, Johnson, & Nabel, 1999; Indraccolo et al., 2006; Indraccolo et al., 2005; Iqbal Ahmed et al., 2001). *In vivo,* anti-tumor activity has been consistently associated to induction of areas of ischemic necrosis as well as to a marked reduction in the microvessel density (De Bouard et al., 2003; Indraccolo, Gola et al., 2002; Indraccolo et al., 1999; Indraccolo et al., 2006; Indraccolo et al., 2005; Rozera et al., 1999). The anti-angiogenic activity of class I IFN has been attributed to inhibition of basic fibroblast growth factor (bFGF) overproduction by tumor cells (Singh et al., 1995) or down-regulation of IL-8 and VEGF gene expression (Oliveira, Sciavolino, Lee, & Vilcek, 1992; von Marschall et al., 2003). Moreover, IFN-α has direct transcriptional and functional effects on endothelial cells (Albini et al., 2000; Indraccolo et al., 2007). Anti-vascular effects of IFNα, and especially IFN-γ, may partially depend upon induction of angiostatic chemokines, including CXCL9, CXCL10 and CXCL11 (Angiolillo et al., 1995; Sgadari, Angiolillo, Cherney et al., 1996).

A second cytokine whose effects are recurrently associated with angiogenesis inhibition is IL-12, which was initially reported to inhibit new vessel formation induced by the pro-angiogenic factor bFGF in a mouse corneal vascularization assay (Kerbel & Hawley, 1995), and in Matrigel plug assays in nude mice (Sgadari, Angiolillo, & Tosato, 1996). It has been shown that IFN-γ and, at least in part, CXCL10, appear to play a critical role as mediators of its anti-angiogenic effects (Sgadari, Angiolillo, & Tosato, 1996; Voest et al., 1995). NK cells may contribute to inhibition of angiogenesis by IL-12 not only through the secretion of anti-angiogenic chemokines but apparently also through NK cell-mediated cytotoxicity against endothelial cells (Yao et al., 1999). More recently, however, angiogenesis inhibition was observed in NK cell-depleted mice as well as in IFN-γ(-/-) and CXCR3(-/-) knockout mice, indicating that NK- and/or T cell-initiated IFN-γ-chemokine cascades were not involved in the angiogenesis inhibition observed *in vivo* (Morini et al., 2004). Whatever the mechanism behind, results from all these studies agree on the identification of endothelial cells as a major target of the biological effects of IL-12.

Which Vector for Optimal Treatment?

Most of the currently available viral vectors, including adenoviral, adeno-associated, retroviral, lentiviral, and herpes simplex viral vectors, have been exploited for tumour angiogenesis targeting approaches (Liu & Deisseroth, 2006). All these vector types can be routinely manufactured and purified to high titres, remaining stable and storable for long time periods.

Adenoviral vectors (Ad) are characterized by high gene transfer efficiency and high levels of transgene expression; furthermore, they can infect both dividing and non-dividing cells. However, some drawbacks include the transient expression of the transgene, the existence or rapid induction of neutralizing antibody in humans and the inflammatory and immune response elicited by the vector itself (Liu & Deisseroth, 2006). Ad have often been exploited to deliver single anti-angiogenic factors (examples include angiostatin, endostatin, sFLT-1, Flk-Fc fusion proteins) sometimes with inclusion of EC-specific promoters to limit transgene expression (Brandwijk, Griffioen, & Thijssen, 2007).

Adeno-associated viral vectors (AAV) have also been considered for anti-angiogenic gene therapy approaches. These viral vectors are single-strand DNA, replication-defective viruses. In the absence of a helper virus like the adenovirus, the wild-type AAV genome tends to integrate into the host-cell chromosomal DNA to maintain a latent state. In the presence of the helper virus, however, the AAV genome replicates episomally. Similarly to Ad, AAV can infect both dividing and non dividing cells; however, they generate low-level humoral immune responses. Production of large amounts of clinical grade AAV has remained cumbersome, thus limiting their use in patients.

Retroviral (RV) and lentiviral vectors (LV) have also been used to deliver genes involved in the control of angiogenesis; their distinctive feature is permanent integration of the therapeutic gene into target cells (De Bouard et al., 2003; Hase et al., 2005; Indraccolo, Habeler et al., 2002; Indraccolo et al., 2001; Indraccolo et al., 2006; Indraccolo et al., 2005;

Pfeifer, Kessler, Silletti, Cheresh, & Verma, 2000). RV and LV can be pseudotyped with a variety of envelopes achieving a broad trophism (Shichinohe et al., 2001).

Although DNA vectors, particularly Ad, can have unbeatable efficiency of gene delivery, the requirement of long-term production of anti-angiogenic factors in order to achieve durable control of tumor angiogenesis is better matched by integrating vectors (RV and LV). Which role could be envisioned for these vectors in anti-angiogenic therapy? In our opinion, RV and LV represent excellent tools for ex vivo transduction of hematopoietic cells, which could then be re-infused to tumor-bearing mice and home to tumor deposits. Moreover, LV have improved performance in terms of gene delivery in vivo compared to RV (Indraccolo, Habeler et al., 2002), and they could also be used for transduction of specific cell types following systemic administration, including i.e. hepatocytes or mesothelial cells, in order to convert them into cell factories of the anti-angiogenic protein.

For further information on the features of viral vectors exploited for angiostatic cancer treatment the reader is referred to specialized reviews (Liu & Deisseroth, 2006).

From Understanding the Mechanism of Anti-Tumor Effect to the Design of new Delivery Approaches

In pre-clinical models angiogenesis inhibition has been capable of delaying progression of primary tumors. The key question is, however, how to target micrometastatic foci dispersed into different organs. Engineering selected bone marrow (BM)-derived cells could be, in our opinion, an appropriate answer.

Histologic analysis of tumor sections commonly highlights the presence of a mixed hematopoietic infiltrate into tumors, formed by diverse types of host leukocytes including macrophages, DC, neutrophils, mast cells, and T cells (Balkwill, Charles, & Mantovani, 2005; Coussens & Werb, 2002; Nakayama, Yao, & Tosato, 2004). Upon activation, these tumor-associated leukocytes, especially macrophages, release angiogenic factors, mitogens, proteolytic enzymes, and chemotactic factors, recruiting further inflammatory cells and sustaining tumor growth, invasion and angiogenesis (Yan, Anderson, DeWitte, & Nakada, 2006). In addition, novel subsets of BM-derived cells have recently been identified in tumor-bearing mice (Rehman, Li, Orschell, & March, 2003) and subsequently in patients (Dome et al., 2006; Goon, Lip, Boos, Stonelake, & Blann, 2006) which could contribute to tumor angiogenesis. These include circulating endothelial cells (CEC), endothelial progenitor cells (EPC) and special subsets of monocytes, the so called Tie2-expressing monocytes (TEM) and CD11b+Gr1+ myeloid cells (Okamoto et al., 2005). Although a debate about the origin, the degree of identity and the role of these different cell subsets is currently ongoing (Bertolini, Shaked, Mancuso, & Kerbel, 2006), BM-derived cells recruited to tumors and other sites of angiogenesis, rather than providing a source of building blocks for "postnatal vasculogenesis," seem to promote angiogenesis by secreting or mobilizing growth factors or by physically cooperating with endothelial cells in making new blood vessels, for instance, by drilling "tunnels" in the extracellular matrix and supporting the migration of vascular cells.

Mature hematopoietic cells likely represent the most abundant cells in the body endowed with the ability to migrate into tissues, even in hypoxic conditions, and with the capacity of modifying the extracellular matrix and amplify paracrine signals. Based on these facts, arming selective BM-derived cells with therapeutic genes under the control of cell type-specific promoters (such as Tie2) or hypoxia responsive elements (HRE) could represent a smart way to target disseminated cancer nests. In this regard, pioneer experiments have demonstrated that knockout of TEM genetically tagged by a lentiviral vector encoding the HSV-1 thymidine kinase (TK) gene through ganciclovir administration completely prevented human glioma neovascularization in the mouse brain and induced substantial tumor regression (De Palma et al., 2005). As TEM seem to trigger the early phases of tumor vascularization in murine models (De Palma et al., 2005), they could be used to deliver selected genes (i.e. IFN genes) to micrometastases undergoing the angiogenic switch, thus providing systemic anti-tumor effects. It remains to be seen whether sustained TEM recruitment occurs in established metastasis, which could form the basis for tempting delivery of engineered TEMs also to patients with advanced disease. Finally, since integrating vectors seem to be appropriate for stable manipulation of BM-derived cells, safety concerns need to be addressed and it will be important to carefully consider the risk of insertional mutagenesis in haematopoietic stem cells associated with this approach.

Angiogenesis Inhibitors in Clinical Trials

Although drugs targeting tumor angiogenesis at multiple levels have showed promising anti-tumor activity in mouse models, based on the importance of VEGF in tumor angiogenesis and the amount of data indicating that cancer growth could be inhibited by neutralizing VEGF, a number of agents targeting this pathway are currently in advanced clinical development. We will briefly review clinical results obtained with some of these drugs, including Bevacizumab (Avastin), BAY 43-9006 (Sorafenib), and SU11248 (Sunitinib). Comprehensive information on other ongoing clinical trials with angiogenesis inhibitors is reported in Table II.

Bevacizumab (Avastin)

Bevacizumab, a recombinant humanized monoclonal antibody binding to VEGF-A and its isoforms, was the first anti-angiogenic agent to receive approval by the U.S. FDA in 2004. Its current indication, supported by two pivotal clinical studies involving hundreds of patients (Hurwitz et al., 2004; Kabbinavar et al., 2003), is for use with 5-fluorouracil(5-FU)-irinotecan based chemotherapy (IFL) as first-line treatment in patients with metastatic colorectal cancer. Several clinical parameters including the time to progression (TTP) and the overall response (OR) where significantly better in the bevacizumab groups. Importantly, median survival was 15.6 months with IFL but 20.3 months in the IFL plus bevacizumab group ($p<0.001$). Since bevacizumab approval, further studies continue to demonstrate a clinical benefit in patients with colorectal cancer treated with other chemotherapy combinations, such as 5-FU/LV (Hurwitz et al., 2005) or FOLFOX4 (Giantonio et al., 2007). Not all tumors seem to respond to bevacizumab, however; i.e. bevacizumab did not show activity in metastatic breast cancer in combination with capecitabine, as well as in metastatic clear cell renal carcinoma, a type of cancer which was thought to be a potentially promising target since most cases have increased VEGF expression due to accumulation of the HIF-1α protein (Yang et al., 2003). These results clearly indicate that much has still to be done to identify subsets of patients who would be more likely to benefit from the therapy.

Table II: Anti-angiogenic agents under clinical development

Drug	**Active trials (n)**	**Phase (n)**						
	Drugs that block activators of angiogenesis							
		I	**I-II**	**II**	**II-III**	**III**	**IV**	**n.s.**
Anti-VEGF Antibody (Bevacizumab; Avastin™)	**223**	14						
Bay 43-9006 (Sorafenib tosylate)	**63**	19	20	159	2	20	5	3
SU011248 (Sunitinib malate)	**54**	8	9	32		3		
RAD001 (Everolimus)	**28**	7	4	34		7		1
AZD2171	**23**	4	9	9	1	2		
PTK787/ZK 222584 (Vatalanib)	**15**	3		16	2	1		
GW786034 (Pazopanib)	**14**	7	5	7				
ZD6474	**13**	2		5		2		
AMG-706	**8**	4	1	6		4		
AG-013736	**3**		2	2				
BMS-582664	**3**	2		3				
PI-88	**2**			1				
Suramin	**2**	1		2				
ADH-1 (Exherin™)	**1**	1	1					
CHIR-265	**1**	1						
XL184	**1**	1						
	Drugs that inhibit endothelial cells directly							
Thalidomide	**74**	3	5	44	2	17		3
Lenalidomide	**38**	7	3	18	1	7	1	1
Tamoxifen Citrate	**28**	1		11		14	1	1
LY317615 (Enzastaurin)	**16**	2	1	11		2		
Soy Isoflavone	**6**			6				
ABT-510	**2**	1	1					
Combretastatin A4 Phosphate	**2**	1		1				
NGR-TNF	**1**	1						
Dimethylxanthenone Acetic Acide	**1**			1				
TOTAL	622	90	61	368	8	79	7	9

n.s.; not specified

Additional phase II and III studies are currently being conducted with bevacizumab in breast, ovarial, pancreatic, head and neck, lung cancer, and hematologic malignancies, whose results will further define the role of this antibody in clinical oncology (Zakarija & Soff, 2005).

The wide use of bevacizumab in patients also allowed for more careful evaluation of its toxic effects, which comprise hypertension, proteinuria, but also major hemorrhage, venous thrombosis and gastrointestinal perforations. While some of these complications could have been predicted, others were rather unexpected. In particular, it is currently unknown whether the life-threatening gastro-intestinal perforations observed are related to tumor involvement of the intestinal wall -as sometimes has been documented- or, rather, consequences of blocking physiological activities of VEGF in the gut. In seminal studies, VEGF neutralization or inactivation of the *VEGF* gene have shown dramatic consequences during foetal development or in newborns (Carmeliet et al., 1996; Ferrara et al., 1996); on the other hand, no major toxicities were reported in adult animals (Gerber et al., 1999). It should be stressed, however, that while the short-term side effects of angiogenesis inhibition are pretty well known, the consequences of long-term blockage of the VEGF pathway have still to be fully realized. Given the fact that endothelial cells could be involved in the control of tissue mass, as it has been demonstrated for the liver, the prostate, the bone, and fat tissue (reviewed in: (Folkman, 2007)), it is tempting to speculate that protracted inactivation of key angiogenic factors could lead to EC apoptosis followed by destabilization and increased fragility of some tissues.

BAY 43-9006 (Sorafenib)

Sorafenib is a multitargeted small molecule which acts as inhibitor of multiple kinases, including Raf, VEGFR-2 and VEGFR-3, PDGFR-β, FLT-3, and c-kit (Wilhelm et al., 2004). Due to its dual action, it is capable of inhibiting both tumor angiogenesis and Raf-kinase-dependent tumor cell proliferation. Sorafenib is orally available and relatively well tolerated, the most common side effects being diarrhea, hand-foot syndrome, fatigue, and pancreatitis. This drug has recently received approval for advanced renal cell carcinoma, and phase I and II clinical studies are ongoing in other malignancies including head and neck, lung, pancreatic and prostate cancer.

Sunitinib (Sutent)

Conceptually similar to Sorafenib, Sunitinib is also a small molecule inhibitor of the VEGFR-1, VEGFR-2, PDGFR, c-kit, and FLT3 tyrosine kinases, which recently obtained FDA approval as second-line treatment of gastrointestinal stromal tumors and as a first-line treatment for advanced renal cell carcinoma (Chow & Eckhardt, 2007). Preliminary results from an ongoing phase II clinical studies seem to indicate efficacy of sunitinib in women with anthracycline-resistant and taxane-resistant metastatic breast cancer as well (Chow & Eckhardt, 2007). The therapy is generally well-tolerated, although many patients experienced non-VEGF inhibition-related toxicities, such as neutropenia, diarrhea, nausea, and fatigue. Sunitinib is a successful example of a drug which has both anti-angiogenic and anti-tumor activity. Further examples of drugs originally developed to target a specific oncogenic pathway and later discovered to inhibit production of angiogenic factors include the inhibitors of epidermal growth factor receptor tyrosine kinase erlonitib (Tarceva, Genentech) and cetuximab (Eribitux, Merck) (Kerbel, Viloria-Petit, Klement, & Rak, 2000; Morelli et al., 2006).

Although the clinical efficacy of the above reported angiogenesis-targeting drugs is now recognized, the mechanisms behind the therapeutic effect are controversial. In essence, it has still to be firmly established whether angiogenesis inhibition critically contributes to the overall anti-tumor effect or, alternatively, whether neutralization of VEGF-dependent abnormal vessel permeability with consequent reduction of interstitial pressure and improved delivery of chemotherapeutic drugs is the most important consequence of bevacizumab administration to patients (Kerbel, 2006). It could also be that mechanisms differ depending on the time-point of analysis. Specifically, the vessel normalization effect could be an acute effect and thus take place essentially during the first days after bevacizumab administration. In contrast, long-term VEGF-blockage could compromise the generation of new blood vessels, reduce oxygen and nutrient delivery and thus increase intra-tumor hypoxia. Interestingly, addition of anti-VEGF to standard chemotherapy has partially changed the type of responses detected, with an increase in tumor necrosis and cavitation detected by CT scans (Ferrara & Kerbel, 2005), which occur rather rarely in patients responding to chemotherapy alone and are suggestive of hypoxia-induced tumor cell-death. Even less is known about the modalities of action of so-called second generation anti-angiogenic drugs such as Sunitinib and Sorafenib (Marx, 2005), although periodic imaging of the tumor's blood flow did suggest that at least part of their effects where due to their ability to block angiogenesis (Marx, 2005).

Resistance to Angiogenic Therapy

The original hypothesis formulated by Kerbel in 1991 assumed that targeting tumor vasculature represented a form of therapy " resistant to resistance ". This prediction was based on the intrinsic characteristic of the target, i.e. the endotelial cell, a genetically stable normal diploid cell with a low mutational rate that should have been far less prone to developing mechanisms of resistance than tumor cell (Kerbel, 1991). The possibility to circumvent acquired resistance, a phenomenon commonly encountered with standard anti-cancer agents, generated a body of research and great expectations. Kerbel's hypothesis was soon verified successfully by Brem et al. and Boehm et al., who reported that chronic, intermittent administration of AGM-1470 in one case and endostatin in the other one to mice bearing different kinds of solid tumors did not lead to any traces of acquired resistance resulting in complete regression of the tumors (Boehm, Folkman, Browder, & O'Reilly, 1997; Brem H, 1994; Kerbel, 1997). Encouraging results emerged also by numerous studies that examined the pharmacologic efficacy of bevacizumab and/or A4.6.1, the humanized monoclonal antibody anti-VEGF and its murine equivalent respectively, in various tumors grown in nude mice: anti-VEGF treatment resulted in 25% to 95% tumor growth inhibition compared to controls and in several cases, primary tumor growth inhibition was seen with early- and late-treatment onset (Gerber & Ferrara, 2005).

First results from clinical trials with VEGF neutralizing drugs, however, curtailed this initial enthusiasm. In fact, despite the positive outcome in terms of overall survival, progression-free survival and response rate, cure remained elusive and tumor progression eventually occurred (H. Hurwitz et al., 2004; F. F. Kabbinavar et al., 2005). This and other observations indicated that unexpected mechanisms of resistance could intrinsically exist or eventually develop in patients (Herbst et al., 2005; Miller et al., 2005; Yang et al., 2003).

Moreover, existence of resistance has also been noticed in mouse models, although it initially received less attention, especially when the anti-angiogenic drugs were chronically administered. In one seminal study, VEGF blockage had different outcomes depending on the tumor utilized; in particular, highly vascularized rhabdomyosarcoma xenografts, which produced more VEGF, underwent impressive decrease in the mean vasculature density and their growth was dramatically suppressed, whereas leiomyosarcoma and glioblastoma were much less inhibited, suggesting that they were less dependent on VEGF and their vascularization was possibly supported by alternative factors such as bFGF and aFGF (Kim et al., 1993). Different efficacy of VEGF blockage in diverse tumors was also reported by Rowe et al. who measured nearly complete inhibition of primary tumor growth and lung metastasis in a Wilms tumor model as opposed to neuroblastoma where only a modest growth inhibition and persistence of metastasis were seen, despite similar expression of VEGF (Rowe, Huang, Kayton et al., 2000; Rowe, Huang, Li et al., 2000). Furthermore, chronic treatment of a human neuroblastoma xenografts with the anti-FLK-1 antibody DC101, eventually led to escape from the initial state of dormancy induced by effective angiogenesis inhibition (Klement et al., 2000). Another group reported that treatment with anti-VEGF antibody on late-stage tumors induced a less complete growth inhibition then on early-stage tumors, possibly due to a compensatory production of VEGF by the stroma of the host (Gerber, Kowalski, Sherman, Eberhard, & Ferrara, 2000). In our laboratory, we made similar observations with IFN-α in experimental models of ovarian cancer: efficacy was variable and depended on the particular tumor cell line used as well as on the kinetics of IFN-α administration, being usually more effective as an early treatment option than on established tumors (Indraccolo et al., 2005). 2005 HGT).

The first report that demonstrated acquired tumor resistance to an anti-angiogenic agent was published by Filleur in 2001, and it showed that chronic treatment with TSP1 had only transient inhibitory effects on two different tumor models, a fibrosarcoma and a glioblastoma, that grew progressively due to counterbalancing of TSP1 anti-angiogenic effects through increased secretion of angiogenic factors (Filleur et al., 2001). Hypothetically, the intrinsic heterogenicity of the tumor cell population favoured the emergence of resistant cells, through clonal selection of highly angiogenic clones. This study also uncovered the possibility that the schedule of anti-angiogenic drug delivery, i.e. continuous (Filleur et al., 2001) versus intermittent (Boehm et al., 1997; Brem H, 1994), could determine the onset of resistance. In fact, chronic anti-angiogenic therapy could exert a continuous selective pressure which may favour the emergence of resistance, as compared to intermittent administration of the same drugs.

The principal mechanisms of resistance to angiogenic therapy recognized thus far can be grouped into tumor-cell-related, endothelial cells (EC)-related and stromal-cell-related mechanisms. They are illustrated in Figure 2 and will be commented below.

Tumor-Cell-Related Mechanisms

There are at least 3 mechanisms by which tumor cells can contribute to resistance.

The first one, which is often referred to as "redundancy", is a consequence of the well-known plethora of pro-angiogenic growth factors secreted by tumor cells and consists of the augmented expression of the same or other angiogenic factors in response to anti-angiogenic treatment by tumor cell clones that survive a selection process. Angiogenic redundancy appears to be substantially greater in advanced disease than in early stage tumors (Relf et al., 1997). Hence, even if an angiogenic factor is neutralized, new vessel formation can be sustained by alternative pathways leading to rapid tumor relapse. Two seminal studies about this mechanism deserve further comment. In the first one, Casanovas et al. described a mouse model of pancreatic islet cell cancer wherein VEGFR2 inhibition produced a period of stable disease followed by progression. The supposed hypoxic environment induced by the anti-angiogenic treatment triggered the up-regulation of other pro-angiogenic factors including the FGFs, Ephrin-A1 and Ang1, thus making the VEGF/VEGFR2 pathway dispensable. Treatment of the VEGF-independent tumors by a different anti-angiogenic therapy targeting the FGF receptors, however, brought about tumor regression associated to decreased vessel density (Casanovas, Hicklin, Bergers, & Hanahan, 2005).

In the study by Mizukami et al., partial blockage of VEGF secretion by HIF-1α knock-down reduced tumor volumes and weights but the angiogenic response was preserved by NF-kB-dependent induction of interleukin-8 (Mizukami et al., 2005). Collectively, these two reports imply that targeting multiple pro-angiogenic pathways with distinct complementary mechanisms of action, may improve efficacy – at least if toxicity is not a concern. This could be achieved through introduction of inhibitors of the circumventing pro-angiogenic factors at the time of progression or, alternatively, through the use of cocktails of specific inhibitors or multi-targeted inhibitors such as the anti-angiogenic receptor tyrosine kinase inhibitors (RTKIs), seeking to prevent the angiogenic switch.

Another important concept to consider is that tumors might be "intrinsically" resistant to some anti-angiogenic drugs; in fact each tumor could rely on a particular set of angiogenic factors to sustain angiogenesis, different from other tumors and, moreover, this could vary with the stage of progression, thus making treatment most effective when it is targeted to a specific stage of disease (Bergers, Javaherian, Lo, Folkman, & Hanahan, 1999). In this respect, Giavazzi and colleagues demonstrated in a model of human endometrial adenocarcinoma that FGF2 drives angiogenesis mainly at early time points of tumorigenesis, whereas established tumors become partially independent of FGF2 expression (Giavazzi et al., 2001). These results nicely complement a work by Yoshiji et al. who studied the effects of VEGF suppression on the growth of early- and late-stage xenografts of human breast carcinoma, reporting a drastically slowed growth rate in the former but no inhibition in the latter (Yoshiji, Harris, & Thorgeirsson, 1997).

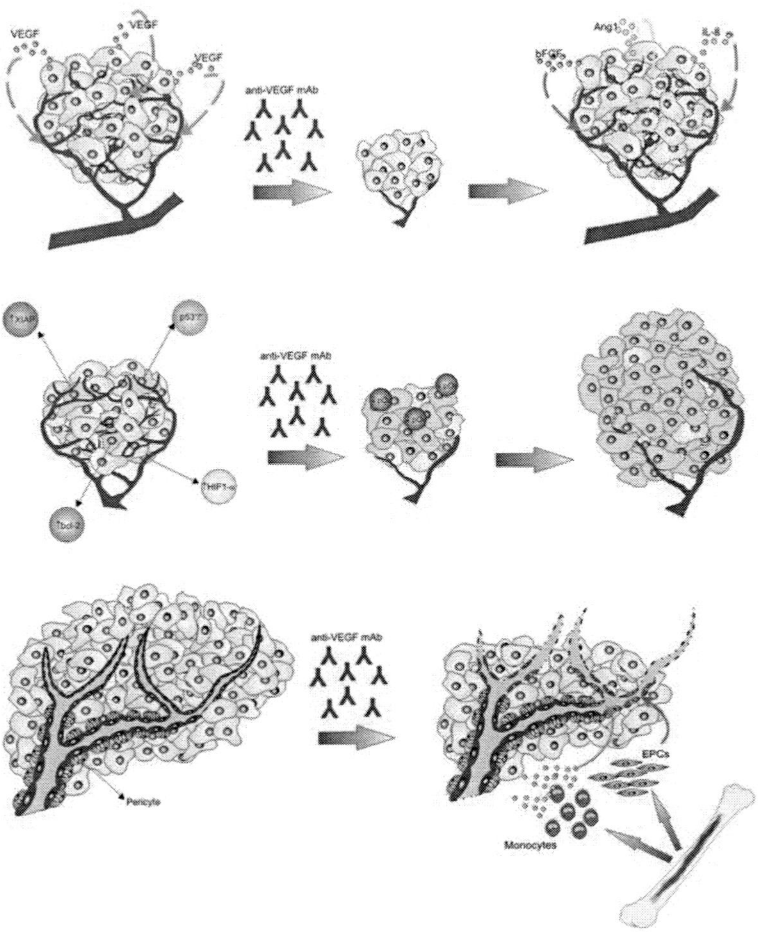

Figure 2. Principal mechanisms of resistance to anti-angiogenic therapy. Both tumor-cell-related and stromal-cell-related mechanisms have been recognized so far. Tumor cells can contribute to resistance by various means: (I) augmented expression of the same or other angiogenic factors by tumor cell clones that survive a selection process (top illustration); (II) selection of tumor cells carrying specific genetic alterations, such as lack of p53, or over-expressig bcl-2, XIAP or HIF-1α, which confer resistance to hypoxia (mid illustration). Another possible explanation of resistance to anti-angiogenic drugs can be ascribed to qualitative modifications in the angiogenic vasculature such as vascular remodelling, defined by progressive replacement of immature with pericyte-covered vessels can diminish efficacy of VEGF-neutralizing drugs. Finally hematopoietic cells (monocytes, EPCs) can bypass VEGF neutralization by release of other angiogenic factors or through their incorporation in the vessel wall (bottom illustration).

There are extensive results demonstrating that tumor cells are heterogeneous in their dependence on adjacent vessels for survival; intuitively, these cells can survive and become selected in hypoxic areas within the tumor mass. Hence, successful anti-angiogenic therapy may further force the selection process by increasing the levels of intra-tumoral hypoxia (Franco et al., 2006), resulting in tumors that gradually become less or completely unresponsive to the therapy. For instance, inactivation of wild-type p53 tumor suppressor gene can render cells less susceptible to apoptosis induced by hypoxic stress in vitro and $p53^{-}/^{-}$ cells-derived tumors are less responsive to treatment with DC101 plus chemotherapy than isogenic p53^{+}/$^{+}$ tumors (Yu, Coomber, & Kerbel, 2002). Moreover, the analysis of tumors derived from 1:1 mixtures of p53^{+}/$^{+}$ and p53^{-}/$^{-}$ cells and treated with the same combination of drugs as above, revealed a dramatic decrease in the proportion of p53 wild type cells that were mainly distributed close to the perfused vasculature (Yu, Rak, Coomber, Hicklin, & Kerbel, 2002). These observations are consistent with the selective advantage of cells lacking p53 due to decreased sensitivity to hypoxia-induced apoptosis. It is likely that p53 alterations represent only one example of the types of genetic lesions that could affect the vascular dependence or hypoxia-sensitivity of tumor cells. In this respect, given its central importance in inducing both pro- or anti-survival signals (Bacon & Harris, 2004), changes in the hypoxia-inducible factor-1α (HIF-1α) pathway could also result in altered cellular responses to hypoxia and survival capacity of tumor cells under stressful conditions (Yu et al., 2001). VEGF may confer resistance by up-regulating anti-apoptotic genes such as bcl-2, A1, XIAP, and survivin in EC (Gerber, Dixit, & Ferrara, 1998; Nor, Christensen, Mooney, & Polverini, 1999; O'Connor et al., 2000; Tran et al., 1999); thus, high local concentrations of VEGF near new blood vessels could antagonize the effects of various drugs, especially those inducing apoptosis of EC. Therefore, one possible approach for the improvement of anti-angiogenic agents could be the combination with inhibitors of oncogene-mediated signals of survival to hypoxic stress or with hypoxic cell cytotoxins.

Endothelial-Cell-Related Mechanisms

One of the possible explanations of heterogeneous responses of tumors to anti-angiogenic drugs can be ascribed to qualitative modifications in the angiogenic vasculature throughout tumor progression. The observation that inhibitors such as TNP-470, that blocks EC proliferation but also smooth-muscle cell migration, reduced mass of end-stage pancreatic tumors otherwise resistant to VEGF-neutralizing factors (Bergers et al., 1999), indirectly suggested the importance of "tumor vascular remodelling". This term describes a process through which the neo-vasculature becomes a stable, mature vessel bed covered by pericytes not easily pruned by EC-targeted treatment. Indeed, pericytes have gained attention as functional and critical contributors to tumor angiogenesis and, therefore, as a potential new target to improve the efficacy of anti-angiogenic therapies. Therapeutic regimes combining SU5416 (which blocks VEGFR) and SU6668 (which blocks PDGFR on pericytes, and, to a lesser extent, FGFR and VEGFR on EC) proved to be more efficacious against all stages of pancreatic islet cells carcinogenesis then either single agent, and combination of the VEGFR inhibitor with another distinctive kinase inhibitor targeting PDGFR (Gleevec) was also able to induce regression of advanced tumors (Bergers, Song, Meyer-Morse, Bergsland, & Hanahan, 2003). The same effect was achieved when PDGF inhibitors were combined with anti-angiogenic chemotherapy regimen that targeted EC (Pietras & Hanahan, 2005); targeting PDGFR signalling disrupted pericytes support, while the anti-angiogenic chemotherapy targeted the sensitized EC, collectively destabilizing the pre-existing tumor vasculature. These data suggest the potential significance of targeting interdependent cellular constituents of the tumor vasculature to significantly impact treatment of well-established solid tumors.

Another phenomenon which has been argued to give raise to resistance to angiogenesis inhibitors is "vasculogenic mimicry". Initially recognized in aggressive melanomas (Maniotis et al., 1999) and then confirmed in other tumors (Hendrix, Seftor, Hess, & Seftor, 2003), the term describes a phenotypic and functional adaptation of tumor cells which acquire some features typical of EC and contribute to the formation of perfused vessels. It has been shown that trans-differentiated tumor cells do not acquire sensitivity to angiogenesis inhibitors (van der Schaft et al., 2004), thus suggesting that tumors presenting vasculogenic mimicry could be resistant to angiogenesis inhibition. Ewing sarcoma, given its abundant vasculogenic structures, may be an ideal model to develop and test therapies designed to counteract vessels formation by attacking tumor cells that take part in the formation of vascular lakes (van der Schaft et al., 2005).

Finally, some recent studies showed that in some human cancers EC exhibit cytogenic abnormalities and are not genetically stable, thus representing a potential further mechanism of resistance. Hida et al. described cytogenetical abnormalities such as aneuploidy with chromosomes and multiple abnormal centrosomes, in murine EC isolated from human tumor xenografts (Hida et al., 2004). Furthermore, Streubel et al. reported that 37% of the microvascular EC in the B-cell lymphomas analysed harboured lymphoma-specific chromosomal translocations (Streubel et al., 2004). These findings could be considered on one hand as further evidence of the " vasculogenic mimicry" described above but, on the other hand reinforce the evidence that tumor-associated EC could be genetically mutated and thus prone to develop acquired resistance to angiogenesis-targeting drugs.

Stromal-Cell-Related Mechanisms

The microenvironment of tumors comprises different cell types including fibroblasts and bone marrow-derived cells (BMDCs) that can contribute to tumor angiogenesis either by direct incorporation in tumor vasculature or supply of pro-angiogenic factors, thus providing a potential mechanism of escape to some anti-angiogenic treatments. The recruitment of BMDCs might be triggered by ischemia, vascular injury, secretion of chemokines or cytokines like SDF-1, VEGF, IL-1, GM-CSF and G-CSF by tumor cells or by tumor associated fibroblasts (TAFs) (Takahashi et al., 1999) and their homing to the tumor could negatively affect the efficacy of the treatment. Orimo et al. showed that TAFs can contribute to tumor angiogenesis through the release of SDF-1 that, in turn, recruits endothelial progenitor cells into breast carcinomas (Orimo et al., 2005). The relevance of the interaction between SDF-1 and its receptor CXCR4 in relationship to neoangiogenesis was also reported by Guleng et al. who showed that the in vivo neutralization of CXCR4 resulted in attenuation of tumor growth in a mouse model of colon and pancreatic carcinoma by the inhibition of tumor neovascularization (Guleng et al., 2005). A major contribution of TAFs on angiogenesis may be expected in those tumor types where the stromal component is more represented.

One of the main focuses of research in this field are CD11b+Gr1+ cells, including both monocytes and granulocytes recruited from bone marrow to the tumor where they secrete MMP-9 and pro–angiogenic factors (Yang et al., 2004); their role in the induction of angiogenic switch in a transgenic model of β-cell carcinogenesis has recently been elucidated (Nozawa, Chiu, & Hanahan, 2006). De Palma and colleagues identified a small subset of CD11b+ myeloid tumor-infiltrating cells characterized by the expression of the Tie2 angiopoietin receptor (Tie2-expressing monocytes (TEMs)) that represents a hematopoietic lineage of proangiogenic cells, selectively recruited to spontaneous pancreatic and orthotopically growing brain tumors in nude mice, where they promote angiogenesis in a paracrine manner (De Palma et al., 2005).

Although the precise identity of BMDCs is still debated (Jain & Duda, 2003) and their actual contribution to the growing vessels seems to depend substantially on the experimental system employed (De Palma, Venneri, Roca, & Naldini, 2003; Peters et al., 2005; Ruzinova et al., 2003), many agree to consider them as a putative target for anti-angiogenic treatments (Shaked et al., 2005).

Biomarkers for Monitoring Anti-Angiogenic Therapy

Clinical evaluation of anti-angiogenic drugs has been somewhat delayed by the lack of appropriate clinical criteria to measure efficacy. In fact, as anti-angiogenic drugs are generally cytostatic, the objective response rate - a readout commonly used to measure activity of cytotoxic drugs - is a poor estimate of benefit and of other valuable parameters, such as measurement of survival, require long-term observation. Furthermore, concerning dosage of anti-angiogenic drugs, there is evidence that the maximum tolerated dose is not necessarily the most effective one, also in combination regimens (Jain, 2005).

Biomarkers could be useful at different steps, such as (i) the identification of early clinical benefit, (ii) to guide dosage adjustment and (iii) to detect the onset of resistance. The ideal features of a biomarker include cost-effectiveness, low baseline levels in normal population, non-invasive and standardized methods of determination, robustness in the clinical setting, and reproducibility in multiple clinical centers.

Evaluation of microvessel density (MVD) in tumor specimens following staining with anti-CD31 or anti-CD34 mAb was traditionally deemed to be a reliable marker of efficacy of angiogenesis inhibitors. This technique, however, presents several limitations in clinical practice, first of all because of the requirement of serial tumor biopsies and the possibility that the small sample analyzed may not be representative of the entire tumor. Moreover, there is evidence that the survival benefit associated with the combination of bevacizumab with cytotoxic drugs in colorectal cancer does not correlate with significant changes in MVD (Jubb et al., 2006).

Live imaging of the tumor vasculature and its dynamic changes can be achieved by techniques such as dynamic contrast-enhanced magnetic resonance imaging (DCE-MRI) and dynamic computed tomography (CT) that are currently used in many clinical trials with angiogenesis inhibitors (Liu et al., 2005; Morgan et al., 2003; Willett et al., 2004). In contrast to MVD, these imaging modalities provide a functional analysis of the whole tumor vasculature by a relatively non-invasive procedure.

Measurement of plasma levels of angiogenic factors such as VEGF, FGF, IL8, and HGF or quantification of circulating endothelial (CEC) and progenitors cells (CEPs) have also been proposed as possible surrogate markers of the angiogenic process. Variations in VEGF plasma levels have been measured following treatment of cancer patients with different anti-angiogenic agents (Drevs et al., 2005; Faivre et al., 2006; Motzer et al., 2006; Willett et al., 2005); to date, however, the predictive value of plasma VEGF levels has not been fully elucidated and the possible contribution of platelets-associated VEGF to the levels measured raises concerns.

The presence of circulating endothelial cells was demonstrated many years ago in several pathological conditions including cancer (Blann et al., 2005). CEC in great proportions presents a mature, terminally differentiated phenotype and probably originates from vessels turnover; on the other hand, a small subpopulation of cells, termed CEP, presents progenitor-like or stem-like characteristics, derives from bone marrow and potentially contributes to tumor angiogenesis. Both in preclinical and clinical settings there is evidence that the levels of CEC and CEP are modulated by anti-angiogenic therapy (Beaudry et al., 2005; Beerepoot et al., 2004; Mancuso et al., 2006; Shaked et al., 2005; Willett et al., 2004). In general, anti-angiogenic agents produce either a decrease in CEP levels or a transient increase in total CEC numbers. In any case, the fraction of viable CEC is dramatically reduced by anti-angiogenic therapy, and the fraction of apoptotic CEC is proportionally increased. At the time of writing, understanding of the mechanisms that regulate CEC/CEP and their role in angiogenesis is at a very early stage and there is still a lack of consensus on the markers that best define this population and on the more appropriate time to measure them. Moreover, the current studies on CEC/CEP are hindered both by the very small number of cells obtained and by the great variability in their absolute numbers among patients.

Conclusion

Angiogenesis has been shown to play a pivotal role in the development of human malignancies and it may contribute to other molecular mechanisms involved in tumor progression, including regulation of cancer stem cell behaviour. Blocking angiogenesis is an attractive possibility for treating cancer but realistically as a monotherapy it will not be a “magic bullet” for cancer patients. Selection of patients who could best profit from anti-angiogenic treatments would be highly desirable but we currently lack robust and validated predictive markers.

Thus, whatever the means of administration of anti-angiogenic factors –i.e. recombinant proteins versus gene therapy– a major challenge in the field will be to identify, beginning at the pre-clinical level, which molecular or perhaps metabolic features render tumor cells resistant or sensitive to angiogenesis inhibition.

Another open question is how anti-angiogenic treatments, which have already shown clinical efficacy on established disease, will perform in the so-called adjuvant setting. In pre-clinical models anti-angiogenic factors are generally far more effective in preventing tumor growth than causing regression of established tumors: will this also occur in patients? Moreover, should adjuvant treatment show efficacy, will there be any unpredicted side effects due to long-term inhibition of physiologic angiogenesis? With no doubt the coming years will deserve a lot of fascinating discoveries in angiogenesis research; this progress will eventually drive a rational exploitation of anti-angiogenic drugs in cancer patients.

REFERENCES

Albini, A., Marchisone, C., Del Grosso, F., Benelli, R., Masiello, L., Tacchetti, C., et al. (2000). Inhibition of angiogenesis and vascular tumor growth by interferon-producing cells: A gene therapy approach. *Am J Pathol, 156(4)*, 1381-1393.

Angiolillo, A.L., Sgadari, C., Taub, D.D., Liao, F., Farber, J.M., Maheshwari, S., et al. (1995). Human interferon-inducible protein 10 is a potent inhibitor of angiogenesis in vivo. *J Exp Med, 182(1)*, 155-162.

Asahara, T., Murohara, T., Sullivan, A., Silver, M., van der Zee, R., Li, T., et al. (1997). Isolation of putative progenitor endothelial cells for angiogenesis. *Science, 275(5302)*, 964-967.

Bacon, A.L., & Harris, A.L. (2004). Hypoxia-inducible factors and hypoxic cell death in tumour physiology. *Ann Med, 36(7)*, 530-539.

Balkwill, F., Charles, K.A., & Mantovani, A. (2005). Smoldering and polarized inflammation in the initiation and promotion of malignant disease. *Cancer Cell, 7(3)*, 211-217.

Beaudry, P., Force, J., Naumov, G.N., Wang, A., Baker, C.H., Ryan, A., et al. (2005). Differential effects of vascular endothelial growth factor receptor-2 inhibitor ZD6474 on circulating endothelial progenitors and mature circulating endothelial cells: implications for use as a surrogate marker of antiangiogenic activity. *Clin Cancer Res, 11(9)*, 3514-3522.

Beecken, W.D., Fernandez, A., Joussen, A.M., Achilles, E.G., Flynn, E., Lo, K.M., et al. (2001). Effect of antiangiogenic therapy on slowly growing, poorly vascularized tumors in mice. *J Natl Cancer Inst, 93(5)*, 382-387.

Beerepoot, L.V., Mehra, N., Vermaat, J.S., Zonnenberg, B.A., Gebbink, M.F., & Voest, E.E. (2004). Increased levels of viable circulating endothelial cells are an indicator of progressive disease in cancer patients. *Ann Oncol, 15(1)*, 139-145.

Bergers, G., Brekken, R., McMahon, G., Vu, T.H., Itoh, T., Tamaki, K., et al. (2000). Matrix metalloproteinase-9 triggers the angiogenic switch during carcinogenesis. *Nat Cell Biol, 2(10)*, 737-744.

Bergers, G., Javaherian, K., Lo, K.M., Folkman, J., & Hanahan, D. (1999). Effects of angiogenesis inhibitors on multistage carcinogenesis in mice. *Science, 284(5415)*, 808-812.

Bergers, G., Song, S., Meyer-Morse, N., Bergsland, E., & Hanahan, D. (2003). Benefits of targeting both pericytes and endothelial cells in the tumor vasculature with kinase inhibitors. *J Clin Invest, 111(9)*, 1287-1295.

Bertolini, F., Shaked, Y., Mancuso, P., & Kerbel, R.S. (2006). The multifaceted circulating endothelial cell in cancer: towards marker and target identification. *Nat Rev Cancer, 6(11)*, 835-845.

Blann, A.D., Woywodt, A., Bertolini, F., Bull, T.M., Buyon, J.P., Clancy, R.M., et al. (2005). Circulating endothelial cells. Biomarker of vascular disease. *Thromb Haemost, 93(2)*, 228-235.

Boehm, T., Folkman, J., Browder, T., & O'Reilly, M.S. (1997). Antiangiogenic therapy of experimental cancer does not induce acquired drug resistance. *Nature, 390(6658)*, 404-407.

Brandwijk, R.J., Griffioen, A.W., & Thijssen, V.L. (2007). Targeted gene-delivery strategies for angiostatic cancer treatment. *Trends Mol Med, 13(5)*, 200-209.

Brem H, G.F., Budson A, Saunders L, Folkman J (1994). Minimal drug resistance after prolonged anti-angiogenic therapy with AGM-1470. *Surgical Forum XLV*, 674-677.

Carmeliet, P., Ferreira, V., Breier, G., Pollefeyt, S., Kieckens, L., Gertsenstein, M., et al. (1996). Abnormal blood vessel development and lethality in embryos lacking a single VEGF allele. *Nature, 380(6573)*, 435-439.

Casanovas, O., Hicklin, D.J., Bergers, G., & Hanahan, D. (2005). Drug resistance by evasion of antiangiogenic targeting of VEGF signaling in late-stage pancreatic islet tumors. *Cancer Cell, 8(4)*, 299-309.

Chen, Q.R., Zhang, L., Gasper, W., & Mixson, A.J. (2001). Targeting tumor angiogenesis with gene therapy. *Mol Genet Metab, 74(1-2)*, 120-127.

Chow, L.Q., & Eckhardt, S.G. (2007). Sunitinib: from rational design to clinical efficacy. *J Clin Oncol, 25(7)*, 884-896.

Claesson-Welsh, L., Welsh, M., Ito, N., Anand-Apte, B., Soker, S., Zetter, B., et al. (1998). Angiostatin induces endothelial cell apoptosis and activation of focal adhesion kinase independently of the integrin-binding motif RGD. *Proc Natl Acad Sci U S A, 95(10)*, 5579-5583.

Coussens, L.M., Raymond, W.W., Bergers, G., Laig-Webster, M., Behrendtsen, O., Werb, Z., et al. (1999). Inflammatory mast cells up-regulate angiogenesis during squamous epithelial carcinogenesis. *Genes Dev, 13(11)*, 1382-1397.

Coussens, L.M., & Werb, Z. (2002). Inflammation and cancer. *Nature, 420(6917)*, 860-867.

De Bouard, S., Guillamo, J.S., Christov, C., Lefevre, N., Brugieres, P., Gola, E., et al. (2003). Antiangiogenic therapy against experimental glioblastoma using genetically engineered cells producing interferon-alpha, angiostatin, or endostatin. *Hum Genė Ther, 14(9)*, 883-895.

De Palma, M., Venneri, M.A., Galli, R., Sergi Sergi, L., Politi, L.S., Sampaolesi, M., et al. (2005). Tie2 identifies a hematopoietic lineage of proangiogenic monocytes required for tumor vessel formation and a mesenchymal population of pericyte progenitors. *Cancer Cell, 8(3)*, 211-226.

De Palma, M., Venneri, M.A., Roca, C., & Naldini, L. (2003). Targeting exogenous genes to tumor angiogenesis by transplantation of genetically modified hematopoietic stem cells. *Nat Med, 9(6)*, 789-795.

Dell'Eva, R., Pfeffer, U., Indraccolo, S., Albini, A., & Noonan, D. (2002). Inhibition of tumor angiogenesis by angiostatin: from recombinant protein to gene therapy. *Endothelium, 9(1)*, 3-10.

Dome, B., Timar, J., Dobos, J., Meszaros, L., Raso, E., Paku, S., et al. (2006). Identification and clinical significance of circulating endothelial progenitor cells in human non-small cell lung cancer. *Cancer Res, 66(14)*, 7341-7347.

Drevs, J., Zirrgiebel, U., Schmidt-Gersbach, C.I., Mross, K., Medinger, M., Lee, L., et al. (2005). Soluble markers for the assessment of biological activity with PTK787/ZK 222584 (PTK/ZK), a vascular endothelial growth factor receptor (VEGFR) tyrosine kinase inhibitor in patients with advanced colorectal cancer from two phase I trials. *Ann Oncol, 16(4)*, 558-565.

Dvorak, H.F., & Gresser, I. (1989). Microvascular injury in pathogenesis of interferon-induced necrosis of subcutaneous tumors in mice. *J Natl Cancer Inst, 81(7)*, 497-502.

Faivre, S., Delbaldo, C., Vera, K., Robert, C., Lozahic, S., Lassau, N., et al. (2006). Safety, pharmacokinetic, and antitumor activity of SU11248, a novel oral multitarget tyrosine kinase inhibitor, in patients with cancer. *J Clin Oncol, 24(1)*, 25-35.

Ferrara, N., Carver-Moore, K., Chen, H., Dowd, M., Lu, L., O'Shea, K.S., et al. (1996). Heterozygous embryonic lethality induced by targeted inactivation of the VEGF gene. *Nature, 380(6573)*, 439-442.

Ferrara, N., & Kerbel, R.S. (2005). Angiogenesis as a therapeutic target. *Nature, 438(7070)*, 967-974.

Filleur, S., Volpert, O.V., Degeorges, A., Voland, C., Reiher, F., Clezardin, P., et al. (2001). In vivo mechanisms by which tumors producing thrombospondin 1 bypass its inhibitory effects. *Genes Dev, 15(11)*, 1373-1382.

Folkman, J. (1971). Tumor angiogenesis: therapeutic implications. *N Engl J Med, 285(21)*, 1182-1186.

Folkman, J. (1995). Angiogenesis in cancer, vascular, rheumatoid and other disease. *Nat Med, 1(1)*, 27-31.

Folkman, J. (2003). Angiogenesis inhibitors: a new class of drugs. *Cancer Biol Ther, 2(4 Suppl 1)*, S127-133.

Folkman, J. (2006). Antiangiogenesis in cancer therapy--endostatin and its mechanisms of action. *Exp Cell Res, 312(5)*, 594-607.

Folkman, J. (2007). Is angiogenesis an organizing principle in biology and medicine? *J Pediatr Surg, 42(1)*, 1-11.

Franco, M., Man, S., Chen, L., Emmenegger, U., Shaked, Y., Cheung, A.M., et al. (2006). Targeted anti-vascular endothelial growth factor receptor-2 therapy leads to short-term and long-term impairment of vascular function and increase in tumor hypoxia. *Cancer Res, 66(7)*, 3639-3648.

Fukumori, T., Nishitani, M., Naroda, T., Onishi, T., Oka, N., Kanayama, H., et al. (2002). Expression of angiostatin cDNA in a murine renal cell carcinoma suppresses tumor growth in vivo. *Urology, 59(6)*, 973-977.

Gerber, H.P., Dixit, V., & Ferrara, N. (1998). Vascular endothelial growth factor induces expression of the antiapoptotic proteins Bcl-2 and A1 in vascular endothelial cells. *J Biol Chem, 273(21)*, 13313-13316.

Gerber, H.P., & Ferrara, N. (2005). Pharmacology and pharmacodynamics of bevacizumab as monotherapy or in combination with cytotoxic therapy in preclinical studies. *Cancer Res, 65(3)*, 671-680.

Gerber, H.P., Hillan, K.J., Ryan, A.M., Kowalski, J., Keller, G.A., Rangell, L., et al. (1999). VEGF is required for growth and survival in neonatal mice. *Development, 126(6)*, 1149-1159.

Gerber, H.P., Kowalski, J., Sherman, D., Eberhard, D.A., & Ferrara, N. (2000). Complete inhibition of rhabdomyosarcoma xenograft growth and neovascularization requires blockade of both tumor and host vascular endothelial growth factor. *Cancer Res, 60(22)*, 6253-6258.

Giantonio, B.J., Catalano, P.J., Meropol, N.J., O'Dwyer, P.J., Mitchell, E.P., Alberts, S.R., et al. (2007). Bevacizumab in combination with oxaliplatin, fluorouracil, and leucovorin (FOLFOX4) for previously treated metastatic colorectal cancer: results from the Eastern Cooperative Oncology Group Study E3200. *J Clin Oncol, 25(12)*, 1539-1544.

Giavazzi, R., Giuliani, R., Coltrini, D., Bani, M.R., Ferri, C., Sennino, B., et al. (2001). Modulation of tumor angiogenesis by conditional expression of fibroblast growth factor-2 affects early but not established tumors. *Cancer Res, 61(1)*, 309-317.

Goon, P.K., Lip, G.Y., Boos, C.J., Stonelake, P.S., & Blann, A.D. (2006). Circulating endothelial cells, endothelial progenitor cells, and endothelial microparticles in cancer. *Neoplasia, 8(2)*, 79-88.

Griscelli, F., Li, H., Bennaceur-Griscelli, A., Soria, J., Opolon, P., Soria, C., et al. (1998). Angiostatin gene transfer: inhibition of tumor growth in vivo by blockage of endothelial cell proliferation associated with a mitosis arrest. *Proc Natl Acad Sci U S A, 95(11)*, 6367-6372.

Guleng, B., Tateishi, K., Ohta, M., Kanai, F., Jazag, A., Ijichi, H., et al. (2005). Blockade of the stromal cell-derived factor-1/CXCR4 axis attenuates in vivo tumor growth by inhibiting angiogenesis in a vascular endothelial growth factor-independent manner. *Cancer Res, 65(13)*, 5864-5871.

Hanahan, D., & Folkman, J. (1996). Patterns and emerging mechanisms of the angiogenic switch during tumorigenesis. *Cell, 86(3)*, 353-364.

Hanai, J., Dhanabal, M., Karumanchi, S.A., Albanese, C., Waterman, M., Chan, B., et al. (2002). Endostatin causes G1 arrest of endothelial cells through inhibition of cyclin D1. *J Biol Chem, 277(19)*, 16464-16469.

Hase, R., Miyamoto, M., Uehara, H., Kadoya, M., Ebihara, Y., Murakami, Y., et al. (2005). Pigment epithelium-derived factor gene therapy inhibits human pancreatic cancer in mice. *Clin Cancer Res, 11(24 Pt 1)*, 8737-8744.

Hendrix, M.J., Seftor, E.A., Hess, A.R., & Seftor, R.E. (2003). Vasculogenic mimicry and tumour-cell plasticity: lessons from melanoma. *Nat Rev Cancer, 3(6)*, 411-421.

Herbst, R.S., Johnson, D.H., Mininberg, E., Carbone, D.P., Henderson, T., Kim, E.S., et al. (2005). Phase I/II trial evaluating the anti-vascular endothelial growth factor monoclonal antibody bevacizumab in combination with the HER-1/epidermal growth factor receptor tyrosine kinase inhibitor erlotinib for patients with recurrent non-small-cell lung cancer. *J Clin Oncol, 23(11)*, 2544-2555.

Hida, K., Hida, Y., Amin, D.N., Flint, A.F., Panigrahy, D., Morton, C.C., et al. (2004). Tumor-associated endothelial cells with cytogenetic abnormalities. *Cancer Res, 64(22)*, 8249-8255.

Hobson, B., & Denekamp, J. (1984). Endothelial proliferation in tumours and normal tissues: continuous labelling studies. *Br J Cancer, 49(4)*, 405-413.

Holash, J., Wiegand, S.J., & Yancopoulos, G.D. (1999). New model of tumor angiogenesis: dynamic balance between vessel regression and growth mediated by angiopoietins and VEGF. *Oncogene, 18(38)*, 5356-5362.

Hottiger, M.O., Dam, T.N., Nickoloff, B.J., Johnson, T.M., & Nabel, G.J. (1999). Liposome-mediated gene transfer into human basal cell carcinoma. *Gene Ther, 6(12)*, 1929-1935.

Hurwitz, H., Fehrenbacher, L., Novotny, W., Cartwright, T., Hainsworth, J., Heim, W., et al. (2004). Bevacizumab plus irinotecan, fluorouracil, and leucovorin for metastatic colorectal cancer. *N Engl J Med, 350(23)*, 2335-2342.

Hurwitz, H.I., Fehrenbacher, L., Hainsworth, J.D., Heim, W., Berlin, J., Holmgren, E., et al. (2005). Bevacizumab in combination with fluorouracil and leucovorin: an active regimen for first-line metastatic colorectal cancer. *J Clin Oncol, 23(15)*, 3502-3508.

Indraccolo, S. (2004). Undermining tumor angiogenesis by gene therapy: an emerging field. *Curr Gene Ther, 4(3)*, 297-308.

Indraccolo, S., Gola, E., Rosato, A., Minuzzo, S., Habeler, W., Tisato, V., et al. (2002). Differential effects of angiostatin, endostatin and interferon-alpha(1) gene transfer on in vivo growth of human breast cancer cells. *Gene Ther, 9(13)*, 867-878.

Indraccolo, S., Habeler, W., Tisato, V., Stievano, L., Piovan, E., Tosello, V., et al. (2002). Gene transfer in ovarian cancer cells: a comparison between retroviral and lentiviral vectors. *Cancer Res, 62(21)*, 6099-6107.

Indraccolo, S., Minuzzo, S., Gola, E., Habeler, W., Carrozzino, F., Noonan, D., et al. (1999). Generation of expression plasmids for angiostatin, endostatin and TIMP-2 for cancer gene therapy. *Int J Biol Markers, 14(4)*, 251-256.

Indraccolo, S., Morini, M., Gola, E., Carrozzino, F., Habeler, W., Minghelli, S., et al. (2001). Effects of angiostatin gene transfer on functional properties and in vivo growth of Kaposi's sarcoma cells. *Cancer Res, 61(14)*, 5441-5446.

Indraccolo, S., Moserle, L., Tisato, V., Gola, E., Minuzzo, S., Roni, V., et al. (2006). Gene therapy of ovarian cancer with IFN-alpha-producing fibroblasts: comparison of constitutive and inducible vectors. *Gene Ther, 13(12)*, 953-965.

Indraccolo, S., Pfeffer, U., Minuzzo, S., Esposito, G., Roni, V., Mandruzzato, S., et al. (2007). Identification of genes selectively regulated by IFNs in endothelial cells. *J Immunol, 178(2)*, 1122-1135.

Indraccolo, S., Tisato, V., Tosello, V., Habeler, W., Esposito, G., Moserle, L., et al. (2005). Interferon-alpha gene therapy by lentiviral vectors contrasts ovarian cancer growth through angiogenesis inhibition. *Hum Gene Ther, 16(8)*, 957-970.

Iqbal Ahmed, C.M., Johnson, D.E., Demers, G.W., Engler, H., Howe, J.A., Wills, K.N., et al. (2001). Interferon alpha2b gene delivery using adenoviral vector causes inhibition of tumor growth in xenograft models from a variety of cancers. *Cancer Gene Ther, 8(10)*, 788-795.

Isayeva, T., Ren, C., & Ponnazhagan, S. (2005). Recombinant adeno-associated virus 2-mediated antiangiogenic prevention in a mouse model of intraperitoneal ovarian cancer. *Clin Cancer Res, 11(3)*, 1342-1347.

Jain, R.K. (2005). Normalization of tumor vasculature: an emerging concept in antiangiogenic therapy. *Science, 307(5706)*, 58-62.

Jain, R.K., & Duda, D.G. (2003). Role of bone marrow-derived cells in tumor angiogenesis and treatment. *Cancer Cell, 3(6)*, 515-516.

Jin, X., Bookstein, R., Wills, K., Avanzini, J., Tsai, V., LaFace, D., et al. (2001). Evaluation of endostatin antiangiogenesis gene therapy in vitro and in vivo. *Cancer Gene Ther, 8(12)*, 982-989.

Joseph, J.M., Bouquet, C., Opolon, P., Morizet, J., Aubert, G., Rossler, J., et al. (2003). High level of stabilized angiostatin mediated by adenovirus delivery does not impair the growth of human neuroblastoma xenografts. *Cancer Gene Ther, 10(11)*, 859-866.

Jubb, A.M., Hurwitz, H.I., Bai, W., Holmgren, E.B., Tobin, P., Guerrero, A.S., et al. (2006). Impact of vascular endothelial growth factor-A expression, thrombospondin-2 expression, and microvessel density on the treatment effect of bevacizumab in metastatic colorectal cancer. *J Clin Oncol, 24(2)*, 217-227.

Kabbinavar, F., Hurwitz, H.I., Fehrenbacher, L., Meropol, N.J., Novotny, W.F., Lieberman, G., et al. (2003). Phase II, randomized trial comparing bevacizumab plus fluorouracil (FU)/leucovorin (LV) with FU/LV alone in patients with metastatic colorectal cancer. *J Clin Oncol, 21(1)*, 60-65.

Kabbinavar, F.F., Schulz, J., McCleod, M., Patel, T., Hamm, J.T., Hecht, J.R., et al. (2005). Addition of bevacizumab to bolus fluorouracil and leucovorin in first-line metastatic colorectal cancer: results of a randomized phase II trial. *J Clin Oncol, 23(16)*, 3697-3705.

Kerbel, R.S. (1991). Inhibition of tumor angiogenesis as a strategy to circumvent acquired resistance to anti-cancer therapeutic agents. *Bioessays, 13(1)*, 31-36.

Kerbel, R.S. (1997). A cancer therapy resistant to resistance. *Nature, 390(6658)*, 335-336.

Kerbel, R.S. (2006). Antiangiogenic therapy: a universal chemosensitization strategy for cancer? *Science, 312(5777)*, 1171-1175.

Kerbel, R.S., & Hawley, R.G. (1995). Interleukin 12: newest member of the antiangiogenesis club. *J Natl Cancer Inst, 87(8)*, 557-559.

Kerbel, R.S., Viloria-Petit, A., Klement, G., & Rak, J. (2000). 'Accidental' anti-angiogenic drugs. anti-oncogene directed signal transduction inhibitors and conventional chemotherapeutic agents as examples. *Eur J Cancer, 36(10)*, 1248-1257.

Kim, K.J., Li, B., Winer, J., Armanini, M., Gillett, N., Phillips, H.S., et al. (1993). Inhibition of vascular endothelial growth factor-induced angiogenesis suppresses tumour growth in vivo. *Nature, 362(6423)*, 841-844.

Kim, Y.M., Hwang, S., Pyun, B.J., Kim, T.Y., Lee, S.T., Gho, Y.S., et al. (2002). Endostatin blocks vascular endothelial growth factor-mediated signaling via direct interaction with KDR/Flk-1. *J Biol Chem, 277(31)*, 27872-27879.

Klement, G., Baruchel, S., Rak, J., Man, S., Clark, K., Hicklin, D.J., et al. (2000). Continuous low-dose therapy with vinblastine and VEGF receptor-2 antibody induces sustained tumor regression without overt toxicity. *J Clin Invest, 105(8)*, R15-24.

Kong, H.L., & Crystal, R.G. (1998). Gene therapy strategies for tumor antiangiogenesis. *J Natl Cancer Inst, 90(4)*, 273-286.

Liu, G., Rugo, H.S., Wilding, G., McShane, T.M., Evelhoch, J.L., Ng, C., et al. (2005). Dynamic contrast-enhanced magnetic resonance imaging as a pharmacodynamic measure of response after acute dosing of AG-013736, an oral angiogenesis inhibitor, in patients with advanced solid tumors: results from a phase I study. *J Clin Oncol, 23(24)*, 5464-5473.

Liu, Y., & Deisseroth, A. (2006). Tumor vascular targeting therapy with viral vectors. *Blood, 107(8)*, 3027-3033.

Lucas, R., Holmgren, L., Garcia, I., Jimenez, B., Mandriota, S.J., Borlat, F., et al. (1998). Multiple forms of angiostatin induce apoptosis in endothelial cells. *Blood, 92(12)*, 4730-4741.

Lyden, D., Hattori, K., Dias, S., Costa, C., Blaikie, P., Butros, L., et al. (2001). Impaired recruitment of bone-marrow-derived endothelial and hematopoietic precursor cells blocks tumor angiogenesis and growth. *Nat Med, 7(11)*, 1194-1201.

Ma, H.I., Guo, P., Li, J., Lin, S.Z., Chiang, Y.H., Xiao, X., et al. (2002). Suppression of intracranial human glioma growth after intramuscular administration of an adeno-associated viral vector expressing angiostatin. *Cancer Res, 62(3)*, 756-763.

Mancuso, P., Colleoni, M., Calleri, A., Orlando, L., Maisonneuve, P., Pruneri, G., et al. (2006). Circulating endothelial-cell kinetics and viability predict survival in breast cancer patients receiving metronomic chemotherapy. *Blood, 108(2)*, 452-459.

Maniotis, A.J., Folberg, R., Hess, A., Seftor, E.A., Gardner, L.M., Pe'er, J., et al. (1999). Vascular channel formation by human melanoma cells in vivo and in vitro: vasculogenic mimicry. *Am J Pathol, 155(3)*, 739-752.

Marx, J. (2005). Cancer. Encouraging results for second-generation antiangiogenesis drugs. *Science, 308(5726)*, 1248-1249.

Matsumoto, G., Ohmi, Y., & Shindo, J. (2001). Angiostatin gene therapy inhibits the growth of murine squamous cell carcinoma in vivo. *Oral Oncol, 37(4)*, 369-378.

Miller, K.D., Chap, L.I., Holmes, F.A., Cobleigh, M.A., Marcom, P.K., Fehrenbacher, L., et al. (2005). Randomized phase III trial of capecitabine compared with bevacizumab plus capecitabine in patients with previously treated metastatic breast cancer. *J Clin Oncol, 23(4)*, 792-799.

Mizukami, Y., Jo, W.S., Duerr, E.M., Gala, M., Li, J., Zhang, X., et al. (2005). Induction of interleukin-8 preserves the angiogenic response in HIF-1alpha-deficient colon cancer cells. *Nat Med, 11(9)*, 992-997.

Morelli, M.P., Cascone, T., Troiani, T., Tuccillo, C., Bianco, R., Normanno, N., et al. (2006). Anti-tumor activity of the combination of cetuximab, an anti-EGFR blocking monoclonal antibody and ZD6474, an inhibitor of VEGFR and EGFR tyrosine kinases. *J Cell Physiol, 208(2)*, 344-353.

Morgan, B., Thomas, A.L., Drevs, J., Hennig, J., Buchert, M., Jivan, A., et al. (2003). Dynamic contrast-enhanced magnetic resonance imaging as a biomarker for the pharmacological response of PTK787/ZK 222584, an inhibitor of the vascular endothelial growth factor receptor tyrosine kinases, in patients with advanced colorectal cancer and liver metastases: results from two phase I studies. *J Clin Oncol, 21(21)*, 3955-3964.

Morini, M., Albini, A., Lorusso, G., Moelling, K., Lu, B., Cilli, M., et al. (2004). Prevention of angiogenesis by naked DNA IL-12 gene transfer: angioprevention by immunogene therapy. *Gene Ther, 11(3)*, 284-291.

Moser, T.L., Stack, M.S., Asplin, I., Enghild, J.J., Hojrup, P., Everitt, L., et al. (1999). Angiostatin binds ATP synthase on the surface of human endothelial cells. *Proc Natl Acad Sci U S A, 96(6)*, 2811-2816.

Motzer, R.J., Michaelson, M.D., Redman, B.G., Hudes, G.R., Wilding, G., Figlin, R.A., et al. (2006). Activity of SU11248, a multitargeted inhibitor of vascular endothelial growth factor receptor and platelet-derived growth factor receptor, in patients with metastatic renal cell carcinoma. *J Clin Oncol, 24(1)*, 16-24.

Nakayama, T., Yao, L., & Tosato, G. (2004). Mast cell-derived angiopoietin-1 plays a critical role in the growth of plasma cell tumors. *J Clin Invest, 114(9)*, 1317-1325.

Nor, J.E., Christensen, J., Mooney, D.J., & Polverini, P.J. (1999). Vascular endothelial growth factor (VEGF)-mediated angiogenesis is associated with enhanced endothelial cell survival and induction of Bcl-2 expression. *Am J Pathol, 154(2)*, 375-384.

Nozawa, H., Chiu, C., & Hanahan, D. (2006). Infiltrating neutrophils mediate the initial angiogenic switch in a mouse model of multistage carcinogenesis. *Proc Natl Acad Sci U S A, 103(33)*, 12493-12498.

O'Connor, D.S., Schechner, J.S., Adida, C., Mesri, M., Rothermel, A.L., Li, F., et al. (2000). Control of apoptosis during angiogenesis by survivin expression in endothelial cells. *Am J Pathol, 156(2)*, 393-398.

O'Reilly, M.S., Boehm, T., Shing, Y., Fukai, N., Vasios, G., Lane, W.S., et al. (1997). Endostatin: an endogenous inhibitor of angiogenesis and tumor growth. *Cell, 88(2)*, 277-285.

O'Reilly, M.S., Holmgren, L., Chen, C., & Folkman, J. (1996). Angiostatin induces and sustains dormancy of human primary tumors in mice. *Nat Med, 2(6)*, 689-692.

O'Reilly, M.S., Holmgren, L., Shing, Y., Chen, C., Rosenthal, R.A., Moses, M., et al. (1994). Angiostatin: a novel angiogenesis inhibitor that mediates the suppression of metastases by a Lewis lung carcinoma. *Cell, 79(2)*, 315-328.

Okamoto, R., Ueno, M., Yamada, Y., Takahashi, N., Sano, H., Suda, T., et al. (2005). Hematopoietic cells regulate the angiogenic switch during tumorigenesis. *Blood, 105(7)*, 2757-2763.

Oliveira, I.C., Sciavolino, P.J., Lee, T.H., & Vilcek, J. (1992). Downregulation of interleukin 8 gene expression in human fibroblasts: unique mechanism of transcriptional inhibition by interferon. *Proc Natl Acad Sci U S A, 89(19)*, 9049-9053.

Orimo, A., Gupta, P.B., Sgroi, D.C., Arenzana-Seisdedos, F., Delaunay, T., Naeem, R., et al. (2005). Stromal fibroblasts present in invasive human breast carcinomas promote tumor growth and angiogenesis through elevated SDF-1/CXCL12 secretion. *Cell, 121(3)*, 335-348.

Papetti, M., & Herman, I.M. (2002). Mechanisms of normal and tumor-derived angiogenesis. *Am J Physiol Cell Physiol, 282(5)*, C947-970.

Peters, B.A., Diaz, L.A., Polyak, K., Meszler, L., Romans, K., Guinan, E.C., et al. (2005). Contribution of bone marrow-derived endothelial cells to human tumor vasculature. *Nat Med, 11(3)*, 261-262.

Pfeifer, A., Kessler, T., Silletti, S., Cheresh, D.A., & Verma, I.M. (2000). Suppression of angiogenesis by lentiviral delivery of PEX, a noncatalytic fragment of matrix metalloproteinase 2. *Proc Natl Acad Sci U S A, 97(22)*, 12227-12232.

Pietras, K., & Hanahan, D. (2005). A multitargeted, metronomic, and maximum-tolerated dose "chemo-switch" regimen is antiangiogenic, producing objective responses and survival benefit in a mouse model of cancer. *J Clin Oncol, 23(5)*, 939-952.

Ponnazhagan, S., Mahendra, G., Kumar, S., Shaw, D.R., Stockard, C.R., Grizzle, W.E., et al. (2004). Adeno-associated virus 2-mediated antiangiogenic cancer gene therapy: long-term efficacy of a vector encoding angiostatin and endostatin over vectors encoding a single factor. *Cancer Res, 64(5)*, 1781-1787.

Raikwar, S.P., Temm, C.J., Raikwar, N.S., Kao, C., Molitoris, B.A., & Gardner, T.A. (2005). Adenoviral vectors expressing human endostatin-angiostatin and soluble Tie2: enhanced suppression of tumor growth and antiangiogenic effects in a prostate tumor model. *Mol Ther, 12(6)*, 1091-1100.

Rehman, J., Li, J., Orschell, C.M., & March, K.L. (2003). Peripheral blood "endothelial progenitor cells" are derived from monocyte/macrophages and secrete angiogenic growth factors. *Circulation, 107(8)*, 1164-1169.

Relf, M., LeJeune, S., Scott, P.A., Fox, S., Smith, K., Leek, R., et al. (1997). Expression of the angiogenic factors vascular endothelial cell growth factor, acidic and basic fibroblast growth factor, tumor growth factor beta-1, platelet-derived endothelial cell growth factor, placenta growth factor, and pleiotrophin in human primary breast cancer and its relation to angiogenesis. *Cancer Res, 57(5)*, 963-969.

Rowe, D.H., Huang, J., Kayton, M.L., Thompson, R., Troxel, A., O'Toole, K.M., et al. (2000). Anti-VEGF antibody suppresses primary tumor growth and metastasis in an experimental model of Wilms' tumor. *J Pediatr Surg, 35(1)*, 30-32; discussion 32-33.

Rowe, D.H., Huang, J., Li, J., Manley, C., O'Toole, K.M., Stolar, C.J., et al. (2000). Suppression of primary tumor growth in a mouse model of human neuroblastoma. *J Pediatr Surg, 35(6)*, 977-981.

Rozera, C., Carlei, D., Lollini, P.L., De Giovanni, C., Musiani, P., Di Carlo, E., et al. (1999). Interferon (IFN)-beta gene transfer into TS/A adenocarcinoma cells and comparison with IFN-alpha: differential effects on tumorigenicity and host response. *Am J Pathol, 154(4)*, 1211-1222.

Ruzinova, M.B., Schoer, R.A., Gerald, W., Egan, J.E., Pandolfi, P.P., Rafii, S., et al. (2003). Effect of angiogenesis inhibition by Id loss and the contribution of bone-marrow-derived endothelial cells in spontaneous murine tumors. *Cancer Cell, 4(4)*, 277-289.

Scappaticci, F.A. (2002). Mechanisms and future directions for angiogenesis-based cancer therapies. *J Clin Oncol, 20(18)*, 3906-3927.

Scappaticci, F.A., Smith, R., Pathak, A., Schloss, D., Lum, B., Cao, Y., et al. (2001). Combination angiostatin and endostatin gene transfer induces synergistic antiangiogenic activity in vitro and antitumor efficacy in leukemia and solid tumors in mice. *Mol Ther, 3(2)*, 186-196.

Schmitz, V., Wang, L., Barajas, M., Gomar, C., Prieto, J., & Qian, C. (2004). Treatment of colorectal and hepatocellular carcinomas by adenoviral mediated gene transfer of endostatin and angiostatin-like molecule in mice. *Gut, 53(4)*, 561-567.

Scott, K.A., Holdsworth, H., Balkwill, F.R., & Dias, S. (2000). Exploiting changes in the tumour microenvironment with sequential cytokine and matrix metalloprotease inhibitor treatment in a murine breast cancer model. *Br J Cancer, 83(11)*, 1538-1543.

Sedlacek, H.H. (2001). Pharmacological aspects of targeting cancer gene therapy to endothelial cells. *Crit Rev Oncol Hematol, 37(3)*, 169-215.

Sgadari, C., Angiolillo, A.L., Cherney, B.W., Pike, S.E., Farber, J.M., Koniaris, L.G., et al. (1996). Interferon-inducible protein-10 identified as a mediator of tumor necrosis in vivo. *Proc Natl Acad Sci U S A, 93(24)*, 13791-13796.

Sgadari, C., Angiolillo, A.L., & Tosato, G. (1996). Inhibition of angiogenesis by interleukin-12 is mediated by the interferon-inducible protein 10. *Blood, 87(9)*, 3877-3882.

Shaked, Y., Bertolini, F., Man, S., Rogers, M.S., Cervi, D., Foutz, T., et al. (2005). Genetic heterogeneity of the vasculogenic phenotype parallels angiogenesis; Implications for cellular surrogate marker analysis of antiangiogenesis. *Cancer Cell, 7(1)*, 101-111.

Shichinohe, T., Bochner, B.H., Mizutani, K., Nishida, M., Hegerich-Gilliam, S., Naldini, L., et al. (2001). Development of lentiviral vectors for antiangiogenic gene delivery. *Cancer Gene Ther, 8(11)*, 879-889.

Sidky, Y.A., & Borden, E.C. (1987). Inhibition of angiogenesis by interferons: effects on tumor- and lymphocyte-induced vascular responses. *Cancer Res, 47(19)*, 5155-5161.

Sim, B.K., O'Reilly, M.S., Liang, H., Fortier, A.H., He, W., Madsen, J.W., et al. (1997). A recombinant human angiostatin protein inhibits experimental primary and metastatic cancer. *Cancer Res, 57(7)*, 1329-1334.

Singh, R.K., Gutman, M., Bucana, C.D., Sanchez, R., Llansa, N., & Fidler, I.J. (1995). Interferons alpha and beta down-regulate the expression of basic fibroblast growth factor in human carcinomas. *Proc Natl Acad Sci U S A, 92(10)*, 4562-4566.

Soff, G.A. (2000). Angiostatin and angiostatin-related proteins. *Cancer Metastasis Rev, 19(1-2)*, 97-107.

Stack, M.S., Gately, S., Bafetti, L.M., Enghild, J.J., & Soff, G.A. (1999). Angiostatin inhibits endothelial and melanoma cellular invasion by blocking matrix-enhanced plasminogen activation. *Biochem J, 340 (Pt 1)*, 77-84.

Streubel, B., Chott, A., Huber, D., Exner, M., Jager, U., Wagner, O., et al. (2004). Lymphoma-specific genetic aberrations in microvascular endothelial cells in B-cell lymphomas. *N Engl J Med, 351(3)*, 250-259.

Sudhakar, A., Sugimoto, H., Yang, C., Lively, J., Zeisberg, M., & Kalluri, R. (2003). Human tumstatin and human endostatin exhibit distinct antiangiogenic activities mediated by alpha v beta 3 and alpha 5 beta 1 integrins. *Proc Natl Acad Sci U S A, 100(8)*, 4766-4771.

Takahashi, T., Kalka, C., Masuda, H., Chen, D., Silver, M., Kearney, M., et al. (1999). Ischemia- and cytokine-induced mobilization of bone marrow-derived endothelial progenitor cells for neovascularization. *Nat Med, 5(4)*, 434-438.

Tanaka, T., Cao, Y., Folkman, J., & Fine, H.A. (1998). Viral vector-targeted antiangiogenic gene therapy utilizing an angiostatin complementary DNA. *Cancer Res, 58(15)*, 3362-3369.

Tran, J., Rak, J., Sheehan, C., Saibil, S.D., LaCasse, E., Korneluk, R.G., et al. (1999). Marked induction of the IAP family antiapoptotic proteins survivin and XIAP by VEGF in vascular endothelial cells. *Biochem Biophys Res Commun, 264(3)*, 781-788.

Uesato, M., Gunji, Y., Tomonaga, T., Miyazaki, S., Shiratori, T., Matsubara, H., et al. (2004). Synergistic antitumor effect of antiangiogenic factor genes on colon 26 produced by low-voltage electroporation. *Cancer Gene Ther, 11(9)*, 625-632.

van der Schaft, D.W., Hillen, F., Pauwels, P., Kirschmann, D.A., Castermans, K., Egbrink, M.G., et al. (2005). Tumor cell plasticity in Ewing sarcoma, an alternative circulatory system stimulated by hypoxia. *Cancer Res, 65(24)*, 11520-11528.

van der Schaft, D.W., Seftor, R.E., Seftor, E.A., Hess, A.R., Gruman, L.M., Kirschmann, D.A., et al. (2004). Effects of angiogenesis inhibitors on vascular network formation by human endothelial and melanoma cells. *J Natl Cancer Inst, 96(19)*, 1473-1477.

Voest, E.E., Kenyon, B.M., O'Reilly, M.S., Truitt, G., D'Amato, R.J., & Folkman, J. (1995). Inhibition of angiogenesis in vivo by interleukin 12. *J Natl Cancer Inst, 87(8)*, 581-586.

von Marschall, Z., Scholz, A., Cramer, T., Schafer, G., Schirner, M., Oberg, K., et al. (2003). Effects of interferon alpha on vascular endothelial growth factor gene transcription and tumor angiogenesis. *J Natl Cancer Inst, 95(6)*, 437-448.

Wilhelm, S.M., Carter, C., Tang, L., Wilkie, D., McNabola, A., Rong, H., et al. (2004). BAY 43-9006 exhibits broad spectrum oral antitumor activity and targets the RAF/MEK/ERK pathway and receptor tyrosine kinases involved in tumor progression and angiogenesis. *Cancer Res, 64(19)*, 7099-7109.

Willett, C.G., Boucher, Y., di Tomaso, E., Duda, D.G., Munn, L.L., Tong, R.T., et al. (2004). Direct evidence that the VEGF-specific antibody bevacizumab has antivascular effects in human rectal cancer. *Nat Med, 10(2)*, 145-147.

Willett, C.G., Boucher, Y., Duda, D.G., di Tomaso, E., Munn, L.L., Tong, R.T., et al. (2005). Surrogate markers for antiangiogenic therapy and dose-limiting toxicities for bevacizumab with radiation and chemotherapy: continued experience of a phase I trial in rectal cancer patients. *J Clin Oncol, 23(31)*, 8136-8139.

Xu, R., Sun, X., Tse, L.Y., Li, H., Chan, P.C., Xu, S., et al. (2003). Long-term expression of angiostatin suppresses metastatic liver cancer in mice. *Hepatology, 37(6)*, 1451-1460.

Yan, L., Anderson, G.M., DeWitte, M., & Nakada, M.T. (2006). Therapeutic potential of cytokine and chemokine antagonists in cancer therapy. *Eur J Cancer, 42(6)*, 793-802.

Yang, J.C., Haworth, L., Sherry, R.M., Hwu, P., Schwartzentruber, D.J., Topalian, S.L., et al. (2003). A randomized trial of bevacizumab, an anti-vascular endothelial growth factor antibody, for metastatic renal cancer. *N Engl J Med, 349(5)*, 427-434.

Yang, L., DeBusk, L.M., Fukuda, K., Fingleton, B., Green-Jarvis, B., Shyr, Y., et al. (2004). Expansion of myeloid immune suppressor Gr+CD11b+ cells in tumor-bearing host directly promotes tumor angiogenesis. *Cancer Cell, 6(4)*, 409-421.

Yao, L., Sgadari, C., Furuke, K., Bloom, E.T., Teruya-Feldstein, J., & Tosato, G. (1999). Contribution of natural killer cells to inhibition of angiogenesis by interleukin-12. *Blood, 93(5)*, 1612-1621.

Yoshiji, H., Harris, S.R., & Thorgeirsson, U.P. (1997). Vascular endothelial growth factor is essential for initial but not continued in vivo growth of human breast carcinoma cells. *Cancer Res, 57(18)*, 3924-3928.

Yu, J.L., Coomber, B.L., & Kerbel, R.S. (2002). A paradigm for therapy-induced microenvironmental changes in solid tumors leading to drug resistance. *Differentiation, 70(9-10)*, 599-609.

Yu, J.L., Rak, J.W., Carmeliet, P., Nagy, A., Kerbel, R.S., & Coomber, B.L. (2001). Heterogeneous vascular dependence of tumor cell populations. *Am J Pathol, 158(4)*, 1325-1334.

Yu, J.L., Rak, J.W., Coomber, B.L., Hicklin, D.J., & Kerbel, R.S. (2002). Effect of p53 status on tumor response to antiangiogenic therapy. *Science, 295(5559)*, 1526-1528.

Yuan, A., Yang, P.C., Yu, C.J., Chen, W.J., Lin, F.Y., Kuo, S.H., et al. (2000). Interleukin-8 messenger ribonucleic acid expression correlates with tumor progression, tumor angiogenesis, patient survival, and timing of relapse in non-small-cell lung cancer. *Am J Respir Crit Care Med, 162(5)*, 1957-1963.

Zakarija, A., & Soff, G. (2005). Update on angiogenesis inhibitors. *Curr Opin Oncol, 17(6)*, 578-583.

Zetter, B.R. (1998). Angiogenesis and tumor metastasis. *Annu Rev Med, 49*, 407-424.

In: New Gene Therapy and Cancer Research
Editor: Wilma B. Gustafsson, pp. 145-181

ISBN: 978-1-60021-969-6

Chapter IV

VASCULAR TARGETED GENE THERAPY IN CANCER TREATMENT

Michelle A. Hunt, Gabi U. Dachs* and Margaret J. Currie
Angiogenesis Research Group, Department of Pathology, University of Otago, Christchurch, New Zealand.

ABSTRACT

Over two-thirds of clinical trials in gene therapy are directed against cancer. Suicide gene therapy, or gene directed enzyme prodrug therapy (GDEPT), has been tested in 98 clinical trials worldwide, has reached phase III trials and makes up almost 8% of all current gene therapy trials. GDEPT aims to improve the selectivity of chemotherapy by gene transfer, thus enabling target cells to convert non-toxic prodrugs to cytotoxic drugs. A recent, but as yet clinically untested, development is the targeting of tumour blood vessels using gene therapy. Endothelial cells lining tumour blood vessels are an attractive target, since they are readily accessible for systemic administration and relatively minor vascular damage can amplify into macro-regional tumour infarction. This chapter will review the literature on the heterogeneity of endothelial cells, concentrating on tumour-endothelial factors. We will give an update on gene directed enzyme prodrug systems that have reached clinical trials, as well as those that are in the early phase of development, followed by an overview of approaches to target GDEPT to tumour vessels.

ABBREVIATIONS

Ad5	adenovirus serotype 5
araM,	6-methoxypurine arabinoside;

* Correspondence concerning this article should be addressed to: Gabi Dachs, gabi.dachs@otago.ac.nz.

araT, 1-β-D-arabinofuranosylthymine;
BVDU, (E)-5-(2-bromovinyl)-2 -deoxyuridine;
CMBA, N,N-(2-chloroethyl)(2-mesyloxyethyl)aminobenzoic acid;
CMDA, N,N-(2-chloroethyl)(2-mesyloxyethyl)aminobenzoyl-L-glutamic acid;
Daun02, N-[4'-(beta- D-galactopyranosyl)-3'-nitrobenzyloxycarbonyl]daunomycin;
DNA, deoxyribonucleic acid;
dpVP-16, 1,4'-dipiperidine-1'-carboxylate-etoposide;
E. coli, *Escherichia coli*;
eNOS, endothelial nitric oxide synthase;
EO9, 3-hydroxy-5-aziridinyl-1-methyl-(1H-indole-4,7-dione)-propenol;
F-araA, arabinofuranosyl-2-fluoroadenine;
F-dAdo, 2-fluoro-2'-deoxyadenosine;
5-FdUMP, 5-fluoro-2'-deoxyuridine-5'-monophosphate;
5-FdUTP, 5-fluoro-2'-deoxyuridine-5'-triphosphate;
FIAU, 1-(2'-deoxy-2-fluoro-b-D-arabinofuranosyl)-5-iodouracil;
5-FUMP 5-fluorouridine-5'-monophosphate
5-FUTP, 5-fluorouridine-5'-triphosphate;
GM-CSF, granulocyte-macrophage colony-stimulating factor;
HMR-1826, N-(4-b-glucuronyl-3-nitro-benxyloxy-carbonyl)-doxorubicin;
HUVEC human umbilical vein endothelial cell
MeP-dR, 9-(2-deoxy-β-D-ribofuranosyl)-6-methylpurine;
MRI, magnetic resonance imaging;
PABA/NO, O(2)-[2,4-dinitro-5-(N-methyl-N-4-carboxyphenylamino)phenyl]-1-N,N-dimethylamino)diazen-1-ium-1,2-diolate;
PEG, polyethylene glycol;
PET, positron emission tomography;
RNA, ribonucleic acid;
S. cerevisiae, Saccharomyces cerevisiae;
SN-38, 7-ethyl-10-hydroxy-camptothecin;
VEGF, vascular endothelial growth factor;
ZD-2767P, 4-[bis(2-iodoethyl)aminophenyl]-oxycarbonyl-L-glutamic acid.

INTRODUCTION

A functional vascular network is essential for the survival and growth of solid tumours, making blood vessels a key target for therapeutic strategies (Folkman, 1995). Features which make tumour blood vessels particularly attractive for therapeutic interventions are: 1) a single vascular endothelial cell supports the survival of about a thousand tumour cells, providing oxygen and nutrients, as well as a route for metastatic spread, and hence endothelial cell death magnifies the resulting tumour cell death many-fold, 2) endothelial cells in the tumour vasculature are genetically more stable than tumour cells, and hence result in a lower acquisition of treatment resistance, 3) vascular targeting may be tumour-type independent, and hence may represent a universal cancer treatment, and 4) endothelial cells are accessible by systemic administration, thus circumventing the common problem of treatment delivery (Liu & Deisseroth, 2006).

Most of the work in the area has concentrated on the development of anti-angiogenic approaches, hence inhibiting the formation of new blood vessels, and over 60 agents are undergoing clinical testing. An alternative to the anti-angiogenic approach is to target and destroy the existing tumour vasculature (anti-vascular approach), with several small molecule agents in clinical trials. The enthusiasm for anti-angiogenic approaches to cancer therapy is high following the approval by the Food and Drug Administration of the first angiogenesis inhibitor, Bevacizumab. This anti-VEGF agent was shown to significantly prolong the time to progression of disease in patients with metastatic renal cell carcinoma in a randomised, double blind, phase II trial (Yang et al., 2003). It also significantly improved survival in patients with metastatic colorectal cancer (Hurwitz et al., 2004).

Both approaches aim to exploit differences between tumour vessels and the normal vasculature. The differences include: 1) endothelial cells in tumours tend to proliferate more rapidly than in normal tissues, 2) activated tumour endothelial cells show higher expression of certain surface markers than normal cells, 3) tumour vessels tend to be immature compared to the mature normal vasculature, and 4) the tumour vasculature is chaotic with often disrupted basement membrane.

An attractive alternative to small molecule-based anti-angiogenic/anti-vascular approaches is the use of therapeutic gene transfer. Thus far, cancer gene therapy has been designed to destroy the tumour by delivering therapeutic genes to the malignant cells. However, cancer cells in solid tumours are often difficult to access, both for gene and drug delivery. In fact, poor transduction rates and restricted geometry of vector distribution (needle track only) are the major drawbacks of current gene therapy approaches (Rainov, 2000). This hurdle may be overcome by targeting the tumour vasculature, since vascular endothelial cells are easily accessible from the blood.

Therapeutic genes for gene therapy fall into three categories: mutation compensation, genetic immunopotentiation and molecular chemotherapy. In this chapter, emphasis will be placed on molecular chemotherapy. The advantage of this strategy, over the use of a pure cytotoxin, is that every step can be targeted and controlled. Gene directed enzyme prodrug therapy (GDEPT; also known as 'suicide gene therapy'), a form of molecular chemotherapy, requires delivery of an enzyme-encoding transgene to target cells, followed by systemic administration of a prodrug substrate. The enzyme selectively converts the prodrug to a cellular toxin *in situ*, causing cell death.

In GDEPT, enzyme expression can be genetically restricted and gene delivery targeted to certain surface markers to ensure tumour selectivity (Figure 1). In addition, it is also feasible to monitor, non-invasively, the location, magnitude and duration of vector-mediated gene expression. Advances have been made in recent years using PET, MRI and bioluminescent imaging (Shah et al., 2004). Hence, in GDEPT, an extra safety step is the ability to confirm the correct location of the enzyme, which in itself is harmless, prior to prodrug administration.

In the next section we will review the diversity of vascular endothelial cells, and describe the factors specific to tumour endothelial cells, which may be employed to target gene therapy. The subsequent section will review in detail the GDEPT systems which have reached clinical trials, as well as list those still in early development. We will end the review with an overview of those gene therapy systems which have been targeted to the tumour vasculature.

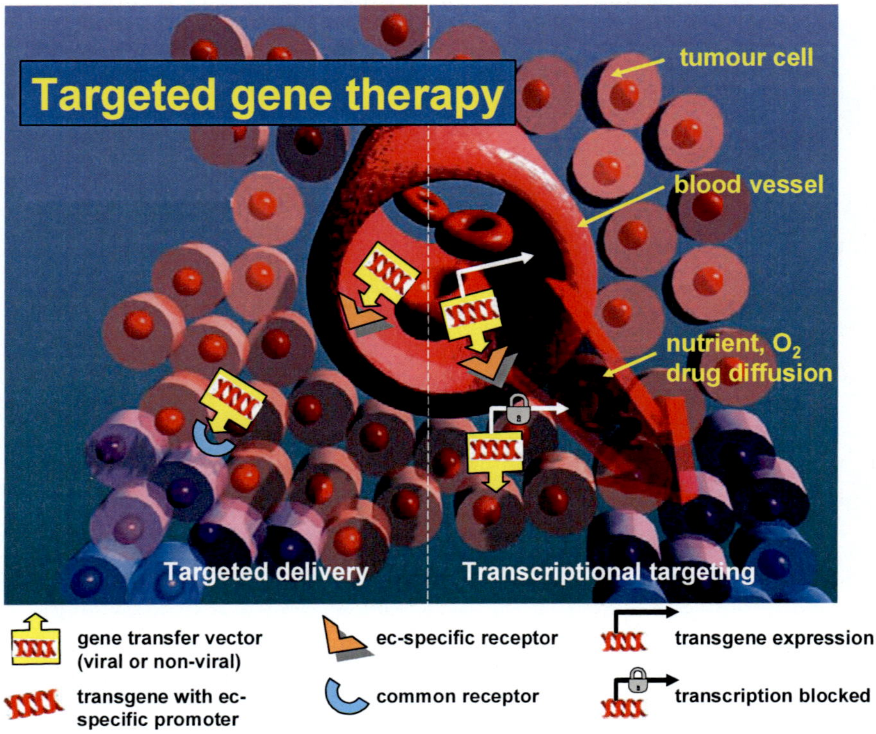

Figure 1. Schematic representation of vascular targeted gene therapy (Adapted from Brandwijk et al., 2007).

ENDOTHELIAL CELL DIVERSITY

The endothelium comprises the inner cellular lining of blood and lymphatic vessels. The endothelial cells (EC) that make up this cellular layer demonstrate remarkable phenotypic diversity and plasticity. Genetic programming, microenvironmental cues (from mural cells, stromal cells and the extracellular matrix) and epigenetic changes all influence EC phenotype (Aird, 2007).

Normal ECs from different blood vessels and microvascular ECs from different anatomical sites can be distinguished based on their unique and characteristic gene expression profiles (Chi et al., 2003; Seaman et al., 2007). Chi et al. (2003) used microarray techniques to evaluate the expression profiles of 53 human endothelial cell lines derived from arteries, veins and microvessels representing 14 distinct locations. They described patterns of gene expression that could distinguish endothelial cells between veins and arteries, large and small vessels, and identify endothelial cells with specialised functional roles (Chi et al., 2003).

Normally in the adult, endothelial cells are 'quiescent'. They do not actively proliferate, and have an average lifespan of more than a year (Aird, 2007). Yet, certain EC populations undergo regular, transient bursts of physiological angiogenesis; for example during corpus luteum formation in the ovary, endometrial regeneration during the female menstrual cycle, pregnancy, and wound healing (Conway & Carmeliet, 2004; Liu & Deisseroth, 2006). Recent studies have demonstrated that gene expression patterns differ in ECs derived from tissues undergoing physiological and pathophysiological angiogenesis (Seaman et al., 2007; van Beijnum et al., 2006).

DISTINGUISHING CHARACTERISTICS OF TUMOUR ENDOTHELIUM

The tumour vasculature is very different from normal vasculature, and tumour vessels are often described as 'immature' (Carmeliet & Jain, 2000; Tozer et al., 2005). Tumour vessel walls are poorly developed, with endothelial cells that are often irregularly shaped and form a discontinuous endothelial cell lining. They are characterized by a structurally abnormal basement membrane, a poor investiture of mural cells (vascular smooth muscle cells and pericytes), and poorly formed connections between pericytes and endothelial cells. These abnormalities in tumour vasculature contribute to increased vascular permeability and the consequent development of high tumour interstitial pressure. Tumour vessel architecture is chaotic and tortuous, and the vessels form complex branching patterns with frequent anastomoses. These features combine to cause tumour blood flow to be irregular and sluggish, with frequent fluxes in directional flow (Tozer et al., 2005). With its poor blood supply, the tumour microenvironment becomes hypoxic (low in oxygen), nutrient starved (low glucose levels), acidic (due to increased lactate production from tumour cells converting to anaerobic glycolysis), and oxidatively stressed (Neri & Bicknell, 2005). In this tumour microenvironment, endothelial cells become uncoupled from their normal extracellular environmental cues and experience phenotypic drift (Aird, 2007). They change from their normal quiescent form to become activated, with ECs demonstrating pro-adhesive, antigen-presenting and pro-coagulant activities (Aird, 2007). Under hypoxic stimulus, the tumour endothelium rapidly proliferates, and new tumour vasculature is formed by processes that include angiogenesis (formation of new blood vessels from existing vessels), vasculogenesis (formation of new blood vessels by recruitment of endothelial precursor cells from the bone marrow), vascular co-option, intussusception (splitting of primary vessels by transcapillary pillars), and vascular mimicry (tumour cells form mosaic vessel with endothelial cells) (Carmeliet & Jain, 2000).

Identification of Molecules Specific to Tumour Endothelium

The safe and effective use of therapeutic modalities against tumour vasculature is dependent on finding strategies that effectively discriminate between normal and tumour-associated vasculature. Despite the enormous phenotypic diversity displayed by ECs, researchers have developed and employed novel methods to identify tumour-specific EC markers (Table 1) that might be used therapeutically.

These methods have included *in vitro* endothelial cell culture in conditions designed to simulate the tumour microenvironment, data-mining and *in silico* analysis of public genomic databases with subsequent validation using molecular expression techniques (Ho et al., 2003; Huminiecki & Bicknell, 2000), Serial Analysis of Gene Expression (SAGE) technology (St Croix et al., 2000), oligonucleotide and cDNA array technologies (Kerbel, 2001), subtractive proteomic mapping of the endothelial surface (Oh et al., 2004), gene-trap expression screening (Hirashima et al., 2004; Stanford et al., 1998), and *in vivo* phage display technology (Balestrieri & Napoli, 2007; Neri & Bicknell, 2005).

However, many of the endothelial-cell specific markers identified by these studies are critical for both physiological and pathophysiological angiogenesis, and clinical side-effects of therapies targeted to these molecules have recently emerged (Carmeliet, 2005; Kramer & Lipp, 2007). In an effort to identify markers that are capable of distinguishing between physiological and pathological angiogenesis, St Croix's group have recently published SAGE analysis of gene expression patterns in ECs derived from the blood vessels of normal murine liver, regenerating liver, and tumour-bearing livers (Seaman et al., 2007). This study revealed that many of the genes over-expressed in physiological angiogenesis were involved in cell-cycle control, whereas those specific to tumour angiogenesis were primarily cell surface molecules making them appealing potential targets for tumour-specific vascular therapy. Several of these (e.g.: CD276, CD137; Table 1) are thought to be involved in regulating inflammatory or autoimmune response (Seaman et al., 2007).

Table 1. Genes over-expressed by the endothelium during angiogenesis

Gene	Comment
Aminopeptidase-N, -A, -P [1,6]	Cell surface proteins upregulated on tumour endothelium.
Annexin A1, Annexin A8 [1]	Annexin 1 is preferentially expressed and accessible on tumour endothelium.
ASPP1 (apoptosis-stimulating protein of p53) [1]	p53 binding protein.
CD24 [1]	Induced by hypoxia in HUVEC.
CD31 (PECAM)-1 [2,3]	Expressed in ECs and hematopoietic cells.
CD59 [4]	Overexpressed in colorectal carcinoma ECs, localised to luminal EC membrane.
CD66 [1]	Upregulated on tumour endothelium.
CD105 (Endoglin) [3,5]	Co-receptor for transforming growth factor β (TGFβ), localised to ECs of normal and tumour tissues, promoter regulated by transcription factor over-expressed in tumour associated vasculature.
CD276 (B7-H3), CD137 (4-1BB) [3]	Murine tumour endothelial markers, involved in regulation of inflammatory or autoimmune responses; CD276 mRNA and protein detected at low levels in tumour cells.
CD133 [5]	Endothelial progenitor cell (EPC) marker.

Table 1. (Continued)

Gene	Comment
Claudin 3, Claudin 5 [1,3]	Claudin 3 induced by hypoxia in HUVEC.
Collagen type Iα1, type IVα1 [4]	Overexpressed on endothelium of colon and breast carcinoma and glioma.
CXCR4 [1]	Induced by hypoxia in HUVEC.
DEL1 (Developmental endothelial locus 1) [1]	Embryonic endothelial-cell-specific adhesion molecule that binds to integrin V3 receptor.
Delta4 [1]	Notch ligand expressed at sites of physiological and tumour angiogenesis, induced by hypoxia and VEGF.
Gene	**Comment**
Ephrin A5, Ephrin A7 [1]	Upregulated on tumour endothelium.
Endomucin [1]	Transmembrane cell surface molecule.
EndoPDI (endothelial-specific protein disulphide isomerase) [1]	Hypoxia-induced gene expressed predominantly by endothelium.
Endothelin-1 and pro-endothelin-1 [5]	Promoter regulated by transcription factor that is over-expressed in tumour associated vasculature.
E-selectin [2,5]	Expressed in activated endothelium; expression largely confined to post-capillary venules.
Fibronectin EDB (extra-domain B) [1]	Abundant in many aggressive solid tumours, vascular or diffuse stromal patterns of expression.
Glut-1 (Glucose transporter-1) [3]	Blood-brain barrier marker expressed on the luminal surface of brain endothelium, hypoxia induced.
HES (Hairy/enhancer of split) [1]	Preferential endothelial expression.
HMGB1 (High-mobility group protein-1) [4]	Secreted cytokine and nonhistone DNA-binding protein, overexpressed in colorectal carcinoma ECs, also expressed in stromal and epithelial cells.
ICAM-1 (intercellular adhesion molecule-1) [2]	Expressed in many vascular and non-vascular cell types.
ICAM-2 (intercellular adhesion molecule-2) [5]	Promoter regulated by transcription factor over-expressed in tumour associated vasculature.
IGFBP7 (Insulin-like growth factor binding protein 7) [4]	Secreted molecule with growth factor modulating function, pan-endothelial marker overexpressed in colorectal carcinoma ECs.
Integrins $\alpha V\beta 3$, $\alpha V\beta 5$ [1,3]	Cell surface molecules that potentiate cell invasion and proliferation.
MMP-1, -2, -3, -9, -10 (Matrix metalloproteinases) [4,6]	Zinc-dependent proteases upregulated on angiogenic endothelial cells.
Myeloperoxidase [1]	Upregulated on tumour endothelium.
Nucleolin [1]	Cell surface molecule recognised by tumour-homing peptide F3. Upregulated on tumour endothelium.
Nrp-1 (Neuropilin-1) [5]	VEGF co-receptor.
PAI-1 (plasminogen activator inhibitor) [2]	Site-specific expression in mice.
P-selectin [2]	Expressed in ECs and megakaryocytes, expressed preferentially in postcapillary venules.
PlGF [3] (Placental Growth Factor)	Important for pathological, but not developmental, angiogenesis. Also present in heart ECs [3].
PLOD1, PLOD2 (procollagen lysyl hydroxylase) [1]	Induced by hypoxia in HUVEC.
ROBO4 (Roundabout-4) [1]	Strongly expressed in developing embryo, only present in adults at sites of active angiogenesis.
TEM1, TEM5, TEM7, TEM8 (Tumour endothelial marker) [1]	TEM1 is identical to endosialin, predominantly expressed by fibroblasts and pericytes associated with tumour vessels.
Tenascin-C [1,3,5]	Extracellular matrix glycoprotein.
Tetranectin [1]	Induced by hypoxia in HUVEC.

Table 1. (Continued)

Gene	Comment
TF [5] (Tissue Factor)	Upregulated in tumour-associated vasculature.
TFPI (Tissue factor pathway inhibitor) [2]	Site-specific expression, primarily in microvascular endothelium.
Thrombomodulin [2]	Expressed in ECs, keratinocytes, trophoblasts and leukocytes.
Tie1, Tie2 [5]	Involved in vascular differentiation, promoter regulated by transcription factor over-expressed in tumour-associated vasculature.
Transferrin receptor [1]	Upregulated in tumour-associated vasculature.
Urokinase receptors [5]	Upregulated in tumour-associated vasculature.
VCAM-1 (Vascular cell adhesion molecule-1) [2]	Expressed in many vascular and non-vascular cell types.
Gene	**Comment**
VE-cadherin (vascular-endothelial cadherin) [2,3]	Localised to ECs of normal and tumour tissues, also expressed in trophoblasts and fetal stem cells.
VEGF	Promotes angiogenesis, increases vascular permeability, contributes to endothelial cell survival, promoter regulated by transcription factor over-expressed in tumour-associated vasculature. Upregulated by hypoxia.
VEGF receptors 1, 2, 3 [5]	VEGFR1 &2 promoters regulated by transcription factors over-expressed in tumour associated vasculature.
Vimentin [4]	Intermediate filament protein, overexpressed in colorectal carcinoma ECs, also detected in normal ECs.
Vitamin D binding protein [1]	Upregulated on tumour endothelium.
vWF (von Willebrand factor) [2]	Expressed predominantly on the venous side of the circulation.

Table was adapted from: Neri and Bicknell, 2005 [1], Aird, 2007 [2], Seaman et al., 2007 [3], van Beijnum et al., 2006 [4], Bazan-Peregrino et al., 2007 [5], Balestieri and Napoli, 2007 [6].

As a further refinement, Griffioen's Group has investigated cancer site-specific tumour endothelial cell markers in colorectal carcinoma (van Beijnum et al., 2006). They used suppression subtractive hybridisation to compare gene expression profiles of ECs isolated from non-angiogenic normal tissues, non-malignant angiogenic placental tissue, and colon carcinoma tissue (van Beijnum et al., 2006). Results from this study demonstrated that genes over-expressed in physiological angiogenesis represent those involved in cellular metabolism and protein regulation (early stage events in angiogenesis), whereas those specific to tumour angiogenesis in colorectal carcinoma were predominantly associated with cytoskeleton organisation and extracellular matrix remodelling (late stage events in angiogenesis). Antibody targeting of four cell-surface expressed or secreted proteins (vimentin, CD59, HMGB1, IGFBP7; Table 1) identified by this study as tumour specific EC markers, inhibited angiogenesis *in vitro* and *in vivo* (van Beijnum et al., 2006). These may thus represent novel factors for targeted gene delivery for gene therapy.

GENE DIRECTED ENZYME PRODRUG THERAPY

Criteria to consider when developing GDEPT strategies include the following: the enzyme should be a monomer, active at physiological pH, and cause rapid and efficient prodrug activation even at low concentrations of the substrate. This requires a prodrug with low Km and high Kcat, and no co-substrate requirements or further catalysis by other enzymes. The prodrug should freely diffuse or be actively transported into target cells, and once converted, a bystander effect (see below) should be observed. The active metabolites should be cell cycle-independent to destroy both cycling and quiescent cells. The half-life of the metabolites should be long enough to allow transport to surrounding cells but short enough to avoid systemic toxicity. Finally, the enzyme-prodrug combination should be able to kill a wide range of tumour cell populations with high differential toxicity. However, it is difficult to design GDEPT systems which meet all of the above criteria.

Inhibition of DNA replication is a common theme among several enzyme-prodrug systems, as tumour cells and associated structures generally have a higher proliferative activity than the relatively quiescent normal tissue (exceptions may include bone marrow, intestinal epithelium and hair follicles; typical tissues known to be affected by chemotherapy treatment). However, inhibition of DNA replication restricts cell kill to the S-phase of the cell cycle, limiting the length of effectiveness of the treatment. In addition, a significant proportion of tumour cells are known to be growth arrested, yet metabolically active. Other enzyme-prodrug combinations that cause inhibition of RNA and protein processing act throughout the cell cycle and are not restricted to proliferating cells, and thus have potential for increased cell kill.

Bystander Effect

GDEPT allows the killing of both transgenic and non-transgenic cells due to the 'bystander effect': the transfer of toxic metabolites from transgenic cells to neighbouring non-transgenic cells, causing cell death. This process is especially important when the delivery of the enzyme-encoding gene to cells shows poor efficiency. Several mechanisms explain the bystander effect, such as the transfer of toxic metabolites by diffusion or active transfer (by apoptotic vesicles or gap junctions), anti-tumour immune stimulation and the transduction of neighbouring tumour endothelial cells (Ram et al., 1993).

Prodrug-activating enzymes can be either of human or foreign origin. Enzymes of non-human origin elicit an immune response, which can be disadvantageous, as it can lead to enzyme inactivation, but could also be beneficial by causing immune-mediated tumour regression (Xu & McLeod, 2001). Introduction of endogenous mammalian enzymes generally does not generate an immune response, but increases the risk of prodrug activation in non-target tissues. Mutation of endogenous enzymes can overcome the potential for systemic toxicity by altering the specificity for prodrug conversion (Xu & McLeod, 2001).

An extended list of novel and proven enzyme-prodrug systems are shown in Table 2; below we discuss the four GDEPT systems which thus far have reached clinical trials (summarised in Figure 2).

Table 2. Enzyme-prodrug systems used in gene therapy

Enzyme (origin)	**Prodrug**	**Released metabolite or cytotoxin**	**Stage of development**	**References**
β-2-alcohol dehydrogenase (human)	Ethanol	Acetaldehyde	*In vivo*	(Savage et al., 2004)
Biphenyl hydrolase-like protein (human)	Val-ACV, Val-GCV	ACV, GCV	*In vitro*	(Kim et al., 2004)
Carboxylesterase (human, rabbit, rat)	Irinotecan Capecitabine Paclitaxel-2-ethylcarbonate dpVP-16	SN-38 5-FU Paclitaxel Etoposide (VP16)	*In vivo*	(Oosterhoff et al., 2003)
Carboxypeptidase A (human, rat)	Methotrexate-α-peptides	Methotrexate	*In vivo*	(Hao et al., 2006)
Carboxypeptidase G2 (*Pseudomonas* R16)	CMDA ZD-2767P Self-immolative prodrugs	CMBA Phenol-bis-iodo nitrogen mustard Alkylating agents, anthracycline antibiotics	*In vivo*	(Davies et al., 2005; Friedlos et al., 2002; Schepelmann et al., 2007)
Cytochrome P450 (Human: CYP2B1, 2B6, 2C8, 2C9, 2C18, 3A), (Rat: CYP2B10), (Rabbit: CYP4B1 ±CYPOR), (Dog: CYP2B11)	Oxazaphosphorines: CPA and IFO Ipomeanol, 2-aminoantracene, dacarbazine, procarbazine Acetaminophen	Alkylating agents (4-hydroxy forms) Toxic metabolites NABQI (*N*-acetyl benzoquinone imine)	Phase I/II (CYP2B1/ IFO, CYP2B6/ CPA)	(Braybrooke et al., 2005; Salmons et al., 2003)
Cytosine deaminase (±UPRT) (*E. coli, S. cerevisiae*)	5-fluorocytosine (5-FC)	5-fluorouracil (5-FU)	Phase I/II (CD/5-FC)	(Freytag et al., 2003; Nemunaitis et al., 2003a; Nemunaitis et al., 2003b; Pandha et al., 1999)
D-Amino acid oxidase (yeast: *Rhodotorula gracilis*)	D-alanine	Hydrogen peroxide	*In vitro*	(Stegman et al., 1998)
Deoxycytidine kinase (human)	Cytosine arabinoside, dFdC	Monophosphorylated forms	*In vivo*	(Manome et al., 1996; Vernejoul et al., 2006)
Deoxyribonucleotide kinase (*Drosophila melanogaster*)	Analogues of pyrimidine and purine 2'-deoxynucleosides e.g. GCV, BVDU, araT	Analogues of pyrimidine and purine 2'-deoxy nucleotide mono phosphorylated forms	*In vitro*	(Kamiya et al., 2006; Zheng et al., 2000)
DT-diaphorase (human, rat)	Bioreductive agents such as EO9	Reduced forms	*In vivo*	(Sharp et al., 2000)
Folylpolyglutamyl synthetase (human)	Edatrexate	Antifolate polyglutamate derivatives	*In vivo*	(Aghi et al., 1999b)
β-Galactosidase (*E. coli*)	Self-immolative prodrugs from anthracycline antibiotics (Daun02)	Anthracycline antibiotics (daunomycin)	*In vitro*	(Farquhar et al., 2002)

Table 2. (Continued)

Enzyme (origin)	**Prodrug**	**Released metabolite or cytotoxin**	**Stage of development**	**References**
β-Glucuronidase (human, *E. coli*, mouse)	Self-immolative doxorubicin prodrug (HMR-1826 with Bax)	Doxorubicin	*In vitro*	(Miller et al., 2004)
Glutathione S-transferase (mouse)	PABA/NO	Nitric oxide	*In vitro*	(Findlay et al., 2004; Townsend et al., 2006)
Horseradish peroxidase (plant: horseradish)	Indole-3-acetic acid and derivatives Acetominophen	3-methylene-2-oxindole NABQI	*In vitro*	(Tupper et al., 2004)
Enzyme (origin)	**Prodrug**	**Released metabolite or cytotoxin**	**Stage of development**	**References**
β-Lactamase (*E. coli*)	Self-immolative cephalosporin prodrugs	Alkylating agents, Vinca alkaloids, anthracycline antibiotics	*In vitro*	(Grant & Smyth, 2004; Svensson et al., 1998)
Linamarase (Cassava plant)	Linamarin	Cyanide	*In vivo*	(Cortes et al., 1998; Link et al., 2006)
Methionine α,γ-lyase (yeast: *Pseudomonas* putida)	Selenomethionine	Methylselenol	*In vivo*	(Gupta et al., 2003; Miki et al., 2001)
NADPH-cytochrome P450 reductase (human)	Tirapazamine, EO9, RSU1069/misonidazole	Reduced metabolites	*In vivo*	(Cowen et al., 2004)
Nitroreductase (*E. coli*)	CB1954 and analogues Self-immolative prodrugs	Alkylating agents (N-acetoxy derivatives) Alkylating agents, pyrazolidines, enediynes	Phase I (NTR/CB1954)	(Palmer et al., 2004)
Penicillin G amidase (*E. coli*)	Modified camptothecin conjugated to PEG	Toxic metabolites	*In vitro*	(Gopin et al., 2006)
Purine nucleoside phosphorylase (*E. coli*)	Purine nucleosides MeP-dR, F-araA, F-dAdo	6-methylpurine 2-fluoroadenine	*In vivo*	(Curlee et al., 2004)
Pyrimidine nucleoside phosphorylase (human)	5'-deoxy-5-fluorouridine	5-FU	*In vivo*	(Nagata et al., 2002)
Thymidine kinase (*Herpes simplex* virus, *Varicella zoster* virus, *Equine herpes* virus)	Modified purine and pyrimidine nucleosides: GCV, E-GCV, ACV, valacyclovir, araM, araT, BVDU FIAU, purine and pyrimidine nucleosides, araM	Monophosphorylated nucleotide analogues Monophosphorylated nucleotide analogues	Phase III (HSV-TK/GCV)	(Immonen et al., 2004; Rainov, 2000)
Thymidine phosphorylase (human)	Pyrimidine analogues e.g. 5'-DFUR	5-fluorodeoxyuridine monophosphate	*In vivo*	(Evrard et al., 1999)
Tyrosinase (human)	Hydroxyphenyl propanol, N-acetyl-4-S-cysteaminylphenol	Toxic metabolites	*In vitro*	(Simonova et al., 2000)

Table 2. (Continued)

Enzyme (origin)	**Prodrug**	**Released metabolite or cytotoxin**	**Stage of development**	**References**
Tyrosine hydroxylase (mouse)	3,4-dihydroxyphenyl carbamate derivative of etoposide	Etoposide	*In vitro*	(Jikai et al., 2003)
Uracil phosphoribosyl transferase (*E. coli*, yeast: *S. cerevisiae*)	5-FU	5-FdUMP	*In vivo*	(Seo et al., 2005; Sunamura et al., 2004)
Xanthine-guanine phosphoribosyl transferase (*E. coli*)	6-thiopurines	6-thiopurine nucleoside	*In vivo*	(Ono et al., 1997)

Table adapted from (Aghi et al., 2000; Niculescu-Duvaz & Springer, 2004; Portsmouth et al., 2007).

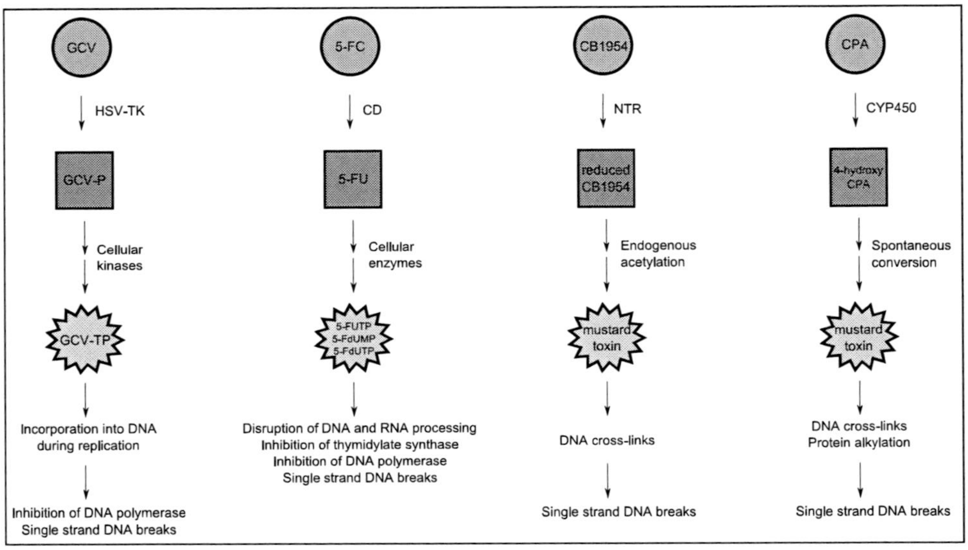

Figure 2. Schematic representation of the mode of action of the four enzyme prodrug systems that have reached clinical testing (Adapted from Dachs et al., 2005).

Herpes Simplex Virus Type 1 Thymidine Kinase with Ganciclovir

Herpes simplex virus type 1 thymidine kinase (HSV-TK) with ganciclovir (GCV) has been tested as a gene therapy system for over 20 years (Moolten, 1986) and has reached phase III clinical trials (Immonen et al., 2004; Rainov, 2000). GCV is an acyclic guanosine analogue used to treat viral infections, including *Herpes simplex* virus. GCV is phosphorylated by HSV-TK to a monophosphate (GCV-MP), and cellular kinases complete the conversion to the active triphosphate, GCV-TP (Portsmouth et al., 2007). GCV-TP is structurally similar to 2'-deoxyguanosine triphosphate and is incorporated into DNA during replication, causing inhibition of DNA polymerase, rapid chain termination and the formation of single strand breaks, leading to cell death during S-phase (Balzarini et al., 1993) (Figure 2).

Human cells express both cytosolic (TK1) and mitochondrial (TK2) TK enzymes but these endogenous enzymes have limited ability to convert GCV compared to HSV-TK (Aghi et al., 2000). In fact, Kuriyama et al. (1999a) showed that stable expression of the HSV-TK gene could increase cellular sensitivity to GCV by up to 2000-fold in a mouse hepatocarcinoma cell line.

The bystander effect induced by the HSV-TK/GCV combination relies on gap junction-dependent transfer of GCV-MP to neighbouring non-transgenic cells where it is converted to active GCV-TP by cellular kinases, causing cell death (Mesnil & Yamasaki, 2000). Aside from gap junctions, immune-mediated effects and soluble factors also contribute to enhanced tumour cell destruction. Death of transgenic tumour cells can stimulate recognition of tumour antigens leading to local inflammation and immune-mediated death of non-transgenic tumour cells, which is thought to be a major factor in the success of *in vivo* gene therapy trials (Kuriyama et al., 2004). It is of note that GCV causes immuno-suppression by bone marrow toxicity, which may lead to an underestimation of the involvement of the immune system in mediating a bystander effect.

Studies in animals have shown that the amount of GCV required to destroy a tumour is toxic to normal, metabolically active but non-proliferating tissues, leading to side effects such as leukopenia, immunosuppression, diarrhoea, liver dysfunction and increased mortality (van der Eb et al., 1998). This process involves accumulation of GCV in the mitochondria and possible inhibition of mitochondrial DNA polymerases (van der Eb et al., 2003). However, phase I human clinical trials of the HSV-TK/GCV combination have not reported major adverse effects in dose escalation studies (Portsmouth et al., 2007). The maximum tolerated dose in humans is much lower than in animals (Greco & Dachs, 2001) which may account for differences in adverse effects.

Because of its toxicity, efforts are underway to develop derivatives of GCV and mutants of HSV-TK. HSV-TK is able to convert a number of substrates, such as the thymidine nucleoside analogue, araT (Aghi et al., 2000), BVDU (an inhibitor of thymidylate synthetase) (De Clercq, 2005), and an elaidic acid ester derivative of GCV, E-GCV (which requires intracellular esterases for conversion to GCV, leading to increased length of GCV exposure) (Balzarini et al., 1998). Long-circulating liposome-encapsulated GCV also causes extended release of GCV over a longer time period. It was three-fold more effective in inhibiting tumour growth compared to standard GCV administration *in vivo* (Kajiwara et al., 2007).

Another interesting diversion from the HSV-TK/GCV combination is the use of mutant *Drosophila melanogaster* deoxyribonucleoside kinase engineered to convert GCV (Solaroli et al., 2007). However, osteosarcoma cells were still 100-fold more sensitive to the HSV-TK/GCV combination compared to mutant nucleoside kinase/GCV and further development of this novel strategy is required.

HSV-TK has a higher affinity for its natural substrate, thymidine, than for GCV. Research has therefore focused on the creation of HSV-TK mutants to increase substrate specificity for GCV and hence allow the use of lower doses of the potentially immunosuppressive agent. Several drug-specific mutant HSV-TK proteins have been created by remodelling the active (nucleoside binding) site (Black et al., 2001; Black et al., 1996). An increase of 5 to 300-fold in cellular sensitivity has been reported for these mutants (Black et al., 2001; Wiewrodt et al., 2003). In addition, Kokoris et al. (2000) identified six mutants of HSV-TK that show increased substrate specificity towards acyclovir (ACV), another nucleoside analogue.

Fusion of guanylate kinase to HSV-TK mediated increased cell killing with GCV, via increased conversion of GCV-MP to the diphosphate GCV-DP, aiding in the conversion to the toxic metabolite, GCV-TP (Willmon et al., 2006).

Glioblastomas (and other high-grade malignancies) often have low expression of the major gap junction protein, connexin (Mesnil, 2002), which alters their susceptibility to the gap junction-mediated bystander effect of the HSV-TK/GCV combination. In an attempt to overcome this hurdle, HSV-TK has been fused with an arginine-rich repeat peptide from HSV-2 US11, resulting in intercellular spread of the TK enzyme (Luo et al., 2007). Alternatively, fusion of proteins with the HSV-1 VP22 protein has been shown to increase intercellular trafficking (Lemken et al., 2007a; Lemken et al., 2007b).

Results from clinical trials in humans thus far have not lived up to expectations. Follow-up of selected patients from a phase I trial to assess dosing and safety in malignant pleural mesothelioma treated with one high dose of adenovirus-delivered HSV-TK concluded that it was safe and led to long-term response and survival in two patients (Sterman et al., 2005). A non-randomised trial tested both retroviral and adenoviral transfer of HSV-TK in glioma patients, indicating that patients treated with adenoviral vector delivery had increased survival compared to retroviral delivery and controls (Sandmair et al., 2000). Most retroviruses are only able to transduce replicating cells by virtue of the fact that they insert their genetic material into the host cell genome.

In the first transcriptionally targeted gene therapy clinical trial, Hinata et al. (2006) used the HSV-TK gene under control of the osteocalcin promoter, and in combination with valacyclovir, to treat advanced prostate cancer patients in a phase I/II trial. Adenoviral delivery was used. Oral valacyclovir (the L-valine ester of ACV) has better bioavailability and gives higher plasma concentrations of ACV, with a reduced dosing regimen, compared to oral ACV administration (Beutner, 1995). Oral valacyclovir therefore increases patient compliance and is a cheaper and effective alternative to intravenous ACV. The authors reported on the outcomes of three patients treated with low dose viral vector, one of which showed a partial response. Fujita et al. (2006) also report the use of the adenoviral-delivered HSV-TK gene with valacyclovir treatment in prostate cancer patients. They measured immune responses to the treatment and found systemic T-cell responses. An immune response was also observed by Ayala et al. (2006), who treated prostate cancer patients in a phase I/II trial with adenoviral-delivered HSV-TK/GCV. Increased apoptosis and decreased microvessel density in tumours was observed.

HSV-TK/GCV has reached Phase III clinical trials, targeting brain tumours. The first trial treated patients with glioblastoma multiforme using retroviral transfer (Rainov, 2000). Although the safety of the procedure was demonstrated, there was a poor rate of delivery of the HSV-TK gene, which only followed the needle track. Overall, the results of the trial were disappointing and showed no difference in time to tumour progression, or overall survival time. In comparison, Immonen et al. (2004) treated patients with malignant glioma with adenoviral-delivered HSV-TK/GCV. They reported a significant increase in survival of the patients (time until death or surgery for recurrence) from 39 to 70 weeks. This was the first report of a randomised, controlled trial showing increased survival of patients treated with HSV-TK/GCV. They attribute the increased survival of patients to use of adenoviral delivery compared to retroviral delivery, hence improving the efficiency of gene transfer and increasing expression of the transgene.

Cytosine Deaminase (CD) with 5-Fluorocytosine (5-FC)

5-fluorouracil (5-FU) is the standard anti-cancer chemotherapeutic agent used to treat colon cancer (and pancreatic, breast, and head and neck cancers to a lesser extent); it has radio-sensitising properties (Zhang et al., 2003). The inherent toxicity of 5-FU can lead to side effects including disruption of the gastrointestinal and haematological systems. 5-fluorocytosine (5-FC) is an anti-fungal agent which is fairly non-toxic to normal human cells and is converted to the toxic 5-FU by cytosine deaminase (CD), an enzyme found in bacteria and fungi. CD from *Saccharomyces cerevisiae* has a higher affinity for 5-FC (22-fold lower Km) compared to the *Escherichia coli* CD (Kievit et al., 1999). Metabolism of 5-FU by intracellular enzymes leads to the production of active metabolites 5-FUTP, 5-FdUMP and 5-FdUTP (Dachs et al., 2005). 5-FUTP incorporates into RNA, disrupts RNA processing and interrupts protein synthesis; 5-FdUMP irreversibly inhibits thymidylate synthase, preventing formation of 2-deoxythymidine 5'-triphosphate, so that 5-FdUTP is incorporated into DNA, causing strand-nicked DNA and inhibition of replication leading to cell death by apoptosis (Kurozumi et al., 2004) (Figure 2). These effects are not cell cycle-specific, but appear dependent on active metabolism, resulting in decreased cytotoxicity under extreme hypoxia *in vitro* (Dachs et al., 2005). However, decreased cytotoxicity has been overcome by targeting the CD/5-FC system to hypoxic regions *in vitro* and *in vivo* using hypoxia-inducible promoters, containing hypoxia-responsive element (HRE) enhancers, to control transgene expression (Chen et al., 2007; Lee et al., 2007; Wang et al., 2005).

In vivo experiments have shown that successful regression of transduced tumour cells may depend on the inherent immunogenicity of the tumour cell line (Kuriyama et al., 1999b). Tumour regression could also be caused by a cytotoxic T cell immune response generated by expression of the CD enzyme alone (Haack et al., 2000).

Uracil phosphoribosyl transferase (UPRT) is a bacterial enzyme that converts uracil to uracil monophosphate (UMP), which contributes to DNA and RNA synthesis. UPRT also converts 5-FU to 5-FUMP and represents the first step in the activation pathway. UPRT has been used to sensitise cells to low concentrations of 5-FU by aiding in its conversion, therefore increasing the cytotoxic effects of 5-FC administration *in vitro* and *in vivo* (Adachi et al., 2000; Koyama et al., 2000). A fusion of the CD and UPRT genes has been created (Chung-Faye et al., 2001; Erbs et al., 2000; Graepler et al., 2005). Adenoviral delivery of a CD/UPRT fusion gene *ex vivo*, into primary tumour cells, isolated from patients with metastatic cancer that have developed resistance to 5-FU, sensitised the cells to treatment with 5-FC (Richard et al., 2007). This effect was evident in both fast and slowly proliferating samples and appeared better than the CD/5-FC combination alone.

Unger et al. (2007) have tested an 'enrichment-eradication' method to increase the bystander effect in tumours. Mice were inoculated with neuroblastoma cells carrying the CD/UPRT fusion gene, and essential *de novo* pyrimidine synthesis in the mice was blocked using N-(phosphonacetyl)-L-aspartate (PALA), followed by cytosine administration. Cells expressing CD/UPRT were able to survive by converting cytosine to UMP via a 'salvage pathway', but non-transgenic tumour cells had reduced survival, thereby enriching the tumour for transgenic cells. The transgenic cells could then be successfully eradicated using 5-FC, leading to a 'near complete' bystander effect and decreased tumour growth *in vivo* (Unger et al., 2007). Although the use of PALA as a blocker of pyrimidine synthesis has potential to cause systemic toxicity, the levels used were not sufficient to cause severe toxicity in the mouse model, and perhaps reflect the fact that no tumour cures were observed *in vivo*.

There is cross-talk between BVDU, an agent used to treat HSV-1 infection and tested as a prodrug for HSV-TK-based GDEPT, and dihydropyrimidine dehydrogenase, an enzyme which degrades 5-FU in the liver. BVDU is reversibly degraded to BVU by thymidine phosphorylase, and BVU directly and irreversibly inhibits dihydropyrimidine dehydrogenase. Therefore, BVDU has been shown to enhance the toxicity of 5-FU, and a CD/5-FC GDEPT system, to give an increased anti-tumour effect (De Clercq, 2005).

To increase the number of cells expressing CD and therefore increasing cell kill, fusion proteins of HSV-1 VP22 with CD have been constructed (Lee et al., 2006; Wybranietz et al., 2001). VP22 or GALV (a glycoprotein from the gibbon ape leukemia virus, which causes cell fusion) were also added to CD/UPRT, increasing cytotoxicity and bystander effects (Lemken et al., 2007a; Simpson et al., 2006).

Alanine-scanning mutagenesis (separately replacing alanine for eleven of the amino acids in the active site of bacterial CD), and random mutagenesis of CD by error-prone polymerase chain reaction (PCR), produced several CD mutants with favorable properties (Mahan et al., 2004a; Mahan et al., 2004b). The mutant CD enzyme D314A has been trialled in human glioma xenografts in mice, with or without ionising radiation treatment, with promising results (Kaliberov et al., 2007).

CD/5-FC has been tested in several Phase I clinical trials. Pandha et al. (1999) reported the first phase I trial to use CD in human patients. CD transgene expression was targeted using the erbB2 promoter. A transgenic plasmid was injected into skin nodules of breast cancer patients. Gene expression was detected, and some lesions regressed following 5-FC administration. Importantly, safety of CD expression was demonstrated.

CD/5-FC, using 18F-labelled 5-FC, has been used for PET imaging (Haberkorn et al., 1996). Recent studies have shown that MRI imaging could predict *in vivo* outcome for the CD/5-FC combination, when the gene was delivered by attenuated *Salmonella typhimurium* (Dubois et al., 2007).

Escherichia Coli Nitroreductase (NTR) with CB1954

CB1954 (2,4-dinitro-5-aziridinylbenzamide) can be reduced efficiently to the toxic metabolite by the rat, or to a lesser extend, the human, DT-diaphorase (Knox et al., 2003; Searle et al., 2004). Other enzymes that convert CB1954 include DT-diaphorase 2 (a latent nitroreductase found in some human tumours) which reduces CB1954 3000 times more effectively than human DT-diaphorase 1 (Knox et al., 2000). It requires dihydronicotinamide riboside (a non-biogenic compound) as a co-substrate. However, the *E. coli* two-electron nitroreductase (NTR) has proved catalytically superior to all mammalian DT-diaphorases. NTR converts CB1954 to the 2- and 4-hydroxy forms by reduction in the presence of the electron donor, NAD(P)H. Subsequent conversion of the 4-hydroxy form by non-enzymatic endogenous acetylation produces 5-(aziridin-1-yl)-4-acetoxyamino-2-nitrobenzamide, a mustard toxin that causes DNA cross-linking (Knox et al., 2003) (Figure 2). Cell death was shown to be cell-cycle independent; thus killing both proliferating and non-proliferating (arrested) cells (Bridgewater et al., 1995). Importantly, the NTR/CB1954 combination is effective during tumour hypoxia, as the conversion to toxin is oxygen-independent. The NTR/CB1954 system has also been shown to sensitise hypoxic cells to radiation (Knox et al., 2003).

The CB1954 metabolite(s) are freely diffusible and give rise to an efficient bystander effect (Bridgewater et al., 1997). The metabolites are much more toxic than the CB1954 prodrug, with a high differential toxicity (Helsby et al., 2004). Rejection of a re-challenge with unmodified tumour cells in mice previously exposed to tumour cells with the NTR/CB1954 combination has been attributed to an immune-mediated bystander effect (Green et al., 2003). However, introduction of mouse GM-CSF to stimulate an immune response in mouse colorectal tumours treated with NTR/CB1954 did not significantly increase survival (Green et al., 2003).

New prodrugs have been designed as *E. coli* NTR substrates, including the chloromustard SN23862, and the bromomustard SN24927, which are more cytotoxic than CB1954 following conversion by NTR (Wilson et al., 2002). The bystander effect of NTR/CB1954 has been quantified in three-dimensional multilayer cell cultures and bystander killing was more effective in multilayers than monolayers (Wilson et al., 2002). SN23862 was more effective in producing a bystander effect than CB1954 in these systems, and bystander killing correlated with the lipophilicity of the prodrug.

Directed evolution by error-prone PCR of the YieF enzyme from *E. coli* was used to identify more potent CB1954-reducing enzymes (Barak et al., 2006). The mutant enzyme in combination with CB1954 was shown to kill human tumour cells much more effectively than the wild-type YieF and NTR enzymes. Similarly, other groups have characterised *E. coli* NTR single and double mutants created by amino acid substitution or identified by SOS response triggering, which showed enhanced efficiency of CB1954 conversion *in vitro* (Grove et al., 2003; Guise et al., 2007; Race et al., 2007). Jackson et al. (2006) substituted unnatural amino acids into NTR and found mutants with 30-fold increased sensitivity to CB1954 *in vitro* compared to wild-type NTR.

NTR with CB1954 has reached Phase I trials in patients with liver cancer (Palmer et al., 2004). Adenoviral delivery of the NTR enzyme by intratumoural injection and administration of a single dose of CB1954 gave no significant side effects, warranting further trials to assess patient response.

Cytochrome P450 (CYP450) with Oxazaphosphorines

Cytochrome P450 (CYP450) enzymes are heme-containing proteins critical for the metabolism of many anti-cancer drugs, and are encoded by about 55 genes in humans (Chiocca & Waxman, 2004). Many different isoforms of the CYP450 enzyme have been used for GDEPT strategies, derived from humans, rats, rabbits and dogs (Table 2). CYP450 isoforms have been used in GDEPT settings to convert cancer chemotherapy prodrugs such as the oxazaphosphorines, cyclophosphamide (CPA) and ifosfamide (IFO), to their 4-hydroxy forms. These undergo spontaneous conversion to a phosphoramide mustard toxin and acrolein in equal proportions. The mustard toxin causes DNA cross-linking and protein alkylation, and ultimately, cell death by apoptosis and necrosis (Roy & Waxman, 2006).

A disadvantage to this GDEPT strategy is the presence of endogenous CYP450 enzymes in humans, especially in the liver, which can cause systemic drug toxicity, therefore making targeting of this system a priority to ensure high metabolite production specifically at the tumour site. Some methods to combat non-specific prodrug activation include: 1) selectively inhibiting endogenous liver CYP450 enzymes (Huang & Waxman, 2001); 2) selectively inhibiting the electron-donating NADPH-cytochrome P450 reductase (CYPOR) in the liver (Huang et al., 2000); or, 3) over-expressing CYPOR in CYP450-transgenic cells. This last approach has not yet been successful, as it lead to reduced CYP2B1 activity towards IFO in cells over-expressing CYPOR in all but one cell line tested (Lengler et al., 2006).

In the CYP450/CPA system, a bystander effect can occur due to diffusion of the soluble 4-hydroxy CPA metabolite to surrounding cells (Ichikawa et al., 2001; Wei et al., 1995). Interestingly, modifying the scheduling of CPA alone has an anti-angiogenic effect by causing apoptosis of tumour-associated endothelial cells and subsequent apoptosis of nearby cancer cells even in CPA-resistant tumours, leading to tumour regression in mice (Browder et al., 2000; Jounaidi & Waxman, 2001).

An immune response to tumour cell death caused by the CYP450/CPA strategy has also been reported, which could be due in part to CPA and its effects on the immune system; CPA at low doses is immune stimulatory but immunosuppressive at high doses (Lord et al., 2007).

There are species-specific and isoform-specific differences in conversion of prodrugs by CYP450 enzymes. The major isoforms of CYP450 that convert CPA and IFO are CYP2B, CYP2C and CYP3A, with the main rat isoform CYP2B1 used for GDEPT (Roy & Waxman, 2006). Rat CYP2B1 shows improved conversion of CPA by 10-fold compared to other rat CYP450 enzymes. Rabbit CYP4B1 has been used with the prodrugs 4-ipomeanol and 2-aminoantracene (Rainov et al., 1998). Human CYP1A2 uses acetaminophen (paracetamol) as its substrate for GDEPT, and has been shown to exhibit a bystander effect with high cytotoxicity *in vitro* (Thatcher et al., 2000).

Mutations of the CYP2B1 enzyme by site-directed mutagenesis lead to an increased substrate specificity of the enzyme for CPA and IFO (Chen et al., 2004). The authors also identified dog CYP2B11 as being up to 8-fold more active than rat CYP2B1 at converting CPA and IFO to their 4-hydroxyl forms.

The CYP450/CPA and CYP450/IFO combinations have both been evaluated in phase I/II clinical trials. Braybrooke et al. (2005) investigated the effects of the human CYP2B6 enzyme on breast cancer and melanoma patients via intratumoral injection of retrovirus and administration of oral CPA. The transgene was detectable in most patients but with limited transduction, and no serious adverse events related to GDEPT were reported. One patient had a partial response to the therapy, and an immune response to the therapy was reported in patients who showed a clinical response. Salmons, Lohr and colleagues investigated the effects of the CYP2B1 enzyme on pancreatic carcinoma patients via transfer of encapsulated allogeneic cells into the vasculature leading to the tumour, followed by IFO administration (Lohr et al., 2001; Lohr et al., 2003; Salmons et al., 2003). Four patients out of 14 showed tumour regression, with increased survival compared to untreated patients (Salmons et al., 2003).

Comparisons of GDEPT systems

Only few studies have been published which directly evaluate enzyme-prodrug systems under the same experimental conditions. Nishihara et al. (1998) compared HSV-TK/GCV, CD/5-FC, NTR/CB1954 and deoxycytidine kinase/cytosine arabinoside in thyroid carcinoma cells and showed that HSV-TK/GCV had the widest therapeutic index, while CD/5-FC and NTR/CB1954 showed a stronger bystander effect.

Combinations of GDEPT Systems

Combinations of enzyme-prodrug systems have been generated to allow a reduction in prodrug dose, to reduce the risk of drug resistance, and to increase efficacy. Combinations of HSV-TK/GCV and CD/5-FC have been tested (TK/CD), and results either reported co-operative (Uckert et al., 1998) or synergistic (Boucher et al., 2006) effects. Boucher et al. (2006) showed that sequential rather than concurrent administration of the prodrugs caused improved anti-tumour effects in tumours transduced with a TK/CD fusion gene. Combinations have also been seen to further sensitise to radiotherapy (Rogulski et al., 2000). Song et al. (2006) combined the TK/CD genes with procaspase-3 in order to increase the apoptotic effect on cell death.

Combinations of HSV-TK/GCV and cytochrome P450 2B1/CPA (TK/CYP450) have been reported to have a synergistic effect, which was reportedly due to GCV-induced damage which inhibited DNA repair of CPA-induced cross-links (Aghi et al., 1999a).

The TK/CD combination has been tested in phase I trials of prostate cancer patients using a replication-competent adenovirus for delivery of the transgenes, with (Freytag et al., 2003) or without (Freytag et al., 2002) radiation therapy. No severe adverse events or dose-limiting toxicities were identified and PSA levels of patients decreased during and after therapy. The trials demonstrated the safety of the approach.

TUMOUR VESSEL TARGETED GENE THERAPY

Several factors identified to be tumour endothelial cell specific have been used to target gene delivery and transcription for gene therapy (Table 3). Alternative gene therapy-based, anti-vascular approaches have utilised delivery of endothelial cells or endothelial progenitor cells. Work by de Palma et al. (2003) has shown tumour-selective homing of bone marrow progenitor cells; these were *ex vivo* transduced with lentivirus vectors carrying Tie2/Tek regulatory elements. In an equivalent method, another study used endothelial progenitor-like cells transduced *ex vivo* by retroviral-mediated transfer of HSV-TK, and showed significant tumour necrosis and lack of systemic toxicity following prodrug administration (Ferrari et al., 2003). Promising results were published by Wei et al. (2004); embryonic progenitor cells were shown to preferentially home to hypoxic lung metastases following intravenous administration in mice (Wei et al., 2004). Specificity was inversely related to tumour perfusion and vascular density, and directly related to tumour hypoxia and VEGF levels.

Table 3. EC specific factors used for transductional and transcriptional targeting

Factor	Ligand used	Promoter used	Transgene
Endoglin	Bi-directional antibody linked to Ad5	Endoglin	Reporter, other
E-selectin	Antibody linked via PEG to Ad5	E-selectin	Reporter, other
ICAM-2		ICAM-2	Reporter
Integrins	RGD linked to Ad5, other viral and non-viral vectors		HSV-TK, reporter, other
PPE-1 (pre-pro-endothelin-1)		PPE-1	HSV-TK, other
Tie1		Tie1	Reporter
Tie2		Tie2	NTR
VE-cadherin		VE-cadherin	HSV-TK
VEGF		HRE elements	HSV-TK, NTR, other
VEGFR-1	VEGF linked to Ad5	VEGFR-1	Reporter
VEGFR-2	Antibody linked to Moloney Murine Leukemia Virus	VEGFR-2	HSV-TK, CD, reporter, other
vWF (von Willebrand Factor)		vWF	HSV-TK

Table adapted from: (Bazan-Peregrino et al., 2007).

A stably NTR-transfected endothelial cell line was either co-injected with tumour cells or injected into tumour-bearing animals (Benouchan et al., 2006). This system could induce a robust bystander killing of tumour cells following CB1954 administration.

Other alternative methods have combined GDEPT with anti-angiogenic factors. Fusion genes, comprising of an anti-angiogenic factor, endostatin, and cytosine deaminase, have been used to successfully induce tumour cell apoptosis and inhibit growth of endothelial cells *in vivo* (Ou-Yang et al., 2006). Jin et al. (2005) used human osteocalcin promoter-targeted, conditionally replicating adenovirus together with an adenoviral vector secreting soluble VEGFR-2 to inhibit growth of prostate cancer models.

Gene delivery, widely accepted as the major hurdle to successful gene therapy, has been addressed in some studies. Radiation-induced eNOS, leading to vascular dilation due to nitric oxide release, resulted in increased tumour blood flow and improved transgene expression following delivery by DNA lipocomplexes (Sonveaux et al., 2007).

Targeted Delivery

Progress has been made in recent years using both viral and non-viral methods to deliver therapeutic genes. Vehicles include viral vectors (retrovirus, adenoviruses, lentiviruses), non-viral vectors (liposomes, naked DNA, polylysine constructs), and cellular vectors (range of mammalian cell types and bacteria) (Brandwijk et al., 2007).

Adenoviral transduction is currently the most successful and widely used gene delivery system. Adenovirus is a double stranded DNA virus which binds initially to the coxsackie and adenovirus receptor (CAR) on the target cell through viral fibre protein, and subsequently enters the cell via the interaction between viral capsid penton proteins and integrins on the target cell. However, many cell types are refractory to adenoviral transduction as they do not express CAR. Combined fibre mutations which block CAR binding (de-targeting) with peptide insertion (re-targeting) have been developed to infect a wide variety of cell types, including EC. Viral tropism has been modified via the insertion of peptides into the adenovirus fibre, and specifically the HI loop of the fibre (Work et al., 2004).

Adenoviral transduction could be rerouted using a bispecific antibody (anti-ACE/anti-Ad capsid) that blocks adenoviral binding to CAR and simultaneously retargets it to the angiotensin-converting enzyme resulted in efficient transgene overexpression in the vasculature of the lung (Miller et al., 2005).

Improved endothelial targeting has been achieved using a chimeric adenoviral construct, consisting of a hybrid Ad5/35 virus, where the serotype 5 fiber was replaced with serotype 35 fiber (Shinozaki et al., 2006). This resulted in retargeting of infection, reducing liver uptake and increasing tumour endothelial cell transduction. The Ad5/35 virus was specifically detected in the angiogenesis-rich border region of solid tumours, and co-localised with CD31 and Flk-1 positive cells.

The αV integrins have been used extensively as EC targets as they are cellular adhesion molecules which show enhanced expression under tumour conditions (Walton et al., 2000). Specifically, the αVβ3 integrin is expressed on proliferating endothelial cells, and αVβ3 and αVβ5 have been implicated in playing a key role in angiogenesis. Hypoxia stimulates expression of both vascular integrins in microvascular endothelial cells, partially through autocrine-paracrine action of VEGF induced by the hypoxic state (Suzuma et al., 1998; Walton et al., 2000).

Studies using both viral and non-viral gene delivery systems have demonstrated the ability of the cyclic arginine-glycine-aspartic acid (RGD-4C) peptide to re-target through αV integrins. Hence, RGD-modified adenoviruses appear to be good candidates for targeting the tumour vasculature, even though they were not initially designed for this purpose. In fact, in intact aorta from spontaneously hypertensive rats, which display enhanced αV integrin expression on dysfunctional endothelium, enhanced levels of transduction were observed using the RGD-modified vector, but not in aorta derived from normotensive control rats (Work et al., 2004). Cationic nanoparticles coupled to an integrin αVβ3-targeting ligand were shown to deliver genes selectively to angiogenic blood vessels in tumour-bearing mice (Hood et al., 2002).

Transcriptional Control

The regulatory elements of the VEGFR-2 and endoglin genes were used to construct conditionally replicating adenovirus vectors to selectively target dividing endothelial cells *in vitro* (Savontaus et al., 2002). However, the VEGFR-2 promoter has also been shown to regulate transgene expression in cells of non-endothelial origin (Szary et al., 2001).

Transcriptional targeting of HSV-TK to the tumour endothelium could be achieved with the use of the pre-pro-endothelin 1 promoter inserted into the long terminal repeat of a retroviral vector (Mavria et al., 2005). In colorectal xenografts, vascular disruption and tumour cell apoptosis was apparent following GCV administration, and could be further increased by combination with irinotecan (a cytotoxic drug used for the treatment of colorectal cancer). Similar targeted results were achieved using recombinant retrovirus with ecotropic envelope (Mavria & Porter, 2001).

Transgenes were successfully targeted to the angiogenic compartment of the tumour vasculature with the use of the Tie2 promoter and enhancer sequences incorporated into lentivirus vectors and administered by intravenous delivery to tumour-bearing animals (De Palma et al., 2003).

Transgenic animals, carrying HSV-TK under VE-cadherin promoter control, showed a marked reduction in tumour vascular density and increased tumour cell death following GCV administration (Dancer et al., 2003).

Conclusion

The vasculature of tumour tissue is different from the normal vasculature. This makes it an ideal target for therapeutic interventions. However, although a range of factors have been identified which are over-expressed in tumour endothelial cells, no single tumour-specific endothelial cell factor has yet been described. Fortunately for gene therapy, several layers of specificity can be added to each other, for example by combining targeted delivery with targeted transcription, which may therefore develop into a highly specific, tumour vascular targeted gene therapy system. However, thus far, highly targeted systems have not equated to highly efficient systems, and work is underway to increase transgene expression in target tissues.

The ability to non-invasively monitor the location and activity of the transgene prior to administration of the prodrug is an added advantage of GDEPT over other therapeutic modalities, and most clinically tested combinations have a PET/MRI-visible, non-toxic prodrug available. Studies have been published that evaluate different suicide gene therapy systems, but results are difficult to compare due to differences in the sensitivity of the target cell type, drug bioavailability and drug stability. Hence, no superior system for vessel targeted gene therapy has been identified yet.

Gene therapy has in recent years undergone a series of set-backs, including a highly publicized patient death (Lehrman, 1999), and acquisition of leukemia leading to halting of several gene therapy trials (Kohn et al., 2003). On the other hand, improved gene delivery resulted in highly promising results in the second HSV-TK/GCV phase III clinical trial (Immonen et al., 2004). In addition, exciting clinical results from small molecule-based vascular disrupting agents have been published (Hurwitz et al., 2004; Yang et al., 2003). Taken together, the future for vascular targeted gene therapy shows great potential.

References

Adachi, Y., Tamiya, T., Ichikawa, T., Terada, K., Ono, Y., Matsumoto, K., Furuta, T., Hamada, H. & Ohmoto, T. (2000). Experimental gene therapy for brain tumors using adenovirus-mediated transfer of cytosine deaminase gene and uracil phosphoribosyltransferase gene with 5-fluorocytosine. *Human Gene Therapy*, *11,* 77-89.

Aghi, M., Chou, T.C., Suling, K., Breakefield, X.O. & Chiocca, E.A. (1999a). Multimodal cancer treatment mediated by a replicating oncolytic virus that delivers the oxazaphosphorine/rat cytochrome P450 2B1 and ganciclovir/herpes simplex virus thymidine kinase gene therapies. *Cancer Res*, *59,* 3861-5.

Aghi, M., Hochberg, F. & Breakefield, X.O. (2000). Prodrug activation enzymes in cancer gene therapy. *J Gene Med*, *2,* 148-64.

Aghi, M., Kramm, C.M. & Breakefield, X.O. (1999b). Folylpolyglutamyl synthetase gene transfer and glioma antifolate sensitivity in culture and in vivo. *J Natl Cancer Inst*, *91,* 1233-41.

Aird, W.C. (2007). Phenotypic heterogeneity of the endothelium: I. Structure, function, and mechanisms. *Circulation Research*, *100,* 158-73.

Ayala, G., Satoh, T., Li, R., Shalev, M., Gdor, Y., Aguilar-Cordova, E., Frolov, A., Wheeler, T.M., Miles, B.J., Rauen, K., Teh, B.S., Butler, E.B., Thompson, T.C. & Kadmon, D. (2006). Biological response determinants in HSV-tk + ganciclovir gene therapy for prostate cancer. *Molecular Therapy: the Journal of the American Society of Gene Therapy*, *13,* 716-28.

Balestrieri, M.L. & Napoli, C. (2007). Novel challenges in exploring peptide ligands and corresponding tissue-specific endothelial receptors. *European Journal of Cancer, 43,* 1242-50.

Balzarini, J., Bohman, C. & De Clercq, E. (1993). Differential mechanism of cytostatic effect of (E)-5-(2-bromovinyl)-2'-deoxyuridine, 9-(1,3-dihydroxy-2-propoxymethyl)guanine, and other antiherpetic drugs on tumor cells transfected by the thymidine kinase gene of herpes simplex virus type 1 or type 2. *Journal of Biological Chemistry, 268,* 6332-7.

Balzarini, J., Degreve, B., Andrei, G., Neyts, J., Sandvold, M., Myhren, F. & de Clercq, E. (1998). Superior cytostatic activity of the ganciclovir elaidic acid ester due to the prolonged intracellular retention of ganciclovir anabolites in herpes simplex virus type 1 thymidine kinase gene-transfected tumor cells. *Gene Therapy, 5,* 419-26.

Barak, Y., Thorne, S.H., Ackerley, D.F., Lynch, S.V., Contag, C.H. & Matin, A. (2006). New enzyme for reductive cancer chemotherapy, YieF, and its improvement by directed evolution. *Molecular Cancer Therapeutics, 5,* 97-103.

Bazan-Peregrino, M., Seymour, L.W. & Harris, A.L. (2007). Gene therapy targeting to tumor endothelium. *Cancer Gene Therapy, 14,* 117-27.

Benouchan, M., Do Nascimento, F., Perret, G.Y. & Colombo, B.M. (2006). Delivery of the bacterial nitroreductase gene into endothelial cells prolongs the survival of tumour-bearing mice by bystander mechanisms. *International Journal of Oncology, 28,* 457-62.

Beutner, K.R. (1995). Valacyclovir: a review of its antiviral activity, pharmacokinetic properties, and clinical efficacy. *Antiviral Res, 28,* 281-90.

Black, M.E., Kokoris, M.S. & Sabo, P. (2001). Herpes simplex virus-1 thymidine kinase mutants created by semi-random sequence mutagenesis improve prodrug-mediated tumor cell killing. *Cancer Research, 61,* 3022-6.

Black, M.E., Newcomb, T.G., Wilson, H.M. & Loeb, L.A. (1996). Creation of drug-specific herpes simplex virus type 1 thymidine kinase mutants for gene therapy. *Proceedings of the National Academy of Sciences of the United States of America, 93,* 3525-9.

Boucher, P.D., Im, M.M., Freytag, S.O. & Shewach, D.S. (2006). A novel mechanism of synergistic cytotoxicity with 5-fluorocytosine and ganciclovir in double suicide gene therapy. *Cancer Research, 66,* 3230-7.

Brandwijk, R.J., Griffioen, A.W. & Thijssen, V.L. (2007). Targeted gene-delivery strategies for angiostatic cancer treatment. *Trends Mol Med, 13,* 200-9.

Braybrooke, J.P., Slade, A., Deplanque, G., Harrop, R., Madhusudan, S., Forster, M.D., Gibson, R., Makris, A., Talbot, D.C., Steiner, J., White, L., Kan, O., Naylor, S., Carroll, M.W., Kingsman, S.M. & Harris, A.L. (2005). Phase I study of MetXia-P450 gene therapy and oral cyclophosphamide for patients with advanced breast cancer or melanoma. *Clinical Cancer Research, 11,* 1512-20.

Bridgewater, J.A., Knox, R.J., Pitts, J.D., Collins, M.K. & Springer, C.J. (1997). The bystander effect of the nitroreductase/CB1954 enzyme/prodrug system is due to a cell-permeable metabolite. *Human Gene Therapy, 8,* 709-17.

Bridgewater, J.A., Springer, C.J., Knox, R.J., Minton, N.P., Michael, N.P. & Collins, M.K. (1995). Expression of the bacterial nitroreductase enzyme in mammalian cells renders them selectively sensitive to killing by the prodrug CB1954. *European Journal of Cancer, 31A,* 2362-70.

Browder, T., Butterfield, C.E., Kraling, B.M., Shi, B., Marshall, B., O'Reilly, M.S. & Folkman, J. (2000). Antiangiogenic scheduling of chemotherapy improves efficacy against experimental drug-resistant cancer. *Cancer Research, 60,* 1878-86.

Carmeliet, P. (2005). Angiogenesis in life, disease and medicine. *Nature, 438,* 932-6.

Carmeliet, P. & Jain, R.K. (2000). Angiogenesis in cancer and other diseases. *Nature, 407,* 249-57.

Chen, C.S., Lin, J.T., Goss, K.A., He, Y.A., Halpert, J.R. & Waxman, D.J. (2004). Activation of the anticancer prodrugs cyclophosphamide and ifosfamide: identification of cytochrome P450 2B enzymes and site-specific mutants with improved enzyme kinetics. *Mol Pharmacol, 65,* 1278-85.

Chen, J.K., Hu, L.J., Wang, D., Lamborn, K.R. & Deen, D.F. (2007). Cytosine deaminase/5-fluorocytosine exposure induces bystander and radiosensitization effects in hypoxic glioblastoma cells in vitro. *Int J Radiat Oncol Biol Phys, 67,* 1538-47.

Chi, J.T., Chang, H.Y., Haraldsen, G., Jahnsen, F.L., Troyanskaya, O.G., Chang, D.S., Wang, Z., Rockson, S.G., van de Rijn, M., Botstein, D. & Brown, P.O. (2003). Endothelial cell diversity revealed by global expression profiling. *Proceedings of the National Academy of Sciences of the United States of America, 100,* 10623-8.

Chiocca, E.A. & Waxman, D.J. (2004). Cytochrome p450-based gene therapies for cancer. *Methods in Molecular Medicine, 90,* 203-22.

Chung-Faye, G.A., Chen, M.J., Green, N.K., Burton, A., Anderson, D., Mautner, V., Searle, P.F. & Kerr, D.J. (2001). In vivo gene therapy for colon cancer using adenovirus-mediated, transfer of the fusion gene cytosine deaminase and uracil phosphoribosyltransferase. *Gene Therapy, 8,* 1547-54.

Conway, E.M. & Carmeliet, P. (2004). The diversity of endothelial cells: a challenge for therapeutic angiogenesis. *Genome Biol, 5,* 207.

Cortes, M.L., de Felipe, P., Martin, V., Hughes, M.A. & Izquierdo, M. (1998). Successful use of a plant gene in the treatment of cancer in vivo. *Gene Therapy, 5,* 1499-507.

Cowen, R.L., Williams, K.J., Chinje, E.C., Jaffar, M., Sheppard, F.C.D., Telfer, B.A., Wind, N.S. & Stratford, I.J. (2004). Hypoxia targeted gene therapy to increase the efficacy of tirapazamine as an adjuvant to radiotherapy: reversing tumor radioresistance and effecting cure. *Cancer Research, 64,* 1396-402.

Curlee, K.V., Parker, W.B. & Sorscher, E.J. (2004). Tumor sensitization to purine analogs by E. coli PNP. *Methods in Molecular Medicine, 90,* 223-45.

Dachs, G.U., Tupper, J. & Tozer, G.M. (2005). From bench to bedside for gene-directed enzyme prodrug therapy of cancer. *Anti-Cancer Drugs, 16,* 349-59.

Dancer, A., Julien, S., Bouillot, S., Pointu, H., Vernet, M. & Huber, P. (2003). Expression of thymidine kinase driven by an endothelial-specific promoter inhibits tumor growth of Lewis lung carcinoma cells in transgenic mice. *Gene Therapy, 10,* 1170-8.

Davies, L.C., Friedlos, F., Hedley, D., Martin, J., Ogilvie, L.M., Scanlon, I.J. & Springer, C.J. (2005). Novel fluorinated prodrugs for activation by carboxypeptidase G2 showing good in vivo antitumor activity in gene-directed enzyme prodrug therapy. *Journal of Medicinal Chemistry, 48,* 5321-8.

De Clercq, E. (2005). (E)-5-(2-bromovinyl)-2'-deoxyuridine (BVDU). *Med Res Rev, 25,* 1-20.

De Palma, M., Venneri, M.A., Roca, C. & Naldini, L. (2003). Targeting exogenous genes to tumor angiogenesis by transplantation of genetically modified hematopoietic stem cells. *Nature Medicine*, *9,* 789-95.

Dubois, L., Dresselaers, T., Landuyt, W., Paesmans, K., Mengesha, A., Wouters, B.G., Van Hecke, P., Theys, J. & Lambin, P. (2007). Efficacy of gene therapy-delivered cytosine deaminase is determined by enzymatic activity but not expression. *British Journal of Cancer*, *96,* 758-61.

Erbs, P., Regulier, E., Kintz, J., Leroy, P., Poitevin, Y., Exinger, F., Jund, R. & Mehtali, M. (2000). In vivo cancer gene therapy by adenovirus-mediated transfer of a bifunctional yeast cytosine deaminase/uracil phosphoribosyltransferase fusion gene. *Cancer Research*, *60,* 3813-22.

Evrard, A., Cuq, P., Robert, B., Vian, L., Pelegrin, A. & Cano, J.P. (1999). Enhancement of 5-fluorouracil cytotoxicity by human thymidine-phosphorylase expression in cancer cells: in vitro and in vivo study. *International Journal of Cancer*, *80,* 465-70.

Farquhar, D., Pan, B.F., Sakurai, M., Ghosh, A., Mullen, C.A. & Nelson, J.A. (2002). Suicide gene therapy using E. coli beta-galactosidase. *Cancer Chemotherapy & Pharmacology*, *50,* 65-70.

Ferrari, N., Glod, J., Lee, J., Kobiler, D. & Fine, H.A. (2003). Bone marrow-derived, endothelial progenitor-like cells as angiogenesis-selective gene-targeting vectors. *Gene Therapy*, *10,* 647-56.

Findlay, V.J., Townsend, D.M., Saavedra, J.E., Buzard, G.S., Citro, M.L., Keefer, L.K., Ji, X. & Tew, K.D. (2004). Tumor cell responses to a novel glutathione S-transferase-activated nitric oxide-releasing prodrug. *Molecular Pharmacology*, *65,* 1070-9.

Folkman, J. (1995). Angiogenesis in cancer, vascular, rheumatoid and other disease. *Nature Medicine*, *1,* 27-31.

Freytag, S.O., Khil, M., Stricker, H., Peabody, J., Menon, M., DePeralta-Venturina, M., Nafziger, D., Pegg, J., Paielli, D., Brown, S., Barton, K., Lu, M., Aguilar-Cordova, E. & Kim, J.H. (2002). Phase I study of replication-competent adenovirus-mediated double suicide gene therapy for the treatment of locally recurrent prostate cancer. *Cancer Research*, *62,* 4968-76.

Freytag, S.O., Stricker, H., Pegg, J., Paielli, D., Pradhan, D.G., Peabody, J., DePeralta-Venturina, M., Xia, X., Brown, S., Lu, M. & Kim, J.H. (2003). Phase I study of replication-competent adenovirus-mediated double-suicide gene therapy in combination with conventional-dose three-dimensional conformal radiation therapy for the treatment of newly diagnosed, intermediate- to high-risk prostate cancer. *Cancer Research*, *63,* 7497-506.

Friedlos, F., Davies, L., Scanlon, I., Ogilvie, L.M., Martin, J., Stribbling, S.M., Spooner, R.A., Niculescu-Duvaz, I., Marais, R. & Springer, C.J. (2002). Three new prodrugs for suicide gene therapy using carboxypeptidase G2 elicit bystander efficacy in two xenograft models. *Cancer Research*, *62,* 1724-9.

Fujita, T., Teh, B.S., Timme, T.L., Mai, W.Y., Satoh, T., Kusaka, N., Naruishi, K., Fattah, E.A., Aguilar-Cordova, E., Butler, E.B. & Thompson, T.C. (2006). Sustained long-term immune responses after in situ gene therapy combined with radiotherapy and hormonal therapy in prostate cancer patients. *International Journal of Radiation Oncology, Biology, Physics*, *65,* 84-90.

Gopin, A., Ebner, S., Attali, B. & Shabat, D. (2006). Enzymatic activation of second-generation dendritic prodrugs: Conjugation of self-immolative dendrimers with poly(ethylene glycol) via click chemistry. *Bioconjug Chem*, *17,* 1432-40.

Graepler, F., Lemken, M.L., Wybranietz, W.A., Schmidt, U., Smirnow, I., Gross, C.D., Spiegel, M., Schenk, A., Graf, H., Lauer, U.A., Vonthein, R., Gregor, M., Armeanu, S., Bitzer, M. & Lauer, U.M. (2005). Bifunctional chimeric SuperCD suicide gene -YCD: YUPRT fusion is highly effective in a rat hepatoma model. *World J Gastroenterol*, *11,* 6910-9.

Grant, J.W. & Smyth, T.P. (2004). Toward the development of a cephalosporin-based dual-release prodrug for use in ADEPT. *J Org Chem*, *69,* 7965-70.

Greco, O. & Dachs, G.U. (2001). Gene directed enzyme/prodrug therapy of cancer: historical appraisal and future prospectives. *Journal of Cellular Physiology*, *187,* 22-36.

Green, N.K., McNeish, I.A., Doshi, R., Searle, P.F., Kerr, D.J. & Young, L.S. (2003). Immune enhancement of nitroreductase-induced cytotoxicity: studies using a bicistronic adenovirus vector. *International Journal of Cancer*, *104,* 104-12.

Grove, J.I., Lovering, A.L., Guise, C., Race, P.R., Wrighton, C.J., White, S.A., Hyde, E.I. & Searle, P.F. (2003). Generation of Escherichia coli nitroreductase mutants conferring improved cell sensitization to the prodrug CB1954. *Cancer Research*, *63,* 5532-7.

Guise, C.P., Grove, J.I., Hyde, E.I. & Searle, P.F. (2007). Direct positive selection for improved nitroreductase variants using SOS triggering of bacteriophage lambda lytic cycle. *Gene Therapy*, *14,* 690-8.

Gupta, A., Miki, K., Xu, M., Yamamoto, N., Moossa, A.R. & Hoffman, R.M. (2003). Combination efficacy of doxorubicin and adenoviral methioninase gene therapy with prodrug selenomethionine. *Anticancer Res*, *23,* 1181-8.

Haack, K., Linnebacher, M., Eisold, S., Zoller, M., von Knebel Doeberitz, M. & Gebert, J. (2000). Induction of protective immunity against syngeneic rat cancer cells by expression of the cytosine deaminase suicide gene. *Cancer Gene Therapy*, *7,* 1357-64.

Haberkorn, U., Oberdorfer, F., Gebert, J., Morr, I., Haack, K., Weber, K., Lindauer, M., van Kaick, G. & Schackert, H.K. (1996). Monitoring gene therapy with cytosine deaminase: in vitro studies using tritiated-5-fluorocytosine. *J Nucl Med*, *37,* 87-94.

Hao, X.K., Liu, J.Y., Yue, Q.H., Wu, G.J., Bai, Y.J. & Yin, Y. (2006). In vitro and in vivo prodrug therapy of prostate cancer using anti-gamma-Sm-scFv/hCPA fusion protein. *Prostate*, *66,* 858-66.

Helsby, N.A., Ferry, D.M., Patterson, A.V., Pullen, S.M. & Wilson, W.R. (2004). 2-Amino metabolites are key mediators of CB 1954 and SN 23862 bystander effects in nitroreductase GDEPT. *British Journal of Cancer*, *90,* 1084-92.

Hinata, N., Shirakawa, T., Terao, S., Goda, K., Tanaka, K., Yamada, Y., Hara, I., Kamidono, S., Fujisawa, M. & Gotoh, A. (2006). Progress report on phase I/II clinical trial of Ad-OC-TK plus VAL therapy for metastatic or locally recurrent prostate cancer: Initial experience at Kobe University. *Int J Urol*, *13,* 834-7.

Hirashima, M., Bernstein, A., Stanford, W.L. & Rossant, J. (2004). Gene-trap expression screening to identify endothelial-specific genes. *Blood*, *104,* 711-8.

Ho, M., Yang, E., Matcuk, G., Deng, D., Sampas, N., Tsalenko, A., Tabibiazar, R., Zhang, Y., Chen, M., Talbi, S., Ho, Y.D., Wang, J., Tsao, P.S., Ben-Dor, A., Yakhini, Z., Bruhn, L. & Quertermous, T. (2003). Identification of endothelial cell genes by combined database mining and microarray analysis. *Physiological Genomics*, *13,* 249-62.

Hood, J.D., Bednarski, M., Frausto, R., Guccione, S., Reisfeld, R.A., Xiang, R. & Cheresh, D.A. (2002). Tumor regression by targeted gene delivery to the neovasculature. *Science*, *296,* 2404-7.

Huang, Z., Raychowdhury, M.K. & Waxman, D.J. (2000). Impact of liver P450 reductase suppression on cyclophosphamide activation, pharmacokinetics and antitumoral activity in a cytochrome P450-based cancer gene therapy model. *Cancer Gene Therapy*, *7,* 1034-42.

Huang, Z. & Waxman, D.J. (2001). Modulation of cyclophosphamide-based cytochrome P450 gene therapy using liver P450 inhibitors. *Cancer Gene Therapy*, *8,* 450-8.

Huminiecki, L. & Bicknell, R. (2000). In silico cloning of novel endothelial-specific genes. *Genome Research*, *10,* 1796-806.

Hurwitz, H., Fehrenbacher, L., Novotny, W., Cartwright, T., Hainsworth, J., Heim, W., Berlin, J., Baron, A., Griffing, S., Holmgren, E., Ferrara, N., Fyfe, G., Rogers, B., Ross, R. & Kabbinavar, F. (2004). Bevacizumab plus irinotecan, fluorouracil, and leucovorin for metastatic colorectal cancer. *N Engl J Med*, *350,* 2335-42.

Ichikawa, T., Petros, W.P., Ludeman, S.M., Fangmeier, J., Hochberg, F.H., Colvin, O.M. & Chiocca, E.A. (2001). Intraneoplastic polymer-based delivery of cyclophosphamide for intratumoral bioconversion by a replicating oncolytic viral vector. *Cancer Research*, *61,* 864-8.

Immonen, A., Vapalahti, M., Tyynela, K., Hurskainen, H., Sandmair, A., Vanninen, R., Langford, G., Murray, N. & Yla-Herttuala, S. (2004). AdvHSV-tk gene therapy with intravenous ganciclovir improves survival in human malignant glioma: a randomised, controlled study. *Molecular Therapy: the Journal of the American Society of Gene Therapy*, *10,* 967-72.

Jackson, J.C., Duffy, S.P., Hess, K.R. & Mehl, R.A. (2006). Improving nature's enzyme active site with genetically encoded unnatural amino acids. *J Am Chem Soc*, *128,* 11124-7.

Jikai, J., Shamis, M., Huebener, N., Schroeder, U., Wrasidlo, W., Wenkel, J., Lange, B., Gaedicke, G., Shabat, D. & Lode, H.N. (2003). Neuroblastoma directed therapy by a rational prodrug design of etoposide as a substrate for tyrosine hydroxylase. *Cancer Letters*, *197,* 219-24.

Jin, F., Xie, Z., Kuo, C.J., Chung, L.W. & Hsieh, C.L. (2005). Cotargeting tumor and tumor endothelium effectively inhibits the growth of human prostate cancer in adenovirus-mediated antiangiogenesis and oncolysis combination therapy. *Cancer Gene Therapy*, *12,* 257-67.

Jounaidi, Y. & Waxman, D.J. (2001). Frequent, moderate-dose cyclophosphamide administration improves the efficacy of cytochrome P-450/cytochrome P-450 reductase-based cancer gene therapy. *Cancer Research*, *61,* 4437-44.

Kajiwara, E., Kawano, K., Hattori, Y., Fukushima, M., Hayashi, K. & Maitani, Y. (2007). Long-circulating liposome-encapsulated ganciclovir enhances the efficacy of HSV-TK suicide gene therapy. *J Control Release*.

Kaliberov, S.A., Market, J.M., Gillespie, G.Y., Krendelchtchikova, V., Della Manna, D., Sellers, J.C., Kaliberova, L.N., Black, M.E. & Buchsbaum, D.J. (2007). Mutation of Escherichia coli cytosine deaminase significantly enhances molecular chemotherapy of human glioma. *Gene Therapy*.

Kamiya, H., Ochiai, H., Harashima, H., Ito, M. & Matsuda, A. (2006). Transient expression of Drosophila melanogaster deoxynucleoside kinase gene enhances cytotoxicity of nucleoside analogs. *Nucleosides Nucleotides Nucleic Acids*, *25,* 553-60.

Kerbel, R.S. (2001). Clinical trials of antiangiogenic drugs: opportunities, problems, and assessment of initial results. *J Clin Oncol*, *19,* 45S-51S.

Kievit, E., Bershad, E., Ng, E., Sethna, P., Dev, I., Lawrence, T.S. & Rehemtulla, A. (1999). Superiority of yeast over bacterial cytosine deaminase for enzyme/prodrug gene therapy in colon cancer xenografts. *Cancer Research*, *59,* 1417-21.

Kim, I., Song, X., Vig, B.S., Mittal, S., Shin, H.C., Lorenzi, P.J. & Amidon, G.L. (2004). A novel nucleoside prodrug-activating enzyme: substrate specificity of biphenyl hydrolase-like protein. *Mol Pharm*, *1,* 117-27.

Knox, R.J., Burke, P.J., Chen, S. & Kerr, D.J. (2003). CB 1954: from the Walker tumor to NQO2 and VDEPT. *Current Pharmaceutical Design*, *9,* 2091-104.

Knox, R.J., Jenkins, T.C., Hobbs, S.M., Chen, S., Melton, R.G. & Burke, P.J. (2000). Bioactivation of 5-(aziridin-1-yl)-2,4-dinitrobenzamide (CB 1954) by human NAD(P)H quinone oxidoreductase 2: a novel co-substrate-mediated antitumor prodrug therapy. *Cancer Research*, *60,* 4179-86.

Kohn, D.B., Sadelain, M. & Glorioso, J.C. (2003). Occurrence of leukaemia following gene therapy of X-linked SCID. *Nat Rev Cancer*, *3,* 477-88.

Kokoris, M.S., Sabo, P. & Black, M.E. (2000). In vitro evaluation of mutant HSV-1 thymidine kinases for suicide gene therapy. *Anticancer Res*, *20,* 959-63.

Koyama, F., Sawada, H., Hirao, T., Fujii, H., Hamada, H. & Nakano, H. (2000). Combined suicide gene therapy for human colon cancer cells using adenovirus-mediated transfer of escherichia coli cytosine deaminase gene and Escherichia coli uracil phosphoribosyltransferase gene with 5-fluorocytosine. *Cancer Gene Therapy*, *7,* 1015-22.

Kramer, I. & Lipp, H.P. (2007). Bevacizumab, a humanized anti-angiogenic monoclonal antibody for the treatment of colorectal cancer. *J Clin Pharm Ther*, *32,* 1-14.

Kuriyama, S., Kikukawa, M., Masui, K., Okuda, H., Nakatani, T., Akahane, T., Mitoro, A., Tominaga, K., Tsujinoue, H., Yoshiji, H., Okamoto, S., Fukui, H. & Ikenaka, K. (1999a). Cancer gene therapy with HSV-tk/GCV system depends on T-cell-mediated immune responses and causes apoptotic death of tumor cells in vivo. *Int J Cancer*, *83,* 374-80.

Kuriyama, S., Kikukawa, M., Masui, K., Okuda, H., Nakatani, T., Sakamoto, T., Yoshiji, H., Fukui, H., Ikenaka, K., Mullen, C.A. & Tsujii, T. (1999b). Cytosine deaminase/5-fluorocytosine gene therapy can induce efficient anti-tumor effects and protective immunity in immunocompetent mice but not in athymic nude mice. *Int J Cancer*, *81,* 592-7.

Kuriyama, S., Tsujinoue, H. & Yoshiji, H. (2004). Immune response to suicide gene therapy. *Methods in Molecular Medicine*, *90,* 353-69.

Kurozumi, K., Tamiya, T., Ono, Y., Otsuka, S., Kambara, H., Adachi, Y., Ichikawa, T., Hamada, H. & Ohmoto, T. (2004). Apoptosis induction with 5-fluorocytosine/cytosine deaminase gene therapy for human malignant glioma cells mediated by adenovirus. *J Neurooncol*, *66,* 117-27.

Lee, C.H., Wu, C.L. & Shiau, A.L. (2007). Hypoxia-induced cytosine deaminase gene expression for cancer therapy. *Human Gene Therapy*, *18,* 27-38.

Lee, K.C., Hamstra, D.A., Bullarayasamudram, S., Bhojani, M.S., Moffat, B.A., Dornfeld, K.J., Ross, B.D. & Rehemtulla, A. (2006). Fusion of the HSV-1 tegument protein vp22 to cytosine deaminase confers enhanced bystander effect and increased therapeutic benefit. *Gene Therapy*, *13,* 127-37.

Lehrman, S. (1999). Virus treatment questioned after gene therapy death. *Nature*, *401,* 517-8.

Lemken, M.L., Graepler, F., Wolf, C., Wybranietz, W.A., Smirnow, I., Schmidt, U., Gregor, M., Bitzer, M. & Lauer, U.M. (2007a). Fusion of HSV-1 VP22 to a bifunctional chimeric SuperCD suicide gene compensates for low suicide gene transduction efficiencies. *Int J Oncol*, *30,* 1153-61.

Lemken, M.L., Wolf, C., Wybranietz, W.A., Schmidt, U., Smirnow, I., Buhring, H.J., Mack, A.F., Lauer, U.M. & Bitzer, M. (2007b). Evidence for intercellular trafficking of VP22 in living cells. *Mol Ther*, *15,* 310-9.

Lengler, J., Omann, M., Duvier, D., Holzmuller, H., Gregor, W., Salmons, B., Gunzburg, W.H. & Renner, M. (2006). Cytochrome P450 reductase dependent inhibition of cytochrome P450 2B1 activity: Implications for gene directed enzyme prodrug therapy. *Biochemical Pharmacology*, *72,* 893-901.

Link, N., Aubel, C., Kelm, J.M., Marty, R.R., Greber, D., Djonov, V., Bourhis, J., Weber, W. & Fussenegger, M. (2006). Therapeutic protein transduction of mammalian cells and mice by nucleic acid-free lentiviral nanoparticles. *Nucleic Acids Res*, *34,* e16.

Liu, Y. & Deisseroth, A. (2006). Tumor vascular targeting therapy with viral vectors. *Blood*, *107,* 3027-33.

Lohr, M., Hoffmeyer, A., Kroger, J., Freund, M., Hain, J., Holle, A., Karle, P., Knofel, W.T., Liebe, S., Muller, P., Nizze, H., Renner, M., Saller, R.M., Wagner, T., Hauenstein, K., Gunzburg, W.H. & Salmons, B. (2001). Microencapsulated cell-mediated treatment of inoperable pancreatic carcinoma. *Lancet*, *357,* 1591-2.

Lohr, M., Kroger, J., Hoffmeyer, A., Freund, M., Hain, J., Holle, A., Knofel, W.T., Liebe, S., Nizze, H., Renner, M., Saller, R., Muller, P., Wagner, T., Hauenstein, K., Salmons, B. & Gunzburg, W.H. (2003). Safety, feasibility and clinical benefit of localized chemotherapy using microencapsulated cells for inoperable pancreatic carcinoma in a phase I/II trial. *Cancer Therapy*, *1,* 121-31.

Lord, R., Nair, S., Schache, A., Spicer, J., Somaihah, N., Khoo, V. & Pandha, H. (2007). Low dose metronomic oral cyclophosphamide for hormone resistant prostate cancer: a phase II study. *J Urol*, *177,* 2136-40; discussion 2140.

Luo, C., Nawa, A., Yamauchi, Y., Kohno, S., Ushijima, Y., Goshima, F., Kikkawa, F. & Nishiyama, Y. (2007). Intercellular trafficking and cytotoxicity of recombinant HSV-1 thymidine kinase fused with HSV-2 US11 RXP repeat peptide. *Virus Genes*, *34,* 263-72.

Mahan, S.D., Ireton, G.C., Knoeber, C., Stoddard, B.L. & Black, M.E. (2004a). Random mutagenesis and selection of Escherichia coli cytosine deaminase for cancer gene therapy. *Protein Engineering, Design & Selection, 17,* 625-33.

Mahan, S.D., Ireton, G.C., Stoddard, B.L. & Black, M.E. (2004b). Alanine-scanning mutagenesis reveals a cytosine deaminase mutant with altered substrate preference. *Biochemistry, 43,* 8957-64.

Manome, Y., Wen, P.Y., Dong, Y., Tanaka, T., Mitchell, B.S., Kufe, D.W. & Fine, H.A. (1996). Viral vector transduction of the human deoxycytidine kinase cDNA sensitizes glioma cells to the cytotoxic effects of cytosine arabinoside in vitro and in vivo. *Nature Medicine, 2,* 567-73.

Mavria, G., Harrington, K.J., Marshall, C.J. & Porter, C.D. (2005). In vivo efficacy of HSV-TK transcriptionally targeted to the tumour vasculature is augmented by combination with cytotoxic chemotherapy. *J Gene Med, 7,* 263-75.

Mavria, G. & Porter, C.D. (2001). Reduced growth in response to ganciclovir treatment of subcutaneous xenografts expressing HSV-tk in the vascular compartment. *Gene Therapy, 8,* 913-20.

Mesnil, M. (2002). Connexins and cancer. *Biol Cell, 94,* 493-500.

Mesnil, M. & Yamasaki, H. (2000). Bystander effect in herpes simplex virus-thymidine kinase/ganciclovir cancer gene therapy: role of gap-junctional intercellular communication. *Cancer Research, 60,* 3989-99.

Miki, K., Xu, M., Gupta, A., Ba, Y., Tan, Y., Al-Refaie, W., Bouvet, M., Makuuchi, M., Moossa, A.R. & Hoffman, R.M. (2001). Methioninase cancer gene therapy with selenomethionine as suicide prodrug substrate. *Cancer Research, 61,* 6805-10.

Miller, S.D., Mohiuddin, I., Cao, X.X., Ozvaran, M.K., Daniel, J.C. & Roy Smythe, W. (2004). Gene therapy for sarcoma utilizing adenoviral transfer of the beta-glucuronidase and bax genes and an anthracyline prodrug. *J Surg Res, 121,* 153-8.

Miller, W.H., Brosnan, M.J., Graham, D., Nicol, C.G., Morecroft, I., Channon, K.M., Danilov, S.M., Reynolds, P.N., Baker, A.H. & Dominiczak, A.F. (2005). Targeting endothelial cells with adenovirus expressing nitric oxide synthase prevents elevation of blood pressure in stroke-prone spontaneously hypertensive rats. *Molecular Therapy: the Journal of the American Society of Gene Therapy, 12,* 321-7.

Moolten, F.L. (1986). Tumor chemosensitivity conferred by inserted herpes thymidine kinase genes: paradigm for a prospective cancer control strategy. *Cancer Research, 46,* 5276-81.

Nagata, T., Nakamori, M., Iwahashi, M. & Yamaue, H. (2002). Overexpression of pyrimidine nucleoside phosphorylase enhances the sensitivity to 5'-deoxy-5-fluorouridine in tumour cells in vitro and in vivo. *European Journal of Cancer, 38,* 712-7.

Nemunaitis, J., Cunningham, C., Senzer, N., Kuhn, J., Cramm, J., Litz, C., Cavagnolo, R., Cahill, A., Clairmont, C. & Sznol, M. (2003a). Pilot trial of genetically modified, attenuated Salmonella expressing the E. coli cytosine deaminase gene in refractory cancer patients. *Cancer Gene Therapy, 10,* 737-44.

Nemunaitis, J., Cunningham, C., Tong, A.W., Post, L., Netto, G., Paulson, A.S., Rich, D., Blackburn, A., Sands, B., Gibson, B., Randlev, B. & Freeman, S. (2003b). Pilot trial of intravenous infusion of a replication-selective adenovirus (ONYX-015) in combination with chemotherapy or IL-2 treatment in refractory cancer patients. *Cancer Gene Ther, 10,* 341-52.

Neri, D. & Bicknell, R. (2005). Tumour vascular targeting. *Nature Reviews Cancer, 5,* 436-46.

Niculescu-Duvaz, I. & Springer, C.J. (2004). Introduction to the background, principles, and state of the art in suicide gene therapy. *Methods in Molecular Medicine, 90,* 1-27.

Nishihara, E., Nagayama, Y., Narimatsu, M., Namba, H., Watanabe, M., Niwa, M. & Yamashita, S. (1998). Treatment of thyroid carcinoma cells with four different suicide gene/prodrug combinations in vitro. *Anticancer Res, 18,* 1521-5.

Oh, P., Li, Y., Yu, J., Durr, E., Krasinska, K.M., Carver, L.A., Testa, J.E. & Schnitzer, J.E. (2004). Subtractive proteomic mapping of the endothelial surface in lung and solid tumours for tissue-specific therapy. *Nature, 429,* 629-35.

Ono, Y., Ikeda, K., Wei, M.X., Harsh, G.R.t., Tamiya, T. & Chiocca, E.A. (1997). Regression of experimental brain tumors with 6-thioxanthine and Escherichia coli gpt gene therapy. *Human Gene Therapy, 8,* 2043-55.

Oosterhoff, D., Witlox, M.A., van Beusechem, V.W., Haisma, H.J., Schaap, G.R., Bras, J., Kruyt, F.A., Molenaar, B., Boven, E., Wuisman, P.I., Pinedo, H.M. & Gerritsen, W.R. (2003). Gene-directed enzyme prodrug therapy for osteosarcoma: sensitization to CPT-11 in vitro and in vivo by adenoviral delivery of a gene encoding secreted carboxylesterase-2. *Molecular Cancer Therapeutics, 2,* 765-71.

Ou-Yang, F., Lan, K.L., Chen, C.T., Liu, J.C., Weng, C.L., Chou, C.K., Xie, X., Hung, J.Y., Wei, Y., Hortobagyi, G.N. & Hung, M.C. (2006). Endostatin-cytosine deaminase fusion protein suppresses tumor growth by targeting neovascular endothelial cells. *Cancer Research, 66,* 378-84.

Palmer, D.H., Mautner, V., Mirza, D., Oliff, S., Gerritsen, W., van der Sijp, J.R., Hubscher, S., Reynolds, G., Bonney, S., Rajaratnam, R., Hull, D., Horne, M., Ellis, J., Mountain, A., Hill, S., Harris, P.A., Searle, P.F., Young, L.S., James, N.D. & Kerr, D.J. (2004). Virus-directed enzyme prodrug therapy: intratumoral administration of a replication-deficient adenovirus encoding nitroreductase to patients with resectable liver cancer. *Journal of Clinical Oncology, 22,* 1546-52.

Pandha, H.S., Martin, L.A., Rigg, A., Hurst, H.C., Stamp, G.W., Sikora, K. & Lemoine, N.R. (1999). Genetic prodrug activation therapy for breast cancer: A phase I clinical trial of erbB-2-directed suicide gene expression. *Journal of Clinical Oncology, 17,* 2180-9.

Portsmouth, D., Hlavaty, J. & Renner, M. (2007). Suicide genes for cancer therapy. *Mol Aspects Med, 28,* 4-41.

Race, P.R., Lovering, A.L., White, S.A., Grove, J.I., Searle, P.F., Wrighton, C.W. & Hyde, E.I. (2007). Kinetic and structural characterisation of Escherichia coli nitroreductase mutants showing improved efficacy for the prodrug substrate CB1954. *J Mol Biol, 368,* 481-92.

Rainov, N.G. (2000). A phase III clinical evaluation of herpes simplex virus type 1 thymidine kinase and ganciclovir gene therapy as an adjuvant to surgical resection and radiation in adults with previously untreated glioblastoma multiforme. *Human Gene Therapy, 11,* 2389-401.

Rainov, N.G., Dobberstein, K.U., Sena-Esteves, M., Herrlinger, U., Kramm, C.M., Philpot, R.M., Hilton, J., Chiocca, E.A. & Breakefield, X.O. (1998). New prodrug activation gene therapy for cancer using cytochrome P450 4B1 and 2-aminoanthracene/4-ipomeanol. *Human Gene Therapy, 9,* 1261-73.

Ram, Z., Culver, K.W., Walbridge, S., Blaese, R.M. & Oldfield, E.H. (1993). In situ retroviral-mediated gene transfer for the treatment of brain tumors in rats. *Cancer Res, 53,* 83-8.

Richard, C., Duivenvoorden, W., Bourbeau, D., Massie, B., Roa, W., Yau, J. & Th'ng, J. (2007). Sensitivity of 5-fluorouracil-resistant cancer cells to adenovirus suicide gene therapy. *Cancer Gene Therapy, 14,* 57-65.

Rogulski, K.R., Wing, M.S., Paielli, D.L., Gilbert, J.D., Kim, J.H. & Freytag, S.O. (2000). Double suicide gene therapy augments the antitumor activity of a replication-competent lytic adenovirus through enhanced cytotoxicity and radiosensitization. *Human Gene Therapy, 11,* 67-76.

Roy, P. & Waxman, D.J. (2006). Activation of oxazaphosphorines by cytochrome P450: application to gene-directed enzyme prodrug therapy for cancer. *Toxicol In Vitro, 20,* 176-86.

Salmons, B., Lohr, M. & Gunzburg, W.H. (2003). Treatment of inoperable pancreatic carcinoma using a cell-based local chemotherapy: results of a phase I/II clinical trial. *J Gastroenterol, 38 Suppl 15,* 78-84.

Sandmair, A.M., Loimas, S., Puranen, P., Immonen, A., Kossila, M., Puranen, M., Hurskainen, H., Tyynela, K., Turunen, M., Vanninen, R., Lehtolainen, P., Paljarvi, L., Johansson, R., Vapalahti, M. & Yla-Herttuala, S. (2000). Thymidine kinase gene therapy for human malignant glioma, using replication-deficient retroviruses or adenoviruses. *Human Gene Therapy, 11,* 2197-205.

Savage, P., Cowburn, P., Clemens, D., Hurley, T., Laguda, B., Martin-Duque, P., Vassaux, G. & Lemoine, N.R. (2004). Suicide gene therapy: conversion of ethanol to acetaldehyde mediated by human beta 2 alcohol dehydrogenase. *Cancer Gene Therapy, 11,* 774-81.

Savontaus, M.J., Sauter, B.V., Huang, T.G. & Woo, S.L.C. (2002). Transcriptional targeting of conditionally replicating adenovirus to dividing endothelial cells. *Gene Therapy, 9,* 972-9.

Schepelmann, S., Ogilvie, L.M., Hedley, D., Friedlos, F., Martin, J., Scanlon, I., Chen, P., Marais, R. & Springer, C.J. (2007). Suicide gene therapy of human colon carcinoma xenografts using an armed oncolytic adenovirus expressing carboxypeptidase G2. *Cancer Research, 67,* 4949-55.

Seaman, S., Stevens, J., Yang, M.Y., Logsdon, D., Graff-Cherry, C. & St Croix, B. (2007). Genes that Distinguish Physiological and Pathological Angiogenesis. *Cancer Cell, 11,* 539-54.

Searle, P.F., Chen, M.J., Hu, L., Race, P.R., Lovering, A.L., Grove, J.I., Guise, C., Jaberipour, M., James, N.D., Mautner, V., Young, L.S., Kerr, D.J., Mountain, A., White, S.A. & Hyde, E.I. (2004). Nitroreductase: a prodrug-activating enzyme for cancer gene therapy. *Clin Exp Pharmacol Physiol, 31,* 811-6.

Seo, E., Abei, M., Wakayama, M., Fukuda, K., Ugai, H., Murata, T., Todoroki, T., Matsuzaki, Y., Tanaka, N., Hamada, H. & Yokoyama, K.K. (2005). Effective gene therapy of biliary tract cancers by a conditionally replicative adenovirus expressing uracil phosphoribosyltransferase: significance of timing of 5-fluorouracil administration. *Cancer Research*, *65,* 546-52.

Shah, K., Jacobs, A., Breakefield, X.O. & Weissleder, R. (2004). Molecular imaging of gene therapy for cancer. *Gene Therapy*, *11,* 1175-87.

Sharp, S.Y., Kelland, L.R., Valenti, M.R., Brunton, L.A., Hobbs, S. & Workman, P. (2000). Establishment of an isogenic human colon tumor model for NQO1 gene expression: application to investigate the role of DT-diaphorase in bioreductive drug activation in vitro and in vivo. *Molecular Pharmacology*, *58,* 1146-55.

Shinozaki, K., Suominen, E., Carrick, F., Sauter, B., Kahari, V.M., Lieber, A., Woo, S.L.C. & Savontaus, M. (2006). Efficient infection of tumor endothelial cells by a capsid-modified adenovirus. *Gene Therapy*, *13,* 52-9.

Simonova, M., Wall, A., Weissleder, R. & Bogdanov, A., Jr. (2000). Tyrosinase mutants are capable of prodrug activation in transfected nonmelanotic cells. *Cancer Research*, *60,* 6656-62.

Simpson, G.R., Han, Z., Liu, B., Wang, Y., Campbell, G. & Coffin, R.S. (2006). Combination of a fusogenic glycoprotein, prodrug activation, and oncolytic herpes simplex virus for enhanced local tumor control. *Cancer Research*, *66,* 4835-42.

Solaroli, N., Johansson, M., Balzarini, J. & Karlsson, A. (2007). Enhanced toxicity of purine nucleoside analogs in cells expressing Drosophila melanogaster nucleoside kinase mutants. *Gene Therapy*, *14,* 86-92.

Song, Y., Kong, B., Ma, D., Qu, X. & Jiang, S. (2006). Procaspase-3 enhances the in vitro effect of cytosine deaminase-thymidine kinase disuicide gene therapy on human ovarian cancer. *Int J Gynecol Cancer*, *16,* 156-64.

Sonveaux, P., Frerart, F., Bouzin, C., Brouet, A., Dewever, J., Jordan, B.F., Gallez, B. & Feron, O. (2007). Irradiation promotes Akt-targeting therapeutic gene delivery to the tumor vasculature. *International Journal of Radiation Oncology, Biology, Physics*, *67,* 1155-62.

St Croix, B., Rago, C., Velculescu, V., Traverso, G., Romans, K.E., Montgomery, E., Lal, A., Riggins, G.J., Lengauer, C., Vogelstein, B. & Kinzler, K.W. (2000). Genes expressed in human tumor endothelium. *Science*, *289,* 1197-202.

Stanford, W.L., Caruana, G., Vallis, K.A., Inamdar, M., Hidaka, M., Bautch, V.L. & Bernstein, A. (1998). Expression trapping: identification of novel genes expressed in hematopoietic and endothelial lineages by gene trapping in ES cells. *Blood*, *92,* 4622-31.

Stegman, L.D., Zheng, H., Neal, E.R., Ben-Yoseph, O., Pollegioni, L., Pilone, M.S. & Ross, B.D. (1998). Induction of cytotoxic oxidative stress by D-alanine in brain tumor cells expressing Rhodotorula gracilis D-amino acid oxidase: a cancer gene therapy strategy. *Human Gene Therapy*, *9,* 185-93.

Sterman, D.H., Recio, A., Vachani, A., Sun, J., Cheung, L., DeLong, P., Amin, K.M., Litzky, L.A., Wilson, J.M., Kaiser, L.R. & Albelda, S.M. (2005). Long-term follow-up of patients with malignant pleural mesothelioma receiving high-dose adenovirus herpes simplex thymidine kinase/ganciclovir suicide gene therapy. *Clinical Cancer Research*, *11,* 7444-53.

Sunamura, M., Hamada, H., Motoi, F., Oonuma, M., Abe, H., Saitoh, Y., Hoshida, T., Ottomo, S., Omura, N. & Matsuno, S. (2004). Oncolytic virotherapy as a novel strategy for pancreatic cancer. *Pancreas*, *28,* 326-9.

Suzuma, K., Takagi, H., Otani, A. & Honda, Y. (1998). Hypoxia and vascular endothelial growth factor stimulate angiogenic integrin expression in bovine retinal microvascular endothelial cells. *Investigative Ophthalmology & Visual Science*, *39,* 1028-35.

Svensson, H.P., Frank, I.S., Berry, K.K. & Senter, P.D. (1998). Therapeutic effects of monoclonal antibody-beta-lactamase conjugates in combination with a nitrogen mustard anticancer prodrug in models of human renal cell carcinoma. *Journal of Medicinal Chemistry*, *41,* 1507-12.

Szary, J., Kalita, K., Przybyszewska, M., Dus, D., Kieda, C., Janik, P. & Szala, S. (2001). KDR promoter can transcriptionally target cytosine deaminase suicide gene to cancer cells of nonendothelial origin. *Anticancer Res*, *21,* 3471-5.

Thatcher, N.J., Edwards, R.J., Lemoine, N.R., Doehmer, J. & Davies, D.S. (2000). The potential of acetaminophen as a prodrug in gene-directed enzyme prodrug therapy. *Cancer Gene Therapy*, *7,* 521-5.

Townsend, D.M., Findlay, V.J., Fazilev, F., Ogle, M., Fraser, J., Saavedra, J.E., Ji, X., Keefer, L.K. & Tew, K.D. (2006). A glutathione S-transferase pi-activated prodrug causes kinase activation concurrent with S-glutathionylation of proteins. *Molecular Pharmacology*, *69,* 501-8.

Tozer, G.M., Kanthou, C. & Baguley, B.C. (2005). Disrupting tumour blood vessels. *Nature Reviews Cancer*, *5,* 423-35.

Tupper, J., Greco, O., Tozer, G.M. & Dachs, G.U. (2004). Analysis of the horseradish peroxidase/indole-3-acetic acid combination in a three-dimensional tumor model. *Cancer Gene Therapy*, *11,* 508-13.

Uckert, W., Kammertons, T., Haack, K., Qin, Z., Gebert, J., Schendel, D.J. & Blankenstein, T. (1998). Double suicide gene (cytosine deaminase and herpes simplex virus thymidine kinase) but not single gene transfer allows reliable elimination of tumor cells in vivo. *Human Gene Therapy*, *9,* 855-65.

Unger, M.M., Wahl, J., Ushmorov, A., Buechele, B., Simmet, T., Debatin, K.M. & Beltinger, C. (2007). Enriching suicide gene bearing tumor cells for an increased bystander effect. *Cancer Gene Therapy*, *14,* 30-8.

van Beijnum, J.R., Dings, R.P., van der Linden, E., Zwaans, B.M., Ramaekers, F.C., Mayo, K.H. & Griffioen, A.W. (2006). Gene expression of tumor angiogenesis dissected: specific targeting of colon cancer angiogenic vasculature. *Blood*, *108,* 2339-48.

van der Eb, M.M., Cramer, S.J., Vergouwe, Y., Schagen, F.H., van Krieken, J.H., van der Eb, A.J., Borel Rinkes, I.H., van de Velde, C.J. & Hoeben, R.C. (1998). Severe hepatic dysfunction after adenovirus-mediated transfer of the herpes simplex virus thymidine kinase gene and ganciclovir administration. *Gene Therapy*, *5,* 451-8.

van der Eb, M.M., Geutskens, S.B., van Kuilenburg, A.B., van Lenthe, H., van Dierendonck, J.H., Kuppen, P.J., van Ormondt, H., van de Velde, C.J., Wanders, R.J., van Gennip, A.H. & Hoeben, R.C. (2003). Ganciclovir nucleotides accumulate in mitochondria of rat liver cells expressing the herpes simplex virus thymidine kinase gene. *J Gene Med*, *5,* 1018-27.

Vernejoul, F., Ghenassia, L., Souque, A., Lulka, H., Drocourt, D., Cordelier, P., Pradayrol, L., Pyronnet, S., Buscail, L. & Tiraby, G. (2006). Gene therapy based on gemcitabine chemosensitization suppresses pancreatic tumor growth. *Molecular Therapy: the Journal of the American Society of Gene Therapy, 14,* 758-67.

Walton, H.L., Corjay, M.H., Mohamed, S.N., Mousa, S.A., Santomenna, L.D. & Reilly, T.M. (2000). Hypoxia induces differential expression of the integrin receptors alpha(vbeta3) and alpha(vbeta5) in cultured human endothelial cells. *Journal of Cellular Biochemistry, 78,* 674-80.

Wang, D., Ruan, H., Hu, L., Lamborn, K.R., Kong, E.L., Rehemtulla, A. & Deen, D.F. (2005). Development of a hypoxia-inducible cytosine deaminase expression vector for gene-directed prodrug cancer therapy. *Cancer Gene Therapy, 12,* 276-83.

Wei, J., Blum, S., Unger, M., Jarmy, G., Lamparter, M., Geishauser, A., Vlastos, G.A., Chan, G., Fischer, K.D., Rattat, D., Debatin, K.M., Hatzopoulos, A.K. & Beltinger, C. (2004). Embryonic endothelial progenitor cells armed with a suicide gene target hypoxic lung metastases after intravenous delivery. *Cancer Cell, 5,* 477-88.

Wei, M.X., Tamiya, T., Rhee, R.J., Breakefield, X.O. & Chiocca, E.A. (1995). Diffusible cytotoxic metabolites contribute to the in vitro bystander effect associated with the cyclophosphamide/cytochrome P450 2B1 cancer gene therapy paradigm. *Clinical Cancer Research, 1,* 1171-7.

Wiewrodt, R., Amin, K., Kiefer, M., Jovanovic, V.P., Kapoor, V., Force, S., Chang, M., Lanuti, M., Black, M.E., Kaiser, L.R. & Albelda, S.M. (2003). Adenovirus-mediated gene transfer of enhanced Herpes simplex virus thymidine kinase mutants improves prodrug-mediated tumor cell killing. *Cancer Gene Therapy, 10,* 353-64.

Willmon, C.L., Krabbenhoft, E. & Black, M.E. (2006). A guanylate kinase/HSV-1 thymidine kinase fusion protein enhances prodrug-mediated cell killing. *Gene Therapy, 13,* 1309-12.

Wilson, W.R., Pullen, S.M., Hogg, A., Helsby, N.A., Hicks, K.O. & Denny, W.A. (2002). Quantitation of bystander effects in nitroreductase suicide gene therapy using three-dimensional cell cultures. *Cancer Research, 62,* 1425-32.

Work, L.M., Ritchie, N., Nicklin, S.A., Reynolds, P.N. & Baker, A.H. (2004). Dual targeting of gene delivery by genetic modification of adenovirus serotype 5 fibers and cell-selective transcriptional control. *Gene Therapy, 11,* 1296-300.

Wybranietz, W.A., Gross, C.D., Phelan, A., O'Hare, P., Spiegel, M., Graepler, F., Bitzer, M., Stahler, P., Gregor, M. & Lauer, U.M. (2001). Enhanced suicide gene effect by adenoviral transduction of a VP22-cytosine deaminase (CD) fusion gene. *Gene Therapy, 8,* 1654-64.

Xu, G. & McLeod, H.L. (2001). Strategies for Enzyme/Prodrug Cancer Therapy. *Clin. Cancer Res., 7,* 3314-3324.

Yang, J.C., Haworth, L., Sherry, R.M., Hwu, P., Schwartzentruber, D.J., Topalian, S.L., Steinberg, S.M., Chen, H.X. & Rosenberg, S.A. (2003). A randomized trial of bevacizumab, an anti-vascular endothelial growth factor antibody, for metastatic renal cancer. *N Engl J Med, 349,* 427-34.

Zhang, Z., Shirakawa, T., Hinata, N., Matsumoto, A., Fujisawa, M., Okada, H., Kamidono, S., Matsuo, M. & Gotoh, A. (2003). Combination with CD/5-FC gene therapy enhances killing of human bladder-cancer cells by radiation. *J Gene Med*, *5,* 860-7.

Zheng, X., Johansson, M. & Karlsson, A. (2000). Retroviral transduction of cancer cell lines with the gene encoding Drosophila melanogaster multisubstrate deoxyribonucleoside kinase. *Journal of Biological Chemistry*, *275,* 39125-9.

In: New Gene Therapy and Cancer Research
Editor: Wilma B. Gustafsson, pp. 183-204
ISBN: 978-1-60021-969-6

Chapter V

CURRENT GENE THERAPY FOR BLADDER CANCER

Kazumasa Matsumoto*[1,*]*, Akira Irie*[2]*, Takefumi Satoh*[1]*,
***Masatsugu Iwamura*[1] *and Shiro Baba*[1]**

[1]Department of Urology, Kitasato University School of Medicine, Japan;
[2]Department of Urology, Kitasato Institution Hospital, Japan.

ABSTRACT

Bladder cancer (transitional cell carcinoma) has been treated with traditional therapeutic alternatives, including transurethral resection, cystectomy, chemotherapy and radiation. Despite these recommended modalities, the therapeutic effect is often insufficient particularly in advanced, recurred, or metastasized diseases. Recently, with the great development of molecular biology with gene transfer methods, cancer gene therapy has become a reality for clinical application. We reviewed the background of and explore gene therapy for bladder cancer and performed a comprehensive literature search with publications.

Gene therapy strategies were broadly categorized as cytotoxic, corrective and immune-modulating gene transfer. A suppressive / corrective gene transfer such as cell cycle regulators is effective in cell culture and animal models, but the clinical realization of specific corrective gene transfer affecting each and every target cell without any detrimental influence on expression of other genes remains a challenge. Cytotoxic gene therapy represents a straightforward approach and is an attractive choice as either monotherapy or in combination with other anticancer therapies. Although this approach showed efficacy in animal models, limitations are the current inability to transduce large percentages of tumor cells and unwanted induction of host immunity to repeat application particularly using viral vector systems. Immunomodulation / cytokine gene

* Correspondence concerning this article should be addressed to: Kazumasa Matsumoto, MD, Department of Urology, Kitasato University School of Medicine, 1-15-1 Kitasato, Sagamihara, Kanagawa, 228-8555, JAPAN. Phone: +81-42-778-8434; Fax: +81-42-778-9374; E-mail address: kazumasa@cd5.so-net.ne.jp.

therapy has the potential of inducing antitumor immunity with possible prevention of metastasis. As most patients ultimately die of metastatic disease, this would represent a major step ahead in anticancer therapy.

Therapeutic gene transfer has proven to be safe and efficacious in pre-clinical studies of bladder cancer using cell cultures and animal models in the previous literatures. Clinical gene therapy trials offer a safe and feasible therapy in an actual clinical scenario; however, it demonstrates only modest antitumor efficacy. Given the current limitations of cancer gene therapy, this progress is promising because of especially considering that the current developments and applications were impossible approximately two decades ago. Further research is warranted for overcoming limitations.

Keywords: gene therapy, bladder cancer.

INTRODUCTION

Bladder cancer is the second most common urological carcinoma, and its incidence is gradually incremental. The overall mortality from this disease has not decreased despite improvements in diagnostic and therapeutic methods. Approximately 70% of bladder cancers are superficial, with the remaining 30% being muscle invasive and/or metastatic lesions at initial diagnosis. Superficial cancers are primarily treated by transurethral resection, but approximately 50% of patients will develop disease recurrence within 5 years. Approximately 30% of these recurrent tumors have higher grade and more aggressive properties than the primary tumors. Intravesical administration of chemotherapeutic agents or BCG vaccine reduces the recurrence of the tumors and is also efficient for the treatment of flat carcinoma in situ (CIS) of the bladder. However, one third of patients will still experience disease recurrence, and some CISs are resistant to intravesical therapy. Surgery, chemotherapy, and radiation are the standard therapeutic options for an attempt to cure patients with cancers. Once disease progression or distant metastases are observed, current cancer therapies have been relatively inadequate for salvage or long-term survival. In addition, today's anticancer therapeutic modalities come at a price because they are relatively nonselective and have detrimental effects on healthy tissues in the body. Novel approaches are desired for the treatment of bladder cancer, especially for both recurrent/treatment-resistant superficial tumors and advanced disease.

With the continuing advances of numerous encouragements in molecular biology, the concept of human gene therapy has become a reality—transferring genetic material into target abnormal cells and expressing proteins of interest in human tissues. Although encouraging results have been demonstrated with gene therapy in certain diseases such as adenosine deaminase (ADA) deficiency (Bordignon et al., 1995), one has to keep in mind that these disease processes are caused by a well-defined or metabolic defect affecting only one or a few genes. In these cases, cure or symptomatic improvement is relatively possible to attain by providing the correct genetic transfer and expressing the physiologic proteins of interest. In recent years, there have been extensive advances in our understanding of the cellular and molecular biology of bladder cancer. Many genetic alterations have been identified, and the pathogenesis appears to involve a multi-step process of carcinogenesis and disease progression. The role of these genetic alterations with respect to carcinogenesis and their relationship to clinical features and outcomes has also been clarified. These advances lead us to apply gene-modulating therapeutic strategies for bladder cancer. Recent advances regarding gene-modulating strategies for the treatment of bladder cancer are reviewed.

DELIVERY SYSTEM OF GENE TRANSFER

Current research in potential delivery systems has focused on two systems: nonviral chemical/physical transfection and viral transduction. The selection of system partially depends on the characteristics of the specific transgene, i.e., the size or molecular weight of the transgenes. Since each vector has its advantages and disadvantages, selection of an adequate system would be crucial.

Generally, virus vectors are more efficacious in regard to gene transduction and are the most common vectors used in human clinical trials. However, these systems introduce a unique question as to the safety of the gene therapy treatment compared to nonvirus vectors. Many of the complicated interactions between the virus and host are not completely understood. The two most widespread virus vector systems used are following two viruses; i.e., adenoviruses and retroviruses.

Adenovirus vectors have been attractive gene transfer vectors because of their ease of handling, ease of producing large amounts of vector, broad host cell range, and high levels of foreign gene expression (Volpers et al., 2004). In addition, adenoviruses infect not only proliferating but also non-dividing cells. However, the duration of gene expression is limited by its nature. In addition, adenoviruses need to bind to the cell surface of the receptor for infection, such as coxsackie adenovirus receptor (CAR)(Bergelson et al., 1997) or CD46 (Gaggar et al., 2003). CAR is a transmembrane glycoprotein and is a receptor for most of the adenovirus groups except for serotype B. Several studies reported that loss or decrease of CAR expression is associated with the biologic aggressiveness of urologic cancer (Matsumoto et al., 2005; Sachs et al., 2002). CD46 plays the role of receptor for both measles and human herpesvirus 6 viruses; thus, this protein is identified with a receptor of adenovirus serotype B (Gaggar et al., 2003). A target cell needs to express sufficient levels of specific receptor to be susceptible adenovirus infection. A recent report has demonstrated the adenoviral transduction efficacy of the wild-type p53 gene in bladder cancer patients (Kuball et al., 2002). In this study, p53-expressing adenovirus was administrated via either intravesical instillation with a transduction-enhancing agent (Big CHAP) or intratumoral injection to bladder cancer patients before their surgical excision. The administration of the adenovirus was confirmed to be safe and feasible, and biological p53 activity was also well documented. Interestingly, the transduction efficacy was reported to be superior in intravesical instillation compared with intratumoral injection.

Transduction of the foreign gene by retrovirus vectors to the nucleus in the target host cell requires the breakdown of the nuclear membranes during mitosis (Merten, 2004). Although retrovirus vectors are not able to infect quiescent cells, infected cells that release a foreign gene transduced by retrovirus over time without being killed themselves are being grafted into the tumor tissue. The retrovirus genome is stably and irreversibly integrated into the host genome at a random location and inherited to progeny cells after being converted to the host genome. This means that the process of inserting virus genetic material might potentially lead to subsequent unexpected transformation by itself. However, retroviral vectors can be produced only at low titers and infectious particles are quite unstable. Lentivirus vectors have become popular and may give us an attractive vehicle to overcome the limitation of transfer into non-dividing cells (Verhoeyen et al., 2004). The lentivirus mechanism allows mitosis-independent nuclear insertion of the foreign gene and transduction of some quiescent cells. However, this vector still has several risks as does the retrovirus vector. Other kinds of recombinant viruses, such as herpes simplex virus, poxvirus, vaccinia virus, and adeno-associated virus, have also been extensively investigated as delivery systems for gene therapy (Lee et al., 1994; Shichinohe et al., 2001; Siemens et al., 2001a).

The nonvirus vector system is an important modality. Although these systems do not possess the implicit risks of virus vectors (e.g., immune response to the foreign gene, use of virus vehicle, and toxicity), they are generally less effective in regard to gene transduction compared to virus vector systems. There is a broad range of techniques involved with nonviral delivery systems, such as particle bombardment, direct injection, lipofection, and receptor-mediated gene delivery. The transduction efficacy of three kinds of nonviral delivery systems, i.e., hemagglutinating virus of Japan liposome, particle gun, and electrotransfection, has been investigated in the bladder of animals (Harimoto et al., 1998). Efficient transduction of therapeutic gene–expressing plasmid into epithelial cells was achieved by all three methods, and transduction to deeper layers was accomplished by particle gun and electrotransfection. Efficient transduction by a cationic liposome via intravesical instillation has also been reported (Horiguchi et al., 2000). Intravesical instillation of plasmid-binding cationic liposome yielded transfection only to bladder cancers, whereas surrounding normal bladder urothelium was not efficiently transfected.

Table 1. Molecular genes related to cancer development and progression in the urinary bladder

Role	Classification	Genes
Tumor proliferation	Oncogenes	ras, fos, myc, erbB-2, CCND1
	Growth factors	EGF, EGFR
	Antiapoptosis	bcl-2, survivin
	Angiogenesis	VEGF, bFGF
	Cell proliferation	Cox-2
Tumor suppression	Suppressor genes	p53, p21, PTEN, ARF, CDKN2A
	Cell cycle regulators	p16, TRAIL, Rb
	Apoptotisis	bax, Fas, gelsolin, TNF
	Cell adhesion	ICAM-1, CCAM-1, CAR, cadherin
Drug resistance	Drug resistance	mdr-1, MRP

bFGF, basic fibroblast growth factor; CAR, coxsackie-adenovirus receptor; CCAM-1, cell-cell adhesion molecule 1; EGF, epidermal growth factor; EGFR, epidermal growth factor receptor; ICAM-1, intercellular adhesion molecule 1; TNF, tumor necrosis factor; TRAIL, tumor necrosis factor–related apoptosis-inducing ligand; VEGF, vascular endothelial growth factor.

CURRENT MOLECULAR GENETICS OF BLADDER CANCER

Numerous genetic alterations have been reported in bladder cancer. It has been proposed that there are two pathways for bladder cancer development and also two distinct disease entities including low-grade superficial tumors and biologically aggressive phenotype of cancers. Most muscle-invasive cancers supposedly develop via epithelial atypia or CIS, not from a precursor superficial bladder cancer. An expected model for bladder cancer development and progression, based on pathologic and molecular findings, has been at least partially elucidated (Lee et al., 2000). In these genetic alterations, numerous specific genes are extensively identified, and their roles in pathogenesis and relationship to clinical outcomes have also been clarified (Table 1). The genetic alterations include activation of the genes that accelerate cancer progression including oncogenes, growth, angiogenic, antiapoptotic and cell cycle–stimulating factors, and inactivation of the genes that inhibit cell proliferation including tumor suppressor and apoptotic genes.

Oncogenic Properties

The ras oncogene was initially identified as the transforming gene of a human bladder cancer cell line. The ras family consists of H-, K-, and N-ras, and all factors are important as components of the signal transduction pathway (Egan et al., 1993). Mutated ras oncogenes activate downstream protein and result in uncontrolled phosphorylation of transcription factors that regulate gene expression. Once a Ras protein is activated, it loses its ability to return to its inactive form and continues to stimulate cell proliferation. The H-ras oncogene has also been reported to stimulate tumor angiogenesis by activation of vascular endothelial growth factor (VEGF) and inactivation of anti-angiogenesis factors (Rak et al., 1995). The fos oncogene, also reacted as the transcription factor, is an early response gene to extracellular mitogenic stimuli, such as growth factors and various oncogenes. The fos protein forms a complex with jun and modulates transcriptional activation of a variety of genes at the activator protein 1 site. This complex plays a critical role in signal transduction and stimulates cell differentiation (Rauscher et al., 1988). The myc oncogene is involved in cell-cycle regulation by activating cell proliferation and differentiation. The overexpression of the myc oncogene has been recognized in up to 60% of bladder cancer (Schmitz-Drager et al., 1997). However, its expression has not been associated with tumor grade or progression (Christoph et al., 1999). The erbB-2 oncogene is a part of the epidermal growth factor receptor (EGFR) family and possesses tyrosine kinase activity. Activation of the erbB-2 gene accelerates cell proliferation. Overexpression of erbB-2 is observed up to 40% of bladder cancers, and activation of erbB-2 is correlated with bladder cancer stage and grade (Moriyama et al., 1991). The proto-oncogene CCND1, which encodes cyclin D1, stimulates cell cycle in the Rb pathway. The overexpression of CCDN1 in bladder cancer and its correlation to early tumor recurrence has been reported (Proctor et al., 1991; Shin et al., 1997). Three oncogenes, int-2, hst1, and bcl-1, are located on the long arm of chromosome 11, a portion of which appears to be amplified in various epithelial tumors, including bladder cancer (Proctor et al., 1991). The int-2 and hst1 genes are members of the fibroblast growth factor family, and bcl-1 is involved in the apoptotic pathway. These genes are thought to be related to bladder cancer carcinogenesis. bcl-2 is well known as an inhibitor of apoptosis, and the overexpression of bcl-2 has been identified in approximately 30% of bladder tumors (King et al., 1996), however, the relationship between the expression of bcl-2 and tumor grade or patient survival remains controversial. Epidermal growth factor (EGF) is a cellular mitogen that is excreted into the urine at high levels and initiates events of cell replication through the EGFR. Over-expression of EGFR is frequently present in patients with bladder cancer and has been shown the association with the cancer stage (Neal et al., 1990).

The process of angiogenesis is one of the important pathogenesis of bladder cancer. The acquisition of angiogenic properties makes cancers more aggressive, leading to cancers that are more invasive and metastatic. The overexpression of various angiogenic factors has been demonstrated in bladder cancer, including VEGF, platelet-derived endothelial growth factor, midkine, and basic fibroblast growth factor (bFGF) (Bochner et al., 1995). The loss of antiangiogenic factors including interferon (IFN)-beta and thrombospondin-1, has also been demonstrated. Cyclooxygenase-2 (COX-2), a prostaglandin-catalyzing enzyme, is related to initiation and progression of various epithelial cancers. Increased expression of COX-2 has been shown in bladder cancer as well and is thought to relate to disease progression (Komhoff et al., 2000).

Suppressor Gene Properties

Alterations in the genetic material encoding for cell cycle regulators known as tumor suppressor genes are commonly shown in a variety of human cancers. Aberrant expression of various tumor suppressor genes has been identified in bladder cancer and is involved in carcinogenesis and progression. Altered expression of p53 has been reported as seen in approximately 50% of bladder cancers (Reznikoff et al., 1996). However, a higher incidence of p53 mutation is observed in muscle-invasive diseases, and a lower incidence of it is seen in superficial disease. Inactivation of p53 can occur by point mutation or sequential deletion at any site, resulting in loss of the wild-type allele of p53. Mutations of the p53 gene and nuclear accumulation of p53 protein are associated with bladder cancer stage and grade. Mutation of the p53 gene is also associated with a higher risk of recurrence after radical cystectomy and with a lower overall survival (Esrig et al., 1994). Functional inactivation of p53 can occur not only by genetic alteration but also by binding to cellular factors such as mdm2 or by alteration of the subcellular localization of the protein. Altered states of p53 function are believed to play an important role in the multi-step of bladder cancer progression. p21 (WAF1/CIP1) protein is a downstream mediator of p53 that inhibits cyclin-dependent activity and causes cell cycle arrest. A recent study indicated that the regulation of p21 is not mediated solely by p53 but also by other pathways (Zhang et al., 1995). The decreased expression of p21 has been reported more frequently in patients with invasive bladder cancer compared with superficial cancers.

Rb is a nuclear phosphoprotein that negatively down-regulates transcription of cell division. Mutation of Rb has been observed in 30% to 40% of invasive bladder cancers. Patients with absent or heterogeneous expression of Rb have decreased survival compared with patients with positive Rb expression (Cordon-Cardo et al., 1992; Logothetis et al., 1992). The p16 (CDKN2) gene is located at 9p21, and deletion of 9p21 has been reported in up to 50% of bladder cancer cases (Czerniak et al., 1999). Deletions of the p16 gene are related to a high recurrence rate of superficial bladder cancer. p16 is an inhibitor of the cyclin/CDK complexes required Rb phosphorylation, and the loss of p16 results in inactivation of Rb. p16 has been thought to be involved in early events in the pathogenesis of bladder cancer (Wu et al., 1996).

Deletions of chromosome 9 are recognized in more than half of bladder cancer patients and are observed in every step of carcinogenesis and disease progression (Hartmann et al., 2002). The chromosome loci at 9p21 are a complex genomic region and encode three distinct negative cell cycle regulators: INK4A/ARF, p15, and p16. Deletion at this region is related to cancer progression. Homozygous deletion of the tumor suppressor PTEN is also seen in approximately 30% of muscle-invasive bladder cancer and is associated with disease progression (Cairns et al., 1998) . Gelsolin, a regulator of the actin cytoskeleton, has tumor suppressive activity and is reduced in bladder cancer progression (Tanaka et al., 1999). Several cell adhesion molecules, such as intercellular adhesion molecule 1, cell-cell adhesion molecule 1 (CCAM-1), coxsackie adenovirus receptor (CAR), and cadherin, act as tumor suppressors. The decreased expression of these genes is identified in invasive bladder cancers but not in superficial diseases and normal urothelium (Okegawa et al., 2002).

Gene Transfer Strategies For Bladder Cancer

Circumstances are more complicated in anti-cancer gene therapy because tumor development involves not only multiple genes in processes such as cell cycle regulation, cell proliferation, loss of adhesion, tumor invasion, transfer to other organs, transplantation, and metastasis, but also because significant genetic heterogeneity exists between individual tumors. There are various strategies for inhibiting cancer growth by modulating molecular-based biological conditions. Reversion of the malignant phenotype by correcting the aberrant expression of the genes related to cell growth is one of the major strategies for cancer gene therapy. Examples include inactivation of oncogenic genes by means of antisense oligonucleotides (ASs), ribozymes (RZs), and dominant negative mutants. Induction of the genes that inhibit tumor growth is another apparent strategy. Immunomodulation therapy is one of the most frequently approved strategies in clinical cancer gene therapy trials, along with various strategies to modify the genetic immune systems. Cytotoxic gene therapy that uses suicide genes or replication-competent, genetically modified viruses has also been excessively investigated both in the laboratory and clinically.

Suppressive / Corrective Gene Transfer

The suppression of oncogenic products has been investigated at many biological information levels, such as DNA synthesis, transcription, and protein, and numerous therapeutic agents have been developed and clinically applied. Use of ASs and RZs may be a simple, specific, and appropriate method of blocking genetic information at the molecular level. AS is a small piece of DNA or RNA designed to be complementary to its target. RZ is a small molecule that possesses specific catalytic activity with an ability to cleave its target. These therapeutic molecules hybridize with their targeted mRNAs and result in interference of the genetic transmission. Since RZs have the capability not only to hybridize with but also to cleave the targeted mRNAs in a specific manner and re-hybridize to the next target one after another, promising efficacy might be expected. Both ASs and RZs can be designed against any gene of interest by modulation of their sequences complementary to the targeted sites. Various targets for ASs and RZs have been investigated in the field of bladder cancer therapy. These targets include oncogenes, antiapoptotic, angiogenic factors, and drug resistance–inducing genes (Irie et al., 1997). While these therapeutic molecules have relatively short sequences, two different methods can be adopted for delivering them to the targeted cells. One is the direct delivery of the synthesized molecules by chemical or mechanical transduction, and the other involves transduction of a transgene-expressing vehicle into the targeted cells.

There are several structures of RZs, such as hammerhead RZ, hairpin RZ, minizyme, and maxizyme. Hammerhead RZ may be the most widely investigated structure for the therapeutic use. In general, a XUX nucleotide triplet (X being any nucleotide) is required for the target of RZ cleavage. For inhibiting the cancer growth by induction of RZ, a hammerhead RZ targeted to H-ras oncogene (a mutation from GGC to GUC) was initially investigated, because this RZ cleaves only the mutated oncogene, the GUC sequence, leaving the normal proto-oncogene, the GGC sequence, unaffected (Koizumi et al., 1989). Unexpected adverse effects regarding the transduction of the exo-delivered nucleotides can be avoided by the specific effect of this RZ. Early studies demonstrated that an anti–H-ras RZ resulted in a decrease of H-ras mRNA and p21-ras protein levels that led to altered morphologic features, cell growth inhibition, and decreased DNA synthesis in vitro (Feng et al., 1995; Tone et al., 1993). Advanced studies demonstrated the antitumor efficacy of a recombinant adenovirus encoding the anti–H-ras RZ in a subcutaneously experimental bladder cancer model established in athymic mice (Irie et al., 1999). Single intratumoral injection of this adenovirus resulted in a significant antitumor effect in a dose-dependent manner, and complete tumor regression was achieved by high-dose instillation of the virus. Higher rates of complete tumor regression were observed by multiple intratumoral injection of this virus with lower dosages.

Because of its ability to activate cell proliferation and tumor growth, the c-fos oncogene is thought to be a suitable suppressive target for the treatment of various cancers. The tumor inhibition efficacy of an anti–c-fos RZ has been demonstrated in a human bladder cancer cell line. Increased expression of an anti-fos RZ decreased DNA synthesis, thereby inhibiting cell growth. An antitumor effect was also reported by an anti–erbB2 RZ against human bladder cancer cells by suppression of both RNA and the encoding protein (Irie et al., 2000). One report demonstrated that the overexpression of erb-B2 was not always required for effective antitumor activity of the anti–erbB-2 RZ (Suzuki et al., 2000). The detailed mechanism of an antitumor effect of the anti–erb-B2 RZ in low-erbB2–expressing cancer cells has not been elucidated. The myc oncogene is an obvious target in various cancers, and AS strategies have been tested against bladder cancer. The enhancement of cis-platinum sensitivity by anti–myc-

AS has also been reported in bladder cancer cells. This effect was caused by the increased intracellular accumulation of cis-platinum by anti–myc-AS (Mizutani et al., 1994). These results demonstrate the potential capability of antioncogene ASs/RZs as therapeutic agents against bladder cancer.

Other genes related to cancer growth have also been chosen as the targets for AS/RZ strategies. Antiapoptotic genes are suitable targets of this strategy. bcl-2 is a major factor for preventing apoptosis, and an anti–bcl-2 AS/RZ has been used for the treatment of various cancers, including bladder cancer (Bilim et al., 2000). The decreased expression of bcl-2 by AS may stimulate apoptotic factors such as bax directly, resulting in the induction of apoptosis. Angiogenic factors, such as VEGF and bFGF, may also be appropriate targets of treatment for bladder cancer. A recent study reported that an anti–bFGF-AS inhibited bladder cancer cell growth both in vitro and in vivo (Inoue et al., 2000). The induction of apoptosis was achieved indirectly through the down-regulation of bFGF and matrix metalloproteinase type 9. AS/RZ approaches have also been applied for reversion of a drug-resistant phenotype by inhibiting the multi-drug resistant gene (mdr-1). Increased expression of the mdr-1 gene has been recognized in various drug-resistant cancer cells after treatment with chemotherapeutic agents. An anti–mdr-1 AS/RZ suppresses the expression of p-glycoprotein, the encoding protein of mdr-1, and results in reversion of the multi-drug-resistant phenotype (Scanlon et al., 1994). Induction of dominant negative mutants is another strategy for inhibition of the signals related to cancer growth by interrupting the correct genetic information. Sufficient antitumor effect of a dominant negative mutant of H-ras oncogene has been demonstrated against bladder cancer cells in vitro and in vivo (Watanabe et al., 2001).

Restoration of tumor suppressor genes into the cancer cells that lack appropriate expression of those genes was an initially proposed modality. However, overexpression of tumor suppressor genes in the cells with their normal functioning status has also been clarified to inhibit cancer growth. p53 plays a crucial role in regulation of cell proliferation and differentiation. Therefore, restoration and/or overexpression of wild-type p53 within cancer cells can cause cell cycle arrest through various pathways. The induction of wild-type p53 has been widely used for the treatment of various cancers, including bladder cancer, not only in the laboratory but also clinically. Laboratory results demonstrated the cell growth inhibition efficacy of adenovirus-mediated p53 transduction against bladder cancer cells, an effect that was partly due to the induction of apoptosis (Irie et al., 2001). Multiple studies using p53 transduction have enabled direct investigations of possible mechanisms of an antitumor effect. Wild-type p53 with adenoviral vectors in orthotopically or intraperitoneally growing murine bladder cancer cells demonstrated the existence of recombinant genetic materials in the transduced cancer tissues (Werthman et al., 1996). The major roles of p53, in general, are induction of apoptosis, cell-cycle regulation, and DNA repair. Additional antitumor effects, including the inhibition of angiogenesis, have also been demonstrated (Bouvet et al., 1998). The mechanism of an antitumor effect by wild-type p53 might be different, at least partially, in various cancer cells because of its molecular state. Some studies have demonstrated that cell cycle arrest was the primary antitumor effect of p53, whereas others have reported that apoptosis was the dominant factor in different cells (Sugrue et al., 1997; Yang et al., 1995). Further investigation of these mechanisms may make p53 transduction strategies more effective and useful in individual patients. p53 has also been reported to increase the sensitivity of cancer cells to irradiation and some DNA-damaging chemotherapeutic agents (Miyake et al., 2000). Combination of p53 transduction and chemotherapy with cisplatin inhibited tumor growth and suppressed the development of lymph node metastases as compared to either treatment alone. p21 is a downstream mediator of p53 and has also been used for cancer treatment. Inhibition of bladder cancer cell growth has been reported by adenovirus-mediated p21 (Hall et al., 2000). This growth suppression was caused primarily by cell cycle arrest but not by the induction of apoptosis.

Transduction of the Rb tumor suppressor gene is the first approved clinical trial of a gene therapy protocol against bladder cancer in the United States. The target of this study is the treatment of resistant bladder cancer with an Rb gene alteration. Adenovirus is used for delivering the wild-type Rb gene by intravesical instillation. Preclinical studies have demonstrated that the wild-type Rb gene arrested cell cycle in the G0/G1 phase by inhibiting the function of growth promoter elements, thereby resulting in tumor growth inhibition (Xu et al., 1996). Another tumor suppressor protein, p16, has been inversely associated with pRB. Expression of p16 inhibited cell growth in $p16^{-}$ pRB^{+} bladder cancer cells but not in $p16^{+}$ pRB^{-} cancer cells (Grim et al., 1997). In addition, chemoresistance was acquired in restored cells after transfer of p16 against both cisplatin and paclitaxel. The p16 gene is also involved in the G1/S regulation of the cell cycle, and an antitumor effect of adenovirus-mediated p16 transduction has been reported (Lee et al., 2001). The antitumor effect of p16 causes a strong G1/S arrest. The therapeutic efficacy of other tumor suppressor genes, such as gelsolin, bax, Fas ligand, and tumor necrosis factor–related apoptosis-inducing ligand, has been reported (Griffith et al., 2000). The tumor suppression by transduction of CCAM-1–expressing adenovirus has also been demonstrated in an orthotopic murine model (Kleinerman et al., 1996).

Cytotoxic Gene Transfer

Cytotoxic gene therapy by induction of suicide genes implies the selective destruction of cancer cells when the prodrugs are selectively activated within targeted cells previously transduced suicide genes. The herpes simplex virus thymidine kinase (HSV-tk) and the prodrug ganciclovir may be the most popular combination today, and clinical trials have been undertaken for the treatment of prostate cancer. This approach has been examined in orthotopic bladder cancer models (Cheon et al., 2002; Sutton et al., 2000). In these studies, orthotopically established bladder cancers in mice were treated by adenovirus-expressing HSV-tk by direct intratumoral injection or transurethral instillation, followed by intraperitoneal administration of ganciclovir. A high rate of HSV-tk transduction was achieved by direct intratumoral injection and resulted in tumor growth reduction and increased survival benefits. Using replicated-deficient adenovirus harboring either the cytomegalovirus (CMV) or Rous sarcoma virus (RSV) promoter, the differential influence of the promoter used to express adenoviral-mediated HSV-tk. Although both vectors had growth inhibition efficacy, CMV-tk demonstrated greater antitumor efficacy as compared to RSV/HSV-tk. CMV/HSV-tk also demonstrated increased treatment-related toxicity (Freund et al., 2000b). In addition, a combination treatment strategy was investigated for enhancement of suicide gene therapy using other therapeutic genes. Although the HSV-tk/ ganciclovir system was combined with adenovirus carrying murine IL-2 for treatment of a murine bladder cancer model, combination therapy showed no improvement over HSV-tk gene therapy alone(Freund et al., 2000a). Connexin (Cx) 26, known as one of the gap junctional intercellular proteins enhanced by the standard effect in HSV-tk gene therapy (Tanaka et al., 2001).

Replication-competent oncolytic viruses that have the capability to specifically lyse targeted cancer cells are being increasingly investigated for cancer treatment. These viruses have the ability to conditionally replicate in a specific manner. One of the most widely investigated viral models is the E1b-deleted adenovirus (ONYX-015), which has the ability to replicate only within cells that lack functional p53 (Heise et al., 1997). Clinical trials using this viral model have been approved in the United States for head and neck cancers. Laboratory results demonstrated an antitumor efficacy of this viral model against bladder cancer cell in vitro. The other investigated oncolytic virus that targets bladder cancer is the herpes simplex virus with a deletion in the gamma 34.5 gene (G207). G207 can replicate only within cells in the activated proliferation/differentiation state, such as cancer cells. Recent reports demonstrated the antitumor efficacy of G207 in experimental bladder cancer models established subcutaneously and in the bladders of mice (Cozzi et al., 2001; Oyama et al., 2000). In this series, the tumors were established orthotopically, and G207 was administered intratumorally, intravenously, or intravesically. Tumor reduction was observed with every administration route without major adverse effects. These results would show that this strategy would have a potential to adjust for the treatment of advanced and metastatic bladder cancer by systemic administration. Since EGFR is overexpressed in various cancers, targeting an oncolytic virus to the EGFR might be a promising option for cancer gene therapy (Hemminki et al., 2001). Antitumor efficacy of oncolytic adenoviruses targeting to EGFR expressing cells and Rb or p53 deficient cells has been shown against bladder cancer (van der Poel et al., 2002).

Recently, replication-competent oncolytic adenoviruses those with cancer-specific promoters have been extensively investigated. Tissue-specific genes would serve as better applications in systematic gene transfers. Uroplakins (UPs) are members of integral membrane proteins including UP Ia, Ib, II, and III (Wu et al., 1994; Yu et al., 1994). UP antibodies stained normal urothelium and primary and metastatic transitional cell carcinoma, without significant binding to any of the nonurotherial cancer and organ tissue (Kaufmann et al., 2000; Moll et al., 1995). These findings suggest that UPs have a potential role as markers for specific identification of urothelium or transitional cell carcinoma. The specific inhibition of bladder cancer growth has been demonstrated by the oncolytic adenovirus, which expresses viral E1A and E1B genes by means of an uroplakin II promoter (Zhang et al., 2002). The 235-bp 5'-fragment, including UP Ib excn 1, has been strongly transcripted in normal and urothelial cancer cell lines (Olsburgh et al., 2002).

Immunomodulation/Cytokine Gene Transfer

The purpose of immunomodulation gene therapy is to enhance the host immunologic response against cancer cells by increasing the antigenicity to cytotoxic lymphocytes (CTLs). Immunomodulation gene therapy strategies involve the administration of cancer cell vaccines genetically modified to express various cytokine genes, vaccination with tumor antigen nucleic acids, or the direct induction of cytokines. Cancer vaccination activates a tumor-specific immune reaction by the induction of genetically engineered cytokine-producing autologous irradiated cancer cells. The advantage of using autologous tumor cells is that they might contain pertinent tumor-specific antigens, allowing for systemic administration. Most studies demonstrate that these kinds of vaccines are efficient for the prevention of a subsequent tumor challenge, but efficacy for tumor reduction remains controversial. It has been thought that these tumor antigens are not efficient enough to trigger a host immune response. Antigen-presenting cells, such as dendritic cells and macrophages, express co-stimulatory molecule B7, but tumor cells usually do not. Therefore, co-transduction of B7 may enhance tumor antigenicity. Vaccination of B7 solely transducted tumor cells has been demonstrated to cause tumor reduction (Fujii et al., 1996). Co-transduction of B7 with major histocompatibility complex molecules and cytokines has also been shown to enhance the antitumor effect compared with transduction of these molecules without B7 (Baskar et al., 1995).

Direct induction of cytokines into cancer cells is another promising option for cancer immunomodulation gene therapy. Various cytokines, such as interleukin (IL) 2, IL-12, granulocyte-macrophage colony-stimulating factor, and interferons, have been used for this strategy. One study has demonstrated the sufficient transfer of an IL-2–expressing plasmid into a preestablished orthotopic mouse bladder tumor via liposomes, which resulted in inhibited tumor growth and prolonged survival (Horiguchi et al., 2000). This antitumor effect was shown to be caused by activation of tumor-specific CTLs. The addition of subsequent B7.1 gene–modified tumor vaccines enhanced this therapeutic effect (Larchian et al., 2000). Antitumor efficacy has also been demonstrated with intratumoral administration of IL-12, when both subunits, p30 and p40, were transfected by adenovirus (Chen et al., 1997). This antitumor efficacy was reduced in mice depleted of CD4+ and CD8+ cells or in nude mice. In addition, cancer treated with IL-12 showed increased IL-12 and IFN-gamma expression and regression of tumor and lung metastases. Another study showed that IL-12 was rejected in a subcutaneous syngeneic mouse model (Yamamoto et al., 1999). Parental cancer cells mixed with IL-12–secreted cells inhibited the growth in the primary site. Increased local production of interferon within a tumor has been shown to inhibit angiogenesis, tumor growth, and metastasis. The therapeutic efficacy of direct transduction of the IFN-gamma gene has been previously demonstrated (Hashimura et al., 1997). In this study, direct injection of IFN-gamma into the same site as the tumor inoculation suppressed tumorigenesis in mice. Some bladder cancer cells produce multiple cytokines, and the growth of these cells can be regulated by nuclear factor kappa B (NFκB). Transduction of the NFκB inhibitor, IkBa, by adenovirus into an NFκB-activated bladder cancer cell line has been shown to inhibit cell growth and induce apoptosis (Sumitomo et al., 1999).

ENHANCEMENT OF GENE TRANSFER IN THE URINARY BLADDER

Effective delivery systems with efficient cellular uptake, specific gene targeting, long-term expression, and minimal toxicity are required for prominent therapeutic efficacy. There are several ways to deliver transgenes into bladder cancer cells. Intratumoral injection and intravesical instillation may achieve successful gene transfer into superficial or locally invasive tumors, and systemic administration would be required for advanced metastatic disease. Bladder is potentially a favorably treatable organ because of its anatomy; i.e., it is easily accessible endoscopically and it may be possible to retain the therapeutic vectors inside the vesical cavity for a long time. However, the glycosaminoglycan (GAG) layer, which overlays the bladder mucosa, may interrupt suitable therapeutic gene transduction, particularly using viral vectors. Several strategies have been adapted to overcome this biological barrier by improving the delivery systems themselves and by disruption of the GAG layer.

Numerous investigations have been undertaken to improve the gene transfer efficacy of bladder cancer cells. For intravesical instillation of therapeutic genes into the bladder, the barrier of the GAG layer may be an obstacle for sufficient transduction of therapeutic genes. Without any other special considerations, the importance of the volume and intravesical pressure has been reported for sufficient gene transduction (Siemens et al., 2001b). Higher instillation pressure with a larger volume of viral vectors resulted in significantly higher transgene expression in the bladder. Another report has demonstrated the difference of viral infectivity, depending on the cancer cell density in vitro. These basic considerations need to be carefully weighed when designing both in vitro and in vivo protocols. The efforts to improve the transduction efficacy in bladder cancer are summarized in Table 2.

Table 2. Molecular genes or agents for enhancing gene transfer in the urinary bladder

Strategies	Mechanism
CAR	Increase adenoviral infectivity
Sodium butyrate	Increase CAR expression
Syn3 polyamide compound	GAG layer disruption
Big CHAP detergent	GAG layer disruption
Hydrochloride	GAG layer disruption
Ethanol	GAG layer disruption
Gelfoam collagen-based matrix	Enhance transgene expression and augment T-cell immunity
Poly-l-lysine	Increase poxvirus infectivity
Oxychlorosene	Increase poxvirus infectivity

CAR, coxsackie adenovirus receptor; GAG, glycosaminoglycan.

Several strategies have been examined for increasing gene transfer efficacy by disruption of the GAG layer in bladder cancer. Some detergents are the well-known material that disrupt GAG layer, and their efficiency and safety have been previously reported (Connor et al.,

2001). Enhanced transgene expression was demonstrated in several detergents, but adverse effects, such as cystitis and stone formation, were also observed. In evaluated detergents, Big CHAP seemed to be the most effective and safe material in the study. The safety and usefulness of Big CHAP have also been demonstrated in a clinical investigation of bladder cancer patients (Kuball et al., 2002). The polyamide compound syn3 has also been demonstrated to increase adenovirus-mediated gene transfer efficacy in bladder cancer (Yamashita et al., 2002). Pretreatment with syn3 caused marked increase of adenoviral infectivity to both normal urothelium and superficial bladder tumors that have little or no CAR expression. Preincubation of the bladder mucosa or tumor cells with chemical agents such as ethanol and hydrochloride has also been shown to increase adenoviral infectivity (Engler et al., 1999; Lin et al., 2002; Shimizu et al., 2001). Co-administration of a Gelfoam collagen-based matrix with adenovirus has been shown to enhance transgene expression and improve CTL activation (Siemens et al., 2001b). The modification of bladder surface by preincubation with oxychlorosene or poly-L-lysine before viral instillation has been demonstrated to improve virus infectivity and transgene expression (Siemens et al., 2001a).

On the other hand, adenoviruses are thought to have tropism for the lower genitourinary epithelium and have been shown to infect epithelial cells with high frequency (Mufson et al., 1976). The gene transfer efficacy of the adenoviral vector expressing a marker gene in vitro and in vivo has been examined, and sufficient infectivity of adenovirus into bladder cancer cells and bladder epithelium has been demonstrated (Bass et al., 1995; Morris et al., 1994; Werthman et al., 1996). However, it has been reported that many bladder cancers, especially in high-grade tumors, lack the expression of CAR (Li et al., 1999). Further investigations have demonstrated the expression of CAR and integrins in bladder cancer and their relationship with adenoviral infectivity (Loskog et al., 2002; Sachs et al., 2002). Since CAR plays an important role in adenoviral infection, decreased CAR expression causes insufficient adenovirus-mediated therapeutic gene transduction. The superior gene transfer efficacy by adenovirus has been reported by co-administration of CAR cDNA (Okegawa et al., 2001). Another report demonstrated the increased expression of CAR by the addition of sodium butyrate (Lee et al., 2001). In this report, the increased CAR expression and the improved adenoviral infectivity have been demonstrated in vitro by preincubation of bladder cancer cells, which lack CAR expression, with sodium butyrate. In addition to CAR expression, other adhesive molecules and factors that influence the integration system would affect the infectivity of adenovirus. Further clarification of the mechanisms of adenoviral infection, including the status of receptors such as CAR and the roles of other related adhesive molecules, would be required to confirm the detailed actions of adenoviral attachment and integration into targeted cells.

Table 3. Current clinical trial of gene therapy for urologic cancer

NIH	Phase	Organ	Gene	Vector	Modality	PI	Institution	Country
9710-219	I	Bladder	p53	Adenovirus	Intravesical	Pagliaro	Univ. of Texas M.D. Anderson Cancer Center	United States
0110-500	I	Bladder	HSV-tk	Adenovirus	Intratumoral	Lerner	Baylor College of Medicine	United States
0304-581	I	Bladder	B7.1 (CD80), GM-CSF	Fowlpox Virus	Intravesical	Wojtowicz	The Cancer Institute of New Jersey	United States

Conclusion

Encouraging results have been demonstrated regarding the antitumor effect of preclinical gene therapy for bladder cancer. To confirm the reliability of gene therapy, a number of clinical trials are currently underway (Table 3). However, the method for delivering the therapeutic genes into targeted cancer cells would be the most significant interruption to overcome for further clinical trials. In addition, due to the complexity of cancer development, it is likely that several approaches will be necessary in cancer gene therapy. Further research is needed to overcome limitations and interruptions to realize the huge potential at stake, with technologies having a possibly comparable impact on all aspects of health and disease. Human knowledge and ingenuity will eventually find better ways to make a novel antitumor treatment including gene therapy an established clinical reality.

References

Baskar, S, Glimcher, L, Nabavi, N, Jones, R T & Ostrand-Rosenberg, S. (1995).Major histocompatibility complex class II+B7-1+ tumor cells are potent vaccines for stimulating tumor rejection in tumor-bearing mice. *J Exp Med*, *181,* 619-629.

Bass, C, Cabrera, G, Elgavish, A, Robert, B, Siegal, G P, Anderson, S C, et al. (1995).Recombinant adenovirus-mediated gene transfer to genitourinary epithelium in vitro and in vivo. *Cancer Gene Ther*, *2,* 97-104.

Bergelson, J M, Cunningham, J A, Droguett, G, Kurt-Jones, E A, Krithivas, A, Hong, J S, et al. (1997).Isolation of a common receptor for Coxsackie B viruses and adenoviruses 2 and 5. *Science*, *275,* 1320-1323.

Bilim, V, Kasahara, T, Noboru, H, Takahashi, K & Tomita, Y. (2000).Caspase involved synergistic cytotoxicity of bcl-2 antisense oligonucleotides and adriamycin on transitional cell cancer cells. *Cancer Lett*, *155,* 191-198.

Bochner, B H, Cote, R J, Weidner, N, Groshen, S, Chen, S C, Skinner, D G, et al. (1995).Angiogenesis in bladder cancer: relationship between microvessel density and tumor prognosis. *J Natl Cancer Inst*, *87,* 1603-1612.

Bordignon, C, Notarangelo, L D, Nobili, N, Ferrari, G, Casorati, G, Panina, P, et al. (1995).Gene therapy in peripheral blood lymphocytes and bone marrow for ADA-immunodeficient patients. *Science*, *270,* 470-475.

Bouvet, M, Ellis, L M, Nishizaki, M, Fujiwara, T, Liu, W, Bucana, C D, et al. (1998).Adenovirus-mediated wild-type p53 gene transfer down-regulates vascular endothelial growth factor expression and inhibits angiogenesis in human colon cancer. *Cancer Res*, *58,* 2288-2292.

Cairns, P, Evron, E, Okami, K, Halachmi, N, Esteller, M, Herman, J G, et al. (1998).Point mutation and homozygous deletion of PTEN/MMAC1 in primary bladder cancers. *Oncogene*, *16,* 3215-3218.

Chen, L, Chen, D, Block, E, O'Donnell, M, Kufe, D W & Clinton, S K. (1997).Eradication of murine bladder carcinoma by intratumor injection of a bicistronic adenoviral vector carrying cDNAs for the IL-12 heterodimer and its inhibition by the IL-12 p40 subunit homodimer. *J Immunol*, *159,* 351-359.

Cheon, J, Moon, D G, Cho, H Y, Park, H S, Kim, J J, Gardner, T A, et al. (2002).Adenovirus-mediated suicide-gene therapy in an orthotopic murine bladder tumor model. *Int J Urol*, *9,* 261-267.

Christoph, F, Schmidt, B, Schmitz-Drager, B J & Schulz, W A. (1999).Over-expression and amplification of the c-myc gene in human urothelial carcinoma. *Int J Cancer*, *84,* 169-173.

Connor, R J, Engler, H, Machemer, T, Philopena, J M, Horn, M T, Sutjipto, S, et al. (2001).Identification of polyamides that enhance adenovirus-mediated gene expression in the urothelium. *Gene Ther*, *8,* 41-48.

Cordon-Cardo, C, Wartinger, D, Petrylak, D, Dalbagni, G, Fair, W R, Fuks, Z, et al. (1992).Altered expression of the retinoblastoma gene product: prognostic indicator in bladder cancer. *J Natl Cancer Inst*, *84,* 1251-1256.

Cozzi, P J, Malhotra, S, McAuliffe, P, Kooby, D A, Federoff, H J, Huryk, B, et al. (2001).Intravesical oncolytic viral therapy using attenuated, replication-competent herpes simplex viruses G207 and Nv1020 is effective in the treatment of bladder cancer in an orthotopic syngeneic model. *Faseb J*, *15,* 1306-1308.

Czerniak, B, Chaturvedi, V, Li, L, Hodges, S, Johnston, D, Roy, J Y, et al. (1999).Superimposed histologic and genetic mapping of chromosome 9 in progression of human urinary bladder neoplasia: implications for a genetic model of multistep urothelial carcinogenesis and early detection of urinary bladder cancer. *Oncogene*, *18,* 1185-1196.

Egan, S E & Weinberg, R A. (1993).The pathway to signal achievement. *Nature*, *365,* 781-783.

Engler, H, Anderson, S C, Machemer, T R, Philopena, J M, Connor, R J, Wen, S F, et al. (1999).Ethanol improves adenovirus-mediated gene transfer and expression to the bladder epithelium of rodents. *Urology*, *53,* 1049-1053.

Esrig, D, Elmajian, D, Groshen, S, Freeman, J A, Stein, J P, Chen, S C, et al. (1994).Accumulation of nuclear p53 and tumor progression in bladder cancer. *N Engl J Med, 331,* 1259-1264.

Feng, M, Cabrera, G, Deshane, J, Scanlon, K J & Curiel, D T. (1995).Neoplastic reversion accomplished by high efficiency adenoviral-mediated delivery of an anti-ras ribozyme. *Cancer Res, 55,* 2024-2028.

Freund, C T, Sutton, M A, Dang, T, Contant, C F, Rowley, D & Lerner, S P. (2000a).Adenovirus-mediated combination suicide and cytokine gene therapy for bladder cancer. *Anticancer Res, 20,* 1359-1365.

Freund, C T, Tong, X W, Block, A, Contant, C F, Kieback, D G, Rowley, D R, et al. (2000b).Adenovirus-mediated suicide gene therapy for bladder cancer: comparison of the cytomegalovirus- and Rous sarcoma virus-promoter. *Anticancer Res, 20,* 2811-2816.

Fujii, H, Inobe, M, Kimura, F, Murata, J, Murakami, M, Onishi, Y, et al. (1996).Vaccination of tumor cells transfected with the B7-1 (CD80) gene induces the anti-metastatic effect and tumor immunity in mice. *Int J Cancer, 66,* 219-224.

Gaggar, A, Shayakhmetov, D M & Lieber, A. (2003).CD46 is a cellular receptor for group B adenoviruses. *Nat Med, 9,* 1408-1412.

Griffith, T S, Anderson, R D, Davidson, B L, Williams, R D & Ratliff, T L. (2000).Adenoviral-mediated transfer of the TNF-related apoptosis-inducing ligand/Apo-2 ligand gene induces tumor cell apoptosis. *J Immunol, 165,* 2886-2894.

Grim, J, D'Amico, A, Frizelle, S, Zhou, J, Kratzke, R A & Curiel, D T. (1997).Adenovirus-mediated delivery of p16 to p16-deficient human bladder cancer cells confers chemoresistance to cisplatin and paclitaxel. *Clin Cancer Res, 3,* 2415-2423.

Hall, M C, Li, Y, Pong, R C, Ely, B, Sagalowsky, A I & Hsieh, J T. (2000).The growth inhibitory effect of p21 adenovirus on human bladder cancer cells. *J Urol, 163,* 1033-1038.

Harimoto, K, Sugimura, K, Lee, C R, Kuratsukuri, K & Kishimoto, T. (1998). In vivo gene transfer methods in the bladder without viral vectors. *Br J Urol, 81,* 870-874.

Hartmann, A, Schlake, G, Zaak, D, Hungerhuber, E, Hofstetter, A, Hofstaedter, F, et al. (2002).Occurrence of chromosome 9 and p53 alterations in multifocal dysplasia and carcinoma in situ of human urinary bladder. *Cancer Res, 62,* 809-818.

Hashimura, T, Ueda, T, Hiura, M, Yoshida, O, Kawabata, K, Watanabe, Y, et al. (1997). [Gene therapy by in vivo interferon-gamma gene transfer to murine bladder tumor]. *Hinyokika Kiyo, 43,* 809-813.

Heise, C, Sampson-Johannes, A, Williams, A, McCormick, F, Von Hoff, D D & Kirn, D H. (1997).ONYX-015, an E1B gene-attenuated adenovirus, causes tumor-specific cytolysis and antitumoral efficacy that can be augmented by standard chemotherapeutic agents. *Nat Med, 3,* 639-645.

Hemminki, A, Dmitriev, I, Liu, B, Desmond, R A, Alemany, R & Curiel, D T. (2001).Targeting oncolytic adenoviral agents to the epidermal growth factor pathway with a secretory fusion molecule. *Cancer Res, 61,* 6377-6381.

Horiguchi, Y, Larchian, W A, Kaplinsky, R, Fair, W R & Heston, W D. (2000).Intravesical liposome-mediated interleukin-2 gene therapy in orthotopic murine bladder cancer model. *Gene Ther, 7,* 844-851.

Inoue, K, Perrotte, P, Wood, C G, Slaton, J W, Sweeney, P & Dinney, C P. (2000).Gene therapy of human bladder cancer with adenovirus-mediated antisense basic fibroblast growth factor. *Clin Cancer Res*, *6,* 4422-4431.

Irie, A, Anderegg, B, Kashani-Sabet, M, Ohkawa, T, Suzuki, T, Halks-Miller, M, et al. (1999).Therapeutic efficacy of an adenovirus-mediated anti-H-ras ribozyme in experimental bladder cancer. *Antisense Nucleic Acid Drug Dev*, *9,* 341-349.

Irie, A, Bouffard, D Y & Scanlon, K J. (1997).Ribozyme-mediated cancer gene therapy. *Int J Urol*, *4,* 329-337.

Irie, A, Kashani-Sabet, M, Scanlon, K J, Uchida, T & Baba, S. (2000).Hammerhead ribozymes as therapeutic agents for bladder cancer. *Mol Urol*, *4,* 61-66.

Irie, A, Uchida, T, Ishida, H, Matsumoto, K, Iwamura, M & Baba, S. (2001).p53 Mutation in bladder cancer patients in Japan and inhibition of growth by in vitro adenovirus-mediated wild-type p53 transduction in bladder cancer cells. *Mol Urol*, *5,* 53-58.

Kaufmann, O, Volmerig, J & Dietel, M. (2000).Uroplakin III is a highly specific and moderately sensitive immunohistochemical marker for primary and metastatic urothelial carcinomas. *Am J Clin Pathol*, *113,* 683-687.

King, E D, Matteson, J, Jacobs, S C & Kyprianou, N. (1996).Incidence of apoptosis, cell proliferation and bcl-2 expression in transitional cell carcinoma of the bladder: association with tumor progression. *J Urol*, *155,* 316-320.

Kleinerman, D I, Dinney, C P, Zhang, W W, Lin, S H, Van, N T & Hsieh, J T. (1996).Suppression of human bladder cancer growth by increased expression of C-CAM1 gene in an orthotopic model. *Cancer Res*, *56,* 3431-3435.

Koizumi, M, Hayase, Y, Iwai, S, Kamiya, H, Inoue, H & Ohtsuka, E. (1989).Design of RNA enzymes distinguishing a single base mutation in RNA. *Nucleic Acids Res*, *17,* 7059-7071.

Komhoff, M, Guan, Y, Shappell, H W, Davis, L, Jack, G, Shyr, Y, et al. (2000).Enhanced expression of cyclooxygenase-2 in high grade human transitional cell bladder carcinomas. *Am J Pathol*, *157,* 29-35.

Kuball, J, Wen, S F, Leissner, J, Atkins, D, Meinhardt, P, Quijano, E, et al. (2002).Successful adenovirus-mediated wild-type p53 gene transfer in patients with bladder cancer by intravesical vector instillation. *J Clin Oncol*, *20,* 957-965.

Larchian, W A, Horiguchi, Y, Nair, S K, Fair, W R, Heston, W D & Gilboa, E. (2000).Effectiveness of combined interleukin 2 and B7.1 vaccination strategy is dependent on the sequence and order: a liposome-mediated gene therapy treatment for bladder cancer. *Clin Cancer Res*, *6,* 2913-2920.

Lee, C T, Seol, J Y, Park, K H, Yoo, C G, Kim, Y W, Ahn, C, et al. (2001).Differential effects of adenovirus-p16 on bladder cancer cell lines can be overcome by the addition of butyrate. *Clin Cancer Res*, *7,* 210-214.

Lee, R & Droller, M J. (2000).The natural history of bladder cancer. Implications for therapy. *Urol Clin North Am*, *27,* 1-13, vii.

Lee, S S, Eisenlohr, L C, McCue, P A, Mastrangelo, M J & Lattime, E C. (1994).Intravesical gene therapy: in vivo gene transfer using recombinant vaccinia virus vectors. *Cancer Res*, *54,* 3325-3328.

Li, Y, Pong, R C, Bergelson, J M, Hall, M C, Sagalowsky, A I, Tseng, C P, et al. (1999).Loss of adenoviral receptor expression in human bladder cancer cells: a potential impact on the efficacy of gene therapy. *Cancer Res*, *59,* 325-330.

Lin, L F, Zhu, G, Yoo, J J, Soker, S, Sukhatme, V P & Atala, A. (2002).A system for the enhancement of adenovirus mediated gene transfer to uro-epithelium. *J Urol*, *168,* 813-818.

Logothetis, C J, Xu, H J, Ro, J Y, Hu, S X, Sahin, A, Ordonez, N, et al. (1992).Altered expression of retinoblastoma protein and known prognostic variables in locally advanced bladder cancer. *J Natl Cancer Inst*, *84,* 1256-1261.

Loskog, A, Hedlund, T, Wester, K, de la Torre, M, Philipson, L, Malmstrom, P U, et al. (2002).Human urinary bladder carcinomas express adenovirus attachment and internalization receptors. *Gene Ther*, *9,* 547-553.

Matsumoto, K, Shariat, S F, Ayala, G E, Rauen, K A & Lerner, S P. (2005).Loss of coxsackie and adenovirus receptor expression is associated with features of aggressive bladder cancer. *Urology*, *66,* 441-446.

Merten, O W. (2004).State-of-the-art of the production of retroviral vectors. *J Gene Med*, *6 Suppl 1,* S105-124.

Miyake, H, Hara, I, Hara, S, Arakawa, S & Kamidono, S. (2000).Synergistic chemosensitization and inhibition of tumor growth and metastasis by adenovirus-mediated P53 gene transfer in human bladder cancer model. *Urology*, *56,* 332-336.

Mizutani, Y, Fukumoto, M, Bonavida, B & Yoshida, O. (1994).Enhancement of sensitivity of urinary bladder tumor cells to cisplatin by c-myc antisense oligonucleotide. *Cancer*, *74,* 2546-2554.

Moll, R, Wu, X R, Lin, J H & Sun, T T. (1995).Uroplakins, specific membrane proteins of urothelial umbrella cells, as histological markers of metastatic transitional cell carcinomas. *Am J Pathol*, *147,* 1383-1397.

Moriyama, M, Akiyama, T, Yamamoto, T, Kawamoto, T, Kato, T, Sato, K, et al. (1991).Expression of c-erbB-2 gene product in urinary bladder cancer. *J Urol*, *145,* 423-427.

Morris, B D, Jr., Drazan, K E, Csete, M E, Werthman, P E, Van Bree, M P, Rosenthal, J T, et al. (1994).Adenoviral-mediated gene transfer to bladder in vivo. *J Urol*, *152,* 506-509.

Mufson, M A & Belshe, R B. (1976).A review of adenoviruses in the etiology of acute hemorrhagic cystitis. *J Urol*, *115,* 191-194.

Neal, D E, Sharples, L, Smith, K, Fennelly, J, Hall, R R & Harris, A L. (1990).The epidermal growth factor receptor and the prognosis of bladder cancer. *Cancer*, *65,* 1619-1625.

Okegawa, T, Li, Y, Pong, R C & Hsieh, J T. (2002).Cell adhesion proteins as tumor suppressors. *J Urol*, *167,* 1836-1843.

Okegawa, T, Pong, R C, Li, Y, Bergelson, J M, Sagalowsky, A I & Hsieh, J T. (2001).The mechanism of the growth-inhibitory effect of coxsackie and adenovirus receptor (CAR) on human bladder cancer: a functional analysis of car protein structure. *Cancer Res*, *61,* 6592-6600.

Olsburgh, J, Weeks, R, Selby, P & Southgate, J. (2002).Human uroplakin lb gene structure and promoter analysis. *Biochim Biophys Acta*, *1576,* 163-170.

Oyama, M, Ohigashi, T, Hoshi, M, Nakashima, J, Tachibana, M, Murai, M, et al. (2000).Intravesical and intravenous therapy of human bladder cancer by the herpes vector G207. *Hum Gene Ther*, *11,* 1683-1693.

Proctor, A J, Coombs, L M, Cairns, J P & Knowles, M A. (1991).Amplification at chromosome 11q13 in transitional cell tumours of the bladder. *Oncogene*, *6,* 789-795.

Rak, J, Mitsuhashi, Y, Bayko, L, Filmus, J, Shirasawa, S, Sasazuki, T, et al. (1995).Mutant ras oncogenes upregulate VEGF/VPF expression: implications for induction and inhibition of tumor angiogenesis. *Cancer Res*, *55,* 4575-4580.

Rauscher, F J, 3rd, Cohen, D R, Curran, T, Bos, T J, Vogt, P K, Bohmann, D, et al. (1988).Fos-associated protein p39 is the product of the jun proto-oncogene. *Science*, *240,* 1010-1016.

Reznikoff, C A, Belair, C D, Yeager, T R, Savelieva, E, Blelloch, R H, Puthenveettil, J A, et al. (1996).A molecular genetic model of human bladder cancer pathogenesis. *Semin Oncol*, *23,* 571-584.

Sachs, M D, Rauen, K A, Ramamurthy, M, Dodson, J L, De Marzo, A M, Putzi, M J, et al. (2002).Integrin alpha(v) and coxsackie adenovirus receptor expression in clinical bladder cancer. *Urology*, *60,* 531-536.

Scanlon, K J, Ishida, H & Kashani-Sabet, M. (1994).Ribozyme-mediated reversal of the multidrug-resistant phenotype. *Proc Natl Acad Sci U S A*, *91,* 11123-11127.

Schmitz-Drager, B J, Schulz, W A, Jurgens, B, Gerharz, C D, van Roeyen, C R, Bultel, H, et al. (1997).c-myc in bladder cancer. Clinical findings and analysis of mechanism. *Urol Res*, *25 Suppl 1,* S45-49.

Shichinohe, T, Bochner, B H, Mizutani, K, Nishida, M, Hegerich-Gilliam, S, Naldini, L, et al. (2001).Development of lentiviral vectors for antiangiogenic gene delivery. *Cancer Gene Ther*, *8,* 879-889.

Shimizu, H, Akasaka, S, Suzuki, S, Akimoto, M & Shimada, T. (2001).Preferential gene transfer to BBN-induced rat bladder tumor by simple instillation of adenoviral vector. *Urology*, *57,* 579-584.

Shin, K Y, Kong, G, Kim, W S, Lee, T Y, Woo, Y N & Lee, J D. (1997).Overexpression of cyclin D1 correlates with early recurrence in superficial bladder cancers. *Br J Cancer*, *75,* 1788-1792.

Siemens, D R, Austin, J C, See, W A, Tartaglia, J & Ratliff, T L. (2001a).Evaluation of gene transfer efficiency by viral vectors to murine bladder epithelium. *J Urol*, *165,* 667-671.

Siemens, D R, Elzey, B D, Lubaroff, D M, Bohlken, C, Jensen, R J, Swanson, A K, et al. (2001b).Cutting edge: restoration of the ability to generate CTL in mice immune to adenovirus by delivery of virus in a collagen-based matrix. *J Immunol*, *166,* 731-735.

Sugrue, M M, Shin, D Y, Lee, S W & Aaronson, S A. (1997).Wild-type p53 triggers a rapid senescence program in human tumor cells lacking functional p53. *Proc Natl Acad Sci U S A*, *94,* 9648-9653.

Sumitomo, M, Tachibana, M, Ozu, C, Asakura, H, Murai, M, Hayakawa, M, et al. (1999).Induction of apoptosis of cytokine-producing bladder cancer cells by adenovirus-mediated IkappaBalpha overexpression. *Hum Gene Ther*, *10,* 37-47.

Sutton, M A, Freund, C T, Berkman, S A, Dang, T D, Kattan, M W, Wheeler, T M, et al. (2000).In vivo adenovirus-mediated suicide gene therapy of orthotopic bladder cancer. *Mol Ther, 2,* 211-217.

Suzuki, T, Anderegg, B, Ohkawa, T, Irie, A, Engebraaten, O, Halks-Miller, M, et al. (2000).Adenovirus-mediated ribozyme targeting of HER-2/neu inhibits in vivo growth of breast cancer cells. *Gene Ther, 7,* 241-248.

Tanaka, M, Fraizer, G C, De La Cerda, J, Cristiano, R J, Liebert, M & Grossman, H B. (2001).Connexin 26 enhances the bystander effect in HSVtk/GCV gene therapy for human bladder cancer by adenovirus/PLL/DNA gene delivery. *Gene Ther, 8,* 139-148.

Tanaka, M, Sazawa, A, Shinohara, N, Kobayashi, Y, Fujioka, Y, Koyanagi, T, et al. (1999).Gelsolin gene therapy by retrovirus producer cells for human bladder cancer in nude mice. *Cancer Gene Ther, 6,* 482-487.

Tone, T, Kashani-Sabet, M, Funato, T, Shitara, T, Yoshida, E, Kashfian, B I, et al. (1993).Suppression of EJ cells tumorigenicity. *In Vivo, 7,* 471-476.

van der Poel, H G, Molenaar, B, van Beusechem, V W, Haisma, H J, Rodriguez, R, Curiel, D T, et al. (2002).Epidermal growth factor receptor targeting of replication competent adenovirus enhances cytotoxicity in bladder cancer. *J Urol, 168,* 266-272.

Verhoeyen, E & Cosset, F L. (2004).Surface-engineering of lentiviral vectors. *J Gene Med, 6 Suppl 1,* S83-94.

Volpers, C & Kochanek, S. (2004).Adenoviral vectors for gene transfer and therapy. *J Gene Med, 6 Suppl 1,* S164-171.

Watanabe, T, Shinohara, N, Sazawa, A, Takimoto, M, Hashimoto, A, Koyanagi, T, et al. (2001).Adenovirus-mediated gene therapy for bladder cancer in an orthotopic model using a dominant negative H-ras mutant. *Int J Cancer, 92,* 712-717.

Werthman, P E, Drazan, K E, Rosenthal, J T, Khalili, R & Shaked, A. (1996).Adenoviral-p53 gene transfer to orthotopic and peritoneal murine bladder cancer. *J Urol, 155,* 753-756.

Wu, Q, Possati, L, Montesi, M, Gualandi, F, Rimessi, P, Morelli, C, et al. (1996).Growth arrest and suppression of tumorigenicity of bladder-carcinoma cell lines induced by the P16/CDKN2 (p16INK4A, MTS1) gene and other loci on human chromosome 9. *Int J Cancer, 65,* 840-846.

Wu, X R, Lin, J H, Walz, T, Haner, M, Yu, J, Aebi, U, et al. (1994).Mammalian uroplakins. A group of highly conserved urothelial differentiation-related membrane proteins. *J Biol Chem, 269,* 13716-13724.

Xu, H J, Zhou, Y, Seigne, J, Perng, G S, Mixon, M, Zhang, C, et al. (1996).Enhanced tumor suppressor gene therapy via replication-deficient adenovirus vectors expressing an N-terminal truncated retinoblastoma protein. *Cancer Res, 56,* 2245-2249.

Yamamoto, T, Arakawa, F, Nakamura, K, Senba, T, Tomita, Y, Ikeda, S, et al. (1999).Enhanced antitumor activity of a combination treatment with a mouse/human chimeric anti-MK-1 antibody and lymphokine-activated killer cells in vitro and in a severe combined immunodeficient mouse xenograft model. *Cancer Immunol Immunother, 48,* 165-171.

Yamashita, M, Rosser, C J, Zhou, J H, Zhang, X Q, Connor, R J, Engler, H, et al. (2002).Syn3 provides high levels of intravesical adenoviral-mediated gene transfer for gene therapy of genetically altered urothelium and superficial bladder cancer. *Cancer Gene Ther*, *9,* 687-691.

Yang, C, Cirielli, C, Capogrossi, M C & Passaniti, A. (1995).Adenovirus-mediated wild-type p53 expression induces apoptosis and suppresses tumorigenesis of prostatic tumor cells. *Cancer Res*, *55,* 4210-4213.

Yu, J, Lin, J H, Wu, X R & Sun, T T. (1994).Uroplakins Ia and Ib, two major differentiation products of bladder epithelium, belong to a family of four transmembrane domain (4TM) proteins. *J Cell Biol*, *125,* 171-182.

Zhang, J, Ramesh, N, Chen, Y, Li, Y, Dilley, J, Working, P, et al. (2002).Identification of human uroplakin II promoter and its use in the construction of CG8840, a urothelium-specific adenovirus variant that eliminates established bladder tumors in combination with docetaxel. *Cancer Res*, *62,* 3743-3750.

Zhang, W, Grasso, L, McClain, C D, Gambel, A M, Cha, Y, Travali, S, et al. (1995).p53-independent induction of WAF1/CIP1 in human leukemia cells is correlated with growth arrest accompanying monocyte/macrophage differentiation. *Cancer Res*, *55,* 668-674.

In: New Gene Therapy and Cancer Research
Editor: Wilma B. Gustafsson, pp. 205-226
ISBN: 978-1-60021-969-6

Chapter VI

GENE AND VIRAL ONCOLYTIC THERAPIES FOR MALIGNANT GLIOMA

Adam M. Sonabend, Ilya V. Ulasov, Karen Dana and Maciej S. Lesniak*

The University of Chicago Brain Tumor Center, The University of Chicago, Chicago, IL, USA

ABSTRACT

Gliomas are the most common form of primary intracranial malignancy, with glioblastoma multiforme (GBM) carrying the worst prognosis. Among all of the novel therapies being explored for this disease, gene and viral oncolytic therapies are becoming a promising alternative. To achieve either a robust transgene expression or efficient viral replication with limited toxicity, a variety of delivery systems are being developed and tested. These include stem cells, viral vectors, liposomes and synthetic polymers. This chapter explores gene therapy and oncolytic viral therapy for malignant gliomas. The rationale for vector development and transgene selection is explored. Special attention is placed on modifications made to adenoviral oncolytic vectors in order to render them specific for gliomas. In addition, we discuss the results of novel treatment strategies, with a special emphasis on the results obtained in human clinical trials.

* Correspondence concerning this article should be addressed to: Maciej S. Lesniak Section of Neurosurgery, The University of Chicago Pritzker School of Medicine, 5841 South Maryland Ave, MC 3026, Chicago, IL 60637; Tel (773) 834-4757 Fax (773) 834-2608; Email: mlesniak@surgery.bsd.uchicago.edu.

INTRODUCTION

High-grade gliomas like glioblastoma multiforme (WHO grade IV glioma) (GBM) are one of the most common and aggressive forms of primary brain cancer [1,2]. In spite of aggressive treatments such as surgical debulking, radiotherapy and adjuvant chemotherapy [3,4], the median survival of patients remains poor [5]. This unfortunate outcome has been attributed to tumor resistance to the available therapy. This resistance is explained by tumor's biological behavior and its location within the central nervous system (CNS). The presence of the blood-brain-barrier limits the penetration of most chemotherapeutic agents to brain tumors [6]. At the same time, the genetic instability of gliomas leads to constant genotypic and phenotypic alterations that culminate in treatment resistance. Taken together, these factors provide a formidable challenge and novel therapies are very much needed to combat this deadly disease.

Some of the experimental treatments currently in development are based on immunotherapy, stem cell therapy, local chemotherapy, and radiotherapy [7-12]. Gene therapy represents an emerging treatment alternative. The fact that brain tumors recur locally and do not present with metastases outside the CNS allows for local delivery of therapeutic vectors [13,14]. To achieve a significant transgene expression and limited toxicity, different delivery systems are being explored. These include stem cells, viral vectors, liposomes and synthetic polymers. In addition, the initial idea of using viruses as delivery vehicles has evolved to include virotherapy. In this setting, the virus is rendered replication competent and is used to actually kill tumor cells. This chapter explores gene therapy and virotherapy for malignant gliomas. Even though many transgenes are explored, gene therapy systems for glioma are mainly discussed under the scope of the vectors employed.

GENE THERAPY

Gene therapy can be defined as the delivery of a gene of interest to tumor cell populations in order to control and/or elicit a cytotoxic effect on the end-target tissue (Figure 1). This principle has been evaluated through multiple approaches. In some cases, the transgene is an enzyme which activates a prodrug that is otherwise non-toxic to cells that don't express it. Herpes simplex virus type 1 (HSV) thymidine kinase (HSV-tk) in combination with ganciclovir (GCV) represent an illustrative example of the latter principle; this system is one of the first and most extensively studied gene therapy approaches in human trials for gliomas [15-19]. In parallel, other strategies for cancer gene therapy attempt to restore the function of a tumor suppressor gene like p53 that is frequently disrupted in a malignancy [20-22]. Other transgenes that have been tested, including interleukins and interferons, are employed to evoke an effective anti-tumor immune response [23-28]. At last, antisense oligonucleotides have also been explored as transgenes since these sequences can shut down oncogenes that play a significant role in the neoplastic phenotype [29-32]. Although many of these modalities appear interesting and complex, only few turn out useful at the bedside.

Since one of the goals of gene therapy is to achieve effective transgene expression, such transgene needs to be delivered to its target cell. This critical step is carried out by the use of vehicles. Mainly, the vehicles used for this purpose include liposomes, synthetic polymers, and of most importance, cells and viruses (Figure 2).

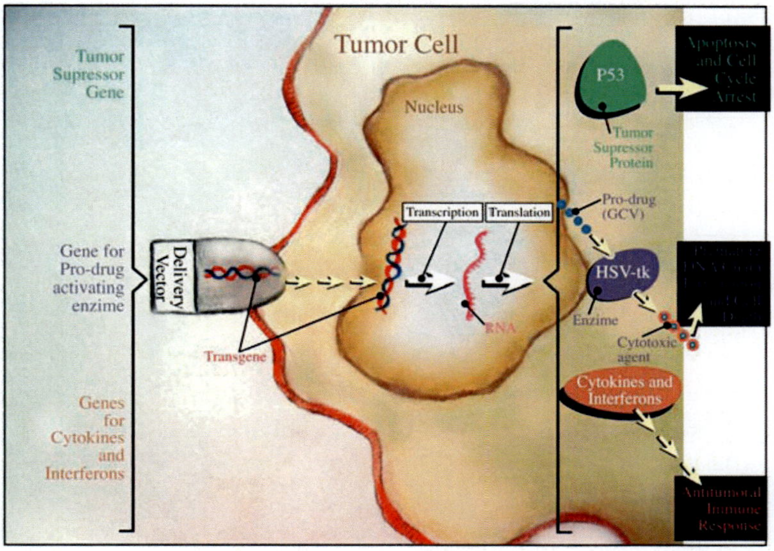

Figure 1.

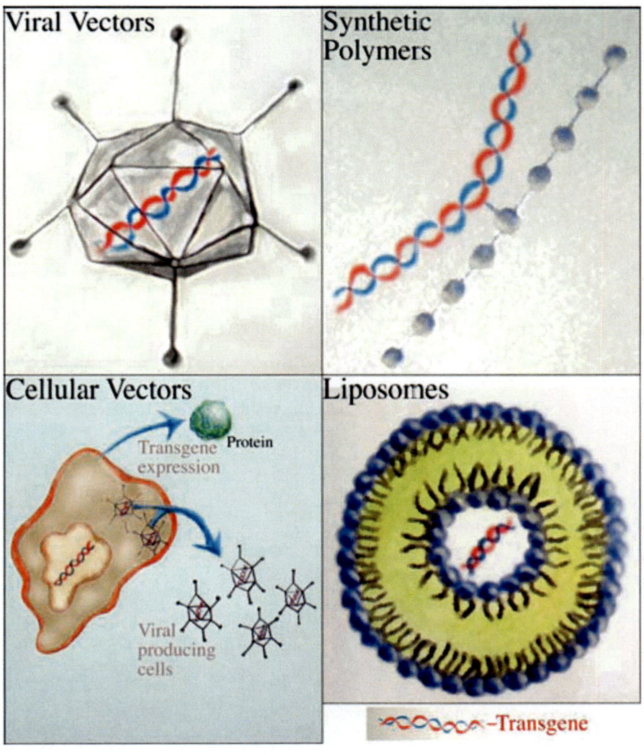

Figure 2.

Liposomes offer considerable advantages for gene therapy. For instance, liposomes are simple and easy to prepare in large quantities and the resulting vectors can easily be sterilized. In addition, liposomes don't have intrinsic toxicity or tissue specificity [27]. On the other hand, recent studies have suggested that with the aid of molecular modifications, liposomes can be further targeted and their transgene delivery capacity can be enhanced [28,33-35]. These vehicles have been used in the clinical setting for gene therapy on malignant brain tumors where some evidence of efficacy in addition to their safety is suggested [27,26,37]. Some scientists believe liposome-based systems are less efficient for gene transfer than viral vectors. On the other hand, the former have the hypothetical advantage of being relatively safe [38]. In any case, liposomes are not likely to surpass viral vectors as tools for most of cancer gene therapy strategies [14]. In the context of the considerable safety that viral vectors have achieved in recent human studies, the main reason for using liposomes seems to be fading away.

Polymer based vehicles facilitate DNA uptake and expression by promoting interaction with cellular membranes, protecting DNA against endogenous nucleases and trafficking plasmid to the nucleus [39,40]. Our group has tested the polyethylenimine, methoxypolyethyleneglycol and cholesterol (PPC) polymer as a vehicle for IL-12 gene transfer in murine model of intracranial glioma. In our study, intracranial injection of this complex was well tolerated and led to IL-12 expression at a therapeutic dose in the brains of tested animals. pmIL-12/PPC treatment of experimental brain tumors significantly prolonged survival of mice with experimental brain tumors [41].

The ideal gene therapy vector for brain tumors includes several features. For instance, selectivity for the desired target, minimal brain toxicity, the capacity to penetrate and diffuse through the tumor, and the ability to remain active in spite of evoking an immune response. For example, cells have been transfected to generate viral particles that can target tumors [15-17,42-44]. This strategy was explored in the first human studies of gene therapy for brain tumors during the 1990's. These pioneer studies consisted of retrovirus (RV) mediated HSV-tk gene therapy delivered by intra-tumoral injections of viral producing cells (VPC) followed by systemic administration of GCV [15-17]. These VPC derive from an embryonic mouse fibroblast cell line [45] and have a limited capacity to deliver viral particles since they are unable to migrate, remaining at the place where they are injected. Surprisingly, other cell carriers offer the capacity to migrate towards tumor cells. In particular, neural stem cells (NSC) are a promising tool to target disseminated tumor cells. NSC have a tropism for infiltrating cancer cells, so they can be used to deliver therapeutic agents directly by chasing the tumor pockets that reside beyond the healthy appearing surgical margin on brain parenchyma [8,46]. Additionally, mesenchymal stem cells could also be used for this purpose since these cells migrate and co-localize with malignant cells in the CNS [47,48].

VIRAL VECTORS

Viruses are naturally occurring gene therapy vehicles. In other words, as part of their reproductive cycle, these particles deliver and achieve transcription of their genome on target cells. A significant number of different viruses have been tested for gene therapy for brain tumors. Some of these include HSV [49-52], RV [15,16,42], measles virus [53], reovirus [54,55], adeno-associated virus [56], Newcastle disease virus (NDV) [57,58], Semliki Forest virus [59], vaccinia virus [60-62], poliovirus [63,64], adenovirus [4,65-70] and Sindbis virus [71].

Initially, non-replicating viral vectors were considered safer since the risk of uncontrolled infection leading to neural and systemic toxicities was conceived as lower when compared to their oncolytic counterparts. Among all of non-replicating vectors, the most exhaustibly studied are replication deficient RV and adenoviruses. Indeed, both of these have been tested in patients with malignant brain tumors.

In the case of RV, these vectors have been shown to be safe for intracranial injection, and for a long time have been a popular vehicle for gene therapy trials for GBM. As described earlier in this chapter, replication deficient RV in combination with VPC were initially used for gene therapy trials. These cells were injected into the tumor cavity and subsequently produced and secreted the vectors.

Some studies have tested a bicistronic RV-based system that carries interleukin-2 and HSV-tk in patients with recurrent GBM. A pilot study with four patients proved varying transgene activity in the tumors of the treated patients. [44]. That study was later extended to a larger population of patients and evaluated safety, feasibility, and biological activity of treatment. This time a total of 12 patients received intra-tumoral injection of VPC followed by intravenous GCV. Treatment was well tolerated with only minor adverse events. Transduction of tumor cells was demonstrated in tumor biopsies. A marked and persistent increase of intra-tumoral and plasma Th1 cytokine levels was demonstrated after treatment injection. Results of that trial suggest that the combined delivery of a suicide and a cytokine gene is safe, it is capable of inducing transgene transduction, it can lead to the activation of systemic cytokine cascade and tumor responses in 50% of cases [43].

Rainov *et al.* conducted a study that challenged the value of RV-based gene therapy for brain tumors; the group used a replication-deficient RV with HSV-tk transgene as insert. The study consisted on a multicenter, randomized, controlled phase III clinical trial [42]. As of today, this is the only published phase III trial evaluating gene therapy for brain tumors. RV vector particles were injected during surgery, followed by systemic treatment with GCV. Unfortunately, clinical outcomes including time to tumor progression, progression-free median survival, median survival, and 12-month survival rates showed no significant differences between treatment and control groups.

RV, although proven safe for intracranial use in the setting of brain tumors, do bare a number of inconveniences that make them inefficient as gene therapy vectors. First, RV have a low transduction efficacy [14,72,73]. Moreover, RV can only integrate into the genomes of replicating cells since they require the dissolution of the nuclear membrane. This fact is relevant since gliomas also contain non-cycling cells [69], implying ineffective transgene expression when these vehicles are used. At last, the low transgene caring capacity (8 kb approximately) and the risk of insertional mutagenesis add to the list of disadvantages of these vectors.

In the context of replication deficient viral vectors, adenoviruses constitute another popular option for gene therapy for brain tumors. Indeed, these vehicles are currently being used in approximately one quarter of all trials for gene therapy [74]. Adenoviruses are efficient and well suited for therapeutic gene delivery. These vectors have the ability to grow as recombinant viruses to high titers and are capable of carrying genes of interest as insertions. In addition, these kind of vectors transduce both dividing and quiescent cells (both kind found in gliomas) [14,75], are efficient with regard to transgene expression and seem to be as safe as RV in human trials [4,76,77]. At last, adenoviruses can be engineered to restrict transduction [65,78] and transgene expression to the desired target cell population [52,79-81]. These features are important in order to decrease toxicity. These features have made adenoviruses one of the most common transgene delivery systems for human gene therapy and a potentially useful therapeutic resource for treatment of brain tumors. When tested in patients with malignant gliomas, non-replicating adenoviruses offer a considerable deal of advantages to RV.

Sandmair *et al.* published the first clinical trial involving adenoviruses as gene therapy vectors for gliomas [76]. The study included 21 patients with primary (n=8) and recurrent (n=13) gliomas that were treated with intra-operative viral injection fallowed by i.v. GCV as adjuvant therapy. In this case, replication-deficient RV-HSV-tk (VPC were injected) and adenoviral vectors with HSV-tk (Ad-HSV-tk) were compared. As controls, one group of patients received Ad-LacZ (no GCV for these patients). Follow up included MRI scans to asses the disease status. No serious secondary effects were reported. Surprisingly, the median survival time of the group treated with Ad-HSV-tk (15 months) was significantly longer than that of RV-HSV-tk (7.4 months) and Ad-LacZ (8.3 months) ($p < 0.012$) [76].

Immonen *et al.*, encouraged by these results, continued the evaluation of Ad-HSV-tk in a phase IIb randomized, controlled trial [13]. For this latter study, 36 patients with operable primary or recurrent malignant glioma were randomized to receive Ad-HSV-tk injection (n=17) followed by i.v. GCV or standard care consisting of radical excision (additional radiotherapy in patients with primary tumors) (n=19). The primary end-point was survival as defined by death or surgery for recurrence. Secondary end-points were all-cause mortality and tumor progression as determined by MRI. Findings were also compared with historical controls (n = 36) from the same unit over 2 years preceding the study. In this study, Ad-HSV-tk treatment produced a clinically and statistically significant increase in mean survival from 39.0 +/- 19.7 to 70.6 +/- 52.9 weeks ($P = 0.0095$). The median survival time increased from 37.7 to 62.4 weeks. The treatment was well tolerated [13].

In spite of having found a certain degree of efficacy with replication-deficient adenoviruses, transgene expression capacity of these vectors appears to be limited. It is believed that in order to achieve a greater therapeutic efficacy, newer vectors need to overcome this challenge. For instance, a phase I clinical trial of p53 gene therapy was performed using a replication-defective adenovirus vector with wild type p53 (Ad-p53, INGN 201) against malignant brain tumors [21]. The vector was stereotactically injected intratumorally via an implanted catheter. Treated tumor specimens were obtained and analyzed. In all patients, exogenous p53 protein was detected within the nuclei of astrocytic tumor cells and transgene expression induced apoptosis of targeted cells. However, with the use of this replication-defective vector, transgene expression was limited to within 5 mm of the injection site. Based on these facts, many scientists favor replication competent vectors over replication defective counterparts. It is thought that due to the fact that the former kind replicates within tumor tissue and has a greater ability to infect and induce transgene expression, these vectors could offer a significant advantage for the treatment of brain tumors. The Ad-p53 cited INGN 201 trial, among other comparative studies suggest this observation [21,82] Nevertheless, these theoretical advantages of oncolytic viruses remain to be proven by efficacy endpoints such as patient survival.

ONCOLYTIC VECTORS FOR GLIOMA

As discussed earlier in this chapter, viruses seem to be prominent vehicles for somatic gene therapy. Most importantly, some viral vectors exhibit oncolytic properties. For this reason, the use of such vectors has been termed as "viral oncolytic therapy", a novel strategy for brain tumors. The cytotoxic feature of these vectors has been related to their ability to replicate in target tissues. In theory, these viruses can expand from the original dose administrated as long as there are tumor cells to sustain their replication. Currently, the oncolytic viral vectors developed for brain tumors are based on measles virus, Newcastle virus, herpes-simplex virus, reovirus and adenovirus. The vectors that have made it to the bedside are based on HSV, NDV and adenoviruses.

In the case of HSV oncolytic vectors, some have been tested in phase I clinical trials where their safety has been proven. Recombinant HSV, with deletion of viral gene coding for ICP34.5 and lacZ insertion into ICP6 (UL39) gene (insertion inactivates viral ribonucleotide reductase) represents one such vector. These deletions render mutant HSV more selective for replication in human gliomas, but also attenuate the viral progeny, decreasing its treatment power [83-85]. HSV 1716 is another vectors. This virus is based on wild type HSV 17 strain, and contains a single deletion in ICP34.5. This vector was also tested in a phase I clinical trial [50] where nine patients with relapsed malignant gliomas received intra-tumoral injections of doses up to $1X10^5$ p.f.u. There were no cases of encephalitis and no adverse clinical symptoms. Of nine patients treated, four remained alive and well 14 to 24 months after the vector's administration [50]. In addition, the same group conducted another phase I study with HSV 1716 in twelve patients with malignant gliomas (same dose of $1X10^5$ p.f.u.) [49]. In this latter study, the authors documented viral replication in tumors resected four to nine days after injection date. HSV DNA was assessed by PCR at the sites of inoculation in ten patients and at distal tumor sites in four. Interestingly, viral replication took place in both HSV-seropositive and -seronegative patients [49]. Overall, only modest results have been obtained with these viruses, but their effectiveness remains to be tested in future trials [49-51].

G207 is yet another example of an HSV-based oncolytic vector. This virus has deletions of both gamma(1)34.5 loci and a lacZ insertion disabling the UL39 gene. With these deletions, HSV no longer produces hemorrhagic, necrotizing encephalitis characteristic of wild-type HSV infection in human CNS [86]. This vector was tested in a dose-escalation phase I study for patients bearing malignant gliomas. The study included 21 patients with recurrent malignant gliomas. Dosage varied from $1x10^6$ plaque forming units (p.f.u.) inoculated at a single site to $3x10^9$ p.f.u. at five sites. No serious adverse effects were attributed to this treatment and no patient developed HSV encephalitis. Radiographic and neuropathologic evidence suggestive of anti-tumor activity and long-term presence of viral DNA was documented in some of the cases [51].

With regard to conditionally replicative adenoviruses (CRAd), vector dl1520, so called ONYX 015 was tested in patients with malignant gliomas. A phase I clinical trial of injection with ONYX 015 into peri-tumoral regions of 24 patients with recurrent malignant gliomas was published [4]. Treatment consisted of intra-cerebral injections of ONYX-015. Patients were assigned into cohort groups to test different doses (n=6 per cohort). Doses varied from $1x10^7$ p.f.u. to $1x10^{10}$ p.f.u. into a total of 10 sites within the resection cavity. None of the 24 patients experienced serious adverse events related to ONYX-015. The median time to progression after treatment with ONYX-015 was 46 days (range 13 to 452 + days). The median survival time was 6.2 months (range 1.3 to 28.0 + months). This trial proved that injection of up to $1x10^{10}$ p.f.u. of ONYX 015 into brain surrounding a resected malignant glioma is safe in humans.

Future Directions: Enhancement of CRAd's Tropism for Brain Tumor Cells

In order to target CRAd, some of the strategies used for the enhancement of viral tropism include the deletion of viral genomic regions that are not required for replication in cancer cells [67-69,87-89], redesigning the adenoviral capsid to promote transduction in neoplastic cells [65-67,78] and transcriptional targeting of viral genes or transgenes using tumor specific promoters [52,79-81,90].

Deletions of Viral Genomic Regions not Required for Replication in Cancer Cells

Non-cancerous cells display an arsenal of antiviral defenses that limit the extent of adenovirus infection. Specifically, to limit the spread of infection, cell cycle regulation and apoptosis are induced on the infected cell. On the other hand, upon infection, adenoviruses express viral proteins that are essential for reproduction and viral replication [91]. For instance, adenoviral E1A proteins provoke host cell induction of S phase by binding and inhibiting retinoblastoma protein (Rb) [92] and by alterations in cyclins A, B1, and E [93]. During S phase, viral DNA synthesis is favored [94]. Often, the same cellular proteins that are implicated in the cell's antiviral mechanisms are deficient in cancer cells as part of the neoplastic phenotype. Some CRAd are designed by deletion of viral genes that antagonize cell's defense and thus, the resulting vectors can only replicate in cancer cells that lack functional antiviral mechanisms. ONYX 015 (addressed earlier in this chapter) has a deletion in the viral genomic region coding E1B 55K. The protein coded in this region binds and inhibits p53, consequently prolonging host cell life and favoring viral progeny [87,89,94]. Apparently, such deletion restricts the replication of ONYX 015 to neoplastic cells with defective p53 pathway [87,89,95,96]. More recently, further investigation suggests that this vector's tropism for cancer cells is also related to a defect in mRNA export from nucleus [97-99].

Following a similar rationale, another oncolytic adenovirus was developed and is undergoing preclinical testing for brain tumors. Ad5-Delta24 is an adenoviral vector that carries a 24-bp deletion in the E1 viral genomic region. This deletion impairs the vector's capacity to interfere with Rb. Nevertheless, Ad5-Delta24 replicates in and destroys cancer cells with deficient Rb pathway [69]. Rb is a tumor suppressor protein with a pathway that is commonly altered in gliomas [100,101]. A hypo-phosphorylated form of Rb controls transition from G1 to S cell phase by binding to E2F transcription factors.

Ad5-Delta24 has been tested *in vivo* in human glioma xenografts in nude mice. A single dose of this vector induced 66.3 % inhibition and multiple injections an 83.8 % inhibition of tumor growth in this model. On the other hand, normal fibroblast or cancer cells with restored Rb activity were resistant to this virus [69] The oncolytic potential of this vector remains to be addressed in clinical studies.

The alteration of adenoviral genome has undesirable consequences that need to be contemplated as well. For instance, besides the functions of E1A and E1B described above, these proteins also perform important roles in adenoviral reproductive machinery. Indeed, E1B 55K protein is involved in transportation of viral mRNA from the nucleus to ribosomes, and this function is impaired in ONYX 015 [1102,103]. Some CRAd show impaired potency and oncolytic properties due to deletions of viral genomic regions such as E1A or E1B. Some of the genes encoded in E3 region have the function of either avoiding or promoting host cell death. Because of these properties, fine tuning of the expression of these genes is essential for generating progeny [104]. Adenoviral vectors with deletions in E3 regions have been proven to induce cell lyses and release their progeny slower than those E3 + in experiments with glioma xenografts [90,105].

Facilitation of Viral Transduction in Neoplastic Cells

Enhancement of viral tropism can be achieved by modification of viral transduction to increase infection of cancerous cells (Figure 3). The entry of adenoviral particles into these cells is mediated by the interaction of specific cell receptors and viral proteins. The transduction process of wild type adenoviruses requires the knob domain of fiber protein binding CAR. This receptor is widely present in most tissues but poorly expressed in gliomas [66,67,106-109] among other malignancies [66,110-113]. On the other hand, brain tumors express a series of alternative receptors. These receptors can be employed to direct viral transduction into gliomas for oncolytic gene therapy. For instance, integrins, molecules that are widely expressed and play an important role in the malignant phenotype of gliomas [109,114,115], can be targeted by modifications in adenoviral capsid. Ad5-Delta24RGD, was designed based on this strategy. This vector has an insertion of an Arg-Gly-Asp (RGD) motif into the fiber knob of vector Delta24 [68]. Such fiber modification enhances viral infection of the target cells by interaction of the inserted motif with αv integrins. Ad5-Delta24RGD led to higher oncolytic activity than that shown by Ad5-Delta24 after infection of glioma cells with low expression of CAR by CAR independent pathways. This vector was tested *in vivo* in nude mice with human malignant glioma IGRG121 xenografts. Intratumoral injection resulted in complete tumor regression in 9 of 10 mice and long-term survival in all treated mice compared to controls. The oncolytic activity of this vector was shown to be enhanced by irradiation such that the same therapeutic effect was achieved when a 10-fold lower viral dose was applied [67].

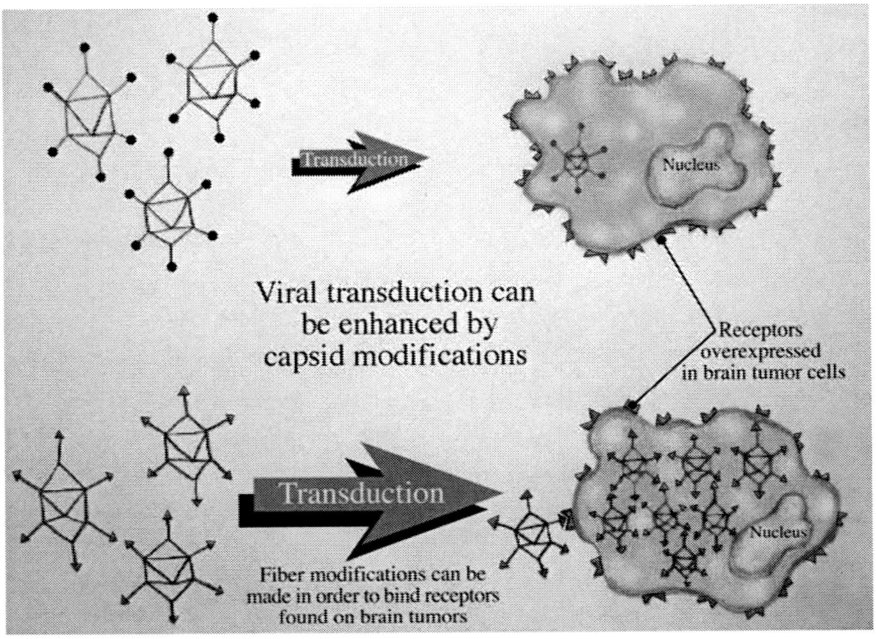

Figure 3.

Another interesting candidate for targeting malignant brain tumors is interleukin-13 receptor alpha2 chain (IL-13Ralpha2). This receptor has been found over-expressed and has been described as a marker of both glial transformation and tumor grade [116-120]. In order to test transductional targeting of gliomas by this receptor, our group constructed a replication-deficient adenoviral vector that possesses an IL-13 ligand on the fiber (LU-13) [120]. Luciferase transduction assays conducted in both primary and passaged glioma cell cultures exhibited at least 10-fold enhanced gene transduction. When tested in vivo, LU-13 showed a 300-fold increase in transgene expression over wild type adenovirus [120].

Epidermal Growth Factor Receptor (EGFR) is another receptor currently been explored for targeting CRAd to brain tumors. This receptor is widely present on high-grade gliomas due to the presence of EGFR gene amplification [121-123]. An advantage for the use of EGFR is that after binding its ligand, it is internalized and activation of phosphatidylinositol 3-OH kinase (PI3K)-dependent pathway takes place [124]. PI3K activation is required for adenovirus entry to host cells [125].

Several approaches for enhancement of viral tropism are based on EGFR. One consists of the development of a bispecific antibody conjugate that interferes with vector binding to cell receptors but retargets virus by binding to EGFR. This antibody promotes preferential adenoviral infection on glioma cells [66]. A different approach is based on the development of an adenoviral vector incapable of binding to host cell's integrins and CAR. Retargeting of this vector is performed by addition of bispecific single-chain antibodies directed to EGFR and adenovirus [65]. Other EGFR targeting strategy consists of an adenovirus that contains a soluble recombinant protein that includes the ectodomain of CAR fused with human EGF (sCAR-EGF fusion protein) [70].

Targeting Viral Genes or Transgenes Using Tumor Specific Promoters

An alternative or complementary approach for improving selectivity of adenoviral infection and oncolysis of gliomas is based on the use of specific promoter elements found active in these tumors. This strategy is based on the fact that the neoplastic phenotype development is accompanied by a series of modifications in gene expression [79,81,90,101,109,114, 121,122,126-129. The neoplastic cells show various activated promoter elements that respond to the abnormal function of transcription factors. These transcription regulatory elements are available as potential tools for targeting transgenes and vectors against gliomas (Figure 4). Some of the promoters about to be described correspond to genes normally expressed in glial cells, others are promoters of genes over-expressed in gliomas, and a third kind correspond to promoters of genes whose expression is up-regulated in endothelial cells of tumor's blood vessels.

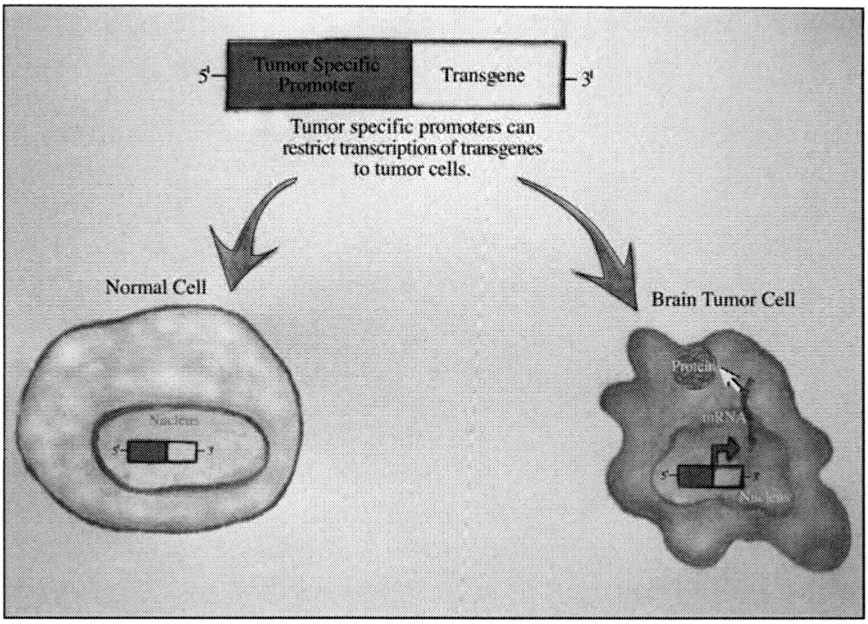

Figure 4.

Tissue specific promoter elements include glial fibrillary acidic protein [79,140,141] or myelin basic protein gene promoter [80,142,143] since these are active in gliomas. In spite of this, such promoters are not ideal for vector targeting because they can also drive the expression of transgenes in normal tissue surrounding the lesion [79,144]. Thus, toxicity might limit their use for targeting brain tumors.

Research in tumor biology has led to the discovery of tumor specific promoter sequences. In many cases these regulate the expression of genes that are essential for the tumors. Telomerase is a representative example of this principle. This promoter is over-expressed in approximately 90% of human cancers [79]. Telomerase has been reported to be active in 10 to 45% of anaplastic astrocytomas and 75 to 89% of GBM tumors, while remaining undetectable in normal brain tissue [133-136]. Telomerase is manly composed by functional or template RNA component and the telomerase catalytic protein subunit. Although controlled by different promoters, both subunits are required for its activity [145,146]. Telomerase promoter elements can be used to target oncolytic viruses as well as other means of gene therapy for gliomas [129,147-149]. Other tumor specific promoters that have been used in the context of CRAd are E2F-1 [81] and midkine [90,138,150-155].

Survivin is a member of the inhibitor-of-apoptosis family inappropriately expressed in astrocytic tumors (79.1%). The expression of this gene correlates with grade and is present in 90% of GBM. The activity of this promoter is enhanced by hypoxia [156], commonly found in rapidly growing tumors like high grade gliomas. Survivin seems to play an important role in the oncogenesis and progression of these tumors [157-159]. This is suggested by its expression pattern and by the fact that patients with survivin-positive astrocytic tumors have significantly shorter overall survival times compared with patients who have survivin-negative tumors [158]. The survivin promoter has already been proven effective for transgene expression in lung cancer [160]. Our group performed a study to compare the activity of survivin, midkine, and CXCR4 tumor-specific promoters for transcriptional targeting of gliomas [161]. Interestingly, in this study the survivin promoter demonstrated the highest level of mRNA expression in primary glioma samples and passaged cell lines. Transcriptional targeting was confirmed by infection of glioma cells with an adenovirus expression vector containing a survivin-driven luciferase reporter gene. Of the tested promoters, minimal level of survivin activity was detected in normal human liver and brain. Finally, as a proof of principle, a novel vector, CRAd-survivin-5/3, with E1a under the control of the survivin promoter, was tested *in vitro* where it exhibited enhanced cytopathic effect against malignant glioma [161].

Conclusions

Malignant brain tumors pose a real therapeutic challenge. Complex tumor biology along with localization to the CNS are two major factors responsible for much of the resistance to current modalities of treatment. Nevertheless, these limitations provide an opportunity for novel therapies, including gene therapy. In this setting, the development of targeting vectors along with the development of novel oncolytic viruses represents a unique opportunity to make an impact on this devastating disease. Although significant progress has been made to date and many of the viruses discussed in this chapter have been found safe in human clinical trials, significant efficacy in a large phase III clinical study has yet to be documented. Our ability to improve the oncolytic potency of viruses while minimizing toxicity to normal and healthy human brain should lay the foundation for the development of the next generation of gene therapy and oncolytic vectors for glioma therapy.

REFERENCES

[1] Annegers, JF, et al., Epidemiologic study of primary intracranial neoplasms. *Arch Neurol*, 1981. 38 (4): 217-9

[2] Louis, DN, Holland, EC and Cairncross, JG, Glioma classification: a molecular reappraisal. *Am J Pathol*, 2001. 159 (3): 779-86

[3] Kleihues, P, et al., The WHO classification of tumors of the nervous system. *J Neuropathol Exp Neurol*, 2002. 61 (3): 215-25; discussion 26-9

[4] Chiocca, EA, et al., A phase I open-label, dose-escalation, multi-institutional trial of injection with an E1B-Attenuated adenovirus, ONYX-015, into the peritumoral region of recurrent malignant gliomas, in the adjuvant setting. *Mol Ther*, 2004. 10 (5): 958-66

[5] Stupp, R, et al., Radiotherapy plus concomitant and adjuvant temozolomide for glioblastoma. *N Engl J Med*, 2005. 352 (10): 987-96

[6] Lesniak, MS and Brem, H, Targeted therapy for brain tumours. *Nat Rev Drug Discov*, 2004. 3 (6): 499-508

[7] Lesniak, MS, Langer, R and Brem, H, Drug delivery to tumors of the central nervous system. *Curr Neurol Neurosci Rep*, 2001. 1 (3): 210-6

[8] Ehtesham, M, Stevenson, CB and Thompson, RC, Stem cell therapies for malignant glioma. *Neurosurg Focus*, 2005. 19 (3): E5

[9] Ehtesham, M, et al., The use of interleukin 12-secreting neural stem cells for the treatment of intracranial glioma. *Cancer Res*, 2002. 62 (20): 5657-63

[10] Liau, LM, et al., Treatment of intracranial gliomas with bone marrow-derived dendritic cells pulsed with tumor antigens. *J Neurosurg*, 1999. 90 (6): 1115-24

[11] Yu, JS, et al., Vaccination with tumor lysate-pulsed dendritic cells elicits antigen-specific, cytotoxic T-cells in patients with malignant glioma. *Cancer Res*, 2004. 64 (14): 4973-9

[12] Yu, JS, et al., Vaccination of malignant glioma patients with peptide-pulsed dendritic cells elicits systemic cytotoxicity and intracranial T-cell infiltration. *Cancer Res*, 2001. 61 (3): 842-7

[13] Immonen, A, et al., AdvHSV-tk gene therapy with intravenous ganciclovir improves survival in human malignant glioma: a randomised, controlled study. *Mol Ther*, 2004. 10 (5): 967-72

[14] Pulkkanen, KJ and Yla-Herttuala, S, Gene therapy for malignant glioma: current clinical status. *Mol Ther*, 2005. 12 (4): 585-98

[15] Oldfield, EH, et al., Gene therapy for the treatment of brain tumors using intra-tumoral transduction with the thymidine kinase gene and intravenous ganciclovir. *Hum Gene Ther*, 1993. 4 (1): 39-69

[16] Raffel, C, et al., Gene therapy for the treatment of recurrent pediatric malignant astrocytomas with in vivo tumor transduction with the herpes simplex thymidine kinase gene/ganciclovir system. *Hum Gene Ther*, 1994. 5 (7): 863-90

[17] Kun, LE, et al., Stereotactic injection of herpes simplex thymidine kinase vector producer cells (PA317-G1Tk1SvNa.7) and intravenous ganciclovir for the treatment of progressive or recurrent primary supratentorial pediatric malignant brain tumors. *Hum Gene Ther*, 1995. 6 (9): 1231-55

[18] Prados, MD, et al., Treatment of progressive or recurrent glioblastoma multiforme in adults with herpes simplex virus thymidine kinase gene vector-producer cells followed by intravenous ganciclovir administration: a phase I/II multi-institutional trial. *J Neurooncol*, 2003. 65 (3): 269-78

[19] Klatzmann, D, et al., A phase I/II study of herpes simplex virus type 1 thymidine kinase "suicide" gene therapy for recurrent glioblastoma. Study Group on Gene Therapy for Glioblastoma. *Hum Gene Ther*, 1998. 9 (17): 2595-604

[20] Geoerger, B, et al., Oncolytic activity of p53-expressing conditionally replicative adenovirus AdDelta24-p53 against human malignant glioma. *Cancer Res*, 2004. 64 (16): 5753-9

[21] Lang, FF, et al., Phase I trial of adenovirus-mediated p53 gene therapy for recurrent glioma: biological and clinical results. *J Clin Oncol*, 2003. 21 (13): 2508-18

[22] Kim, IA, et al., Potential of adenoviral p53 gene therapy and irradiation for the treatment of malignant gliomas. *Int J Oncol*, 2001. 19 (5): 1041-7

[23] Okada, H, et al., Gene therapy of malignant gliomas: a phase I study of IL-4-HSV-TK gene-modified autologous tumor to elicit an immune response. *Hum Gene Ther*, 2000. 11 (4): 637-53

[24] Okada, H, et al., Gene therapy of malignant gliomas: a pilot study of vaccination with irradiated autologous glioma and dendritic cells admixed with IL-4 transduced fibroblasts to elicit an immune response. *Hum Gene Ther*, 2001. 12 (5): 575-95

[25] Kunwar, S, Convection enhanced delivery of IL13-PE38QQR for treatment of recurrent malignant glioma: presentation of interim findings from ongoing phase 1 studies. *Acta Neurochir Suppl*, 2003. 88 105-11

[26] Eck, SL, et al., Treatment of recurrent or progressive malignant glioma with a recombinant adenovirus expressing human interferon-beta (H5.010CMVhIFN-beta): a phase I trial. *Hum Gene Ther*, 2001. 12 (1): 97-113

[27] Yoshida, J, et al., Human gene therapy for malignant gliomas (glioblastoma multiforme and anaplastic astrocytoma) by in vivo transduction with human interferon beta gene using cationic liposomes. *Hum Gene Ther*, 2004. 15 (1): 77-86

[28] Yoshida, J, Mizuno, M and Wakabayashi, T, Interferon-beta gene therapy for cancer: basic research to clinical application. *Cancer Sci*, 2004. 95 (11): 858-65

[29] Ly, A, et al., Human glioma cells transformed by IGF-I triple helix technology show immune and apoptotic characteristics determining cell selection for gene therapy of glioblastoma. *Mol Pathol*, 2001. 54 (4): 230-9

[30] Zhang, Y, et al., MR imaging in rat glioma model and gene therapy using EGFR antisence RNA. *Chin Med J (Engl)*, 1998. 111 (11): 993-7

[31] Andrews, DW, et al., Results of a pilot study involving the use of an antisense oligodeoxynucleotide directed against the insulin-like growth factor type I receptor in malignant astrocytomas. *J Clin Oncol*, 2001. 19 (8): 2189-200

[32] Matsuno, A and Nagashima, T, Specific gene suppression using antisense strategy for growth suppression of glioma. *Med Electron Microsc*, 2004. 37 (3): 158-61

[33] Felgner, PL, et al., Lipofection: a highly efficient, lipid-mediated DNA-transfection procedure. *Proc Natl Acad Sci U S A*, 1987. 84 (21): 7413-7

[34] Felgner, PL, Holm, M and Chan, H, Cationic liposome mediated transfection. *Proc West Pharmacol Soc*, 1989. 32 115-21

[35] Shi, N and Pardridge, WM, Noninvasive gene targeting to the brain. *Proc Natl Acad Sci U S A*, 2000. 97 (13): 7567-72

[36] Jacobs, A, et al., Positron-emission tomography of vector-mediated gene expression in gene therapy for gliomas. *Lancet*, 2001. 358 (9283): 727-9

[37] Voges, J, et al., Imaging-guided convection-enhanced delivery and gene therapy of glioblastoma. *Ann Neurol*, 2003. 54 (4): 479-87

[38] Schatzlein, AG, Non-viral vectors in cancer gene therapy: principles and progress. *Anticancer Drugs*, 2001. 12 (4): 275-304

[39] Anwer, K, et al., Peptide-mediated gene transfer of cationic lipid/plasmid DNA complexes to endothelial cells. *J Drug Target*, 2004. 12 (4): 215-21

[40] Davis, ME, Non-viral gene delivery systems. *Curr Opin Biotechnol*, 2002. 13 (2): 128-31

[41] Sonabend, AM, et al., A Safety and Efficacy Study of Local Delivery of IL-12 Transgene by PPC Polymer in a Model of Experimental Glioma. *Anticancer Drugs*, 2007. Submitted

[42] Rainov, NG, A phase III clinical evaluation of herpes simplex virus type 1 thymidine kinase and ganciclovir gene therapy as an adjuvant to surgical resection and radiation in adults with previously untreated glioblastoma multiforme. *Hum Gene Ther*, 2000. 11 (17): 2389-401

[43] Colombo, F, et al., Combined HSV-TK/IL-2 gene therapy in patients with recurrent glioblastoma multiforme: biological and clinical results. *Cancer Gene Ther*, 2005. 12 (10): 835-48

[44] Palu, G, et al., Gene therapy of glioblastoma multiforme via combined expression of suicide and cytokine genes: a pilot study in humans. *Gene Ther*, 1999. 6 (3): 330-7

[45] Lyons, RM, et al., An improved retroviral vector encoding the herpes simplex virus thymidine kinase gene increases antitumor efficacy in vivo. *Cancer Gene Ther*, 1995. 2 (4): 273-80

[46] Yip, S, et al., Neural stem cell biology may be well suited for improving brain tumor therapies. *Cancer J*, 2003. 9 (3): 189-204

[47] Nakamizo, A, et al., Human bone marrow-derived mesenchymal stem cells in the treatment of gliomas. *Cancer Res*, 2005. 65 (8): 3307-18

[48] Nakamura, K, et al., Antitumor effect of genetically engineered mesenchymal stem cells in a rat glioma model. *Gene Ther*, 2004. 11 (14): 1155-64

[49] Papanastassiou, V, et al., The potential for efficacy of the modified (ICP 34.5(-)) herpes simplex virus HSV1716 following intratumoural injection into human malignant glioma: a proof of principle study. *Gene Ther*, 2002. 9 (6): 398-406

[50] Rampling, R, et al., Toxicity evaluation of replication-competent herpes simplex virus (ICP 34.5 null mutant 1716) in patients with recurrent malignant glioma. *Gene Ther*, 2000. 7 (10): 859-66

[51] Markert, JM, et al., Conditionally replicating herpes simplex virus mutant, G207 for the treatment of malignant glioma: results of a phase I trial. *Gene Ther*, 2000. 7 (10): 867-74

[52] Kambara, H, et al., An oncolytic HSV-1 mutant expressing ICP34.5 under control of a nestin promoter increases survival of animals even when symptomatic from a brain tumor. *Cancer Res*, 2005. 65 (7): 2832-9

[53] Phuong, LK, et al., Use of a vaccine strain of measles virus genetically engineered to produce carcinoembryonic antigen as a novel therapeutic agent against glioblastoma multiforme. *Cancer Res*, 2003. 63 (10): 2462-9

[54] Coffey, MC, et al., Reovirus therapy of tumors with activated Ras pathway. *Science*, 1998. 282 (5392): 1332-4

[55] Yang, WQ, et al., Efficacy and safety evaluation of human reovirus type 3 in immunocompetent animals: racine and nonhuman primates. *Clin Cancer Res*, 2004. 10 (24): 8561-76

[56] Mizuno, M, et al., Adeno-associated virus vector containing the herpes simplex virus thymidine kinase gene causes complete regression of intracerebrally implanted human gliomas in mice, in conjunction with ganciclovir administration. *Jpn J Cancer Res*, 1998. 89 (1): 76-80

[57] Russell, SJ, RNA viruses as virotherapy agents. Cancer Gene Ther, 2002. 9 (12): 961-6

[58] Csatary, LK and Bakacs, T, Use of Newcastle disease virus vaccine (MTH-68/H) in a patient with high-grade glioblastoma. *Jama*, 1999. 281 (17): 1588-9

[59] Ren, H, et al., Immunogene therapy of recurrent glioblastoma multiforme with a liposomally encapsulated replication-incompetent Semliki forest virus vector carrying the human interleukin-12 gene--a phase I/II clinical protocol. *J Neurooncol*, 2003. 64 (1-2): 147-54

[60] Gridley, DS, et al., Evaluation of radiation effects against C6 glioma in combination with vaccinia virus-p53 gene therapy. *Int J Oncol*, 1998. 13 (5): 1093-8

[61] Chen, B, et al., Low-dose vaccinia virus-mediated cytokine gene therapy of glioma. *J Immunother*, 2001. 24 (1): 46-57

[62] Timiryasova, TM, et al., Vaccinia virus-mediated expression of wild-type p53 suppresses glioma cell growth and induces apoptosis. *Int J Oncol*, 1999. 14 (5): 845-54

[63] Gromeier, M, et al., Intergeneric poliovirus recombinants for the treatment of malignant glioma. *Proc Natl Acad Sci U S A*, 2000. 97 (12): 6803-8

[64] Jackson, CA, et al., Repetitive intrathecal injections of poliovirus replicons result in gene expression in neurons of the central nervous system without pathogenesis. *Hum Gene Ther*, 2001. 12 (15): 1827-41

[65] van Beusechem, VW, et al., Efficient and selective gene transfer into primary human brain tumors by using single-chain antibody-targeted adenoviral vectors with native tropism abolished. *J Virol*, 2002. 76 (6): 2753-62

[66] Miller, CR, et al., Differential susceptibility of primary and established human glioma cells to adenovirus infection: targeting via the epidermal growth factor receptor achieves fiber receptor-independent gene transfer. *Cancer Res*, 1998. 58 (24): 5738-48

[67] Lamfers, ML, et al., Potential of the conditionally replicative adenovirus Ad5-Delta24RGD in the treatment of malignant gliomas and its enhanced effect with radiotherapy. *Cancer Res*, 2002. 62 (20): 5736-42

[68] Suzuki, K, et al., A conditionally replicative adenovirus with enhanced infectivity shows improved oncolytic potency. *Clin Cancer Res*, 2001. 7 (1): 120-6

[69] Fueyo, J, et al., A mutant oncolytic adenovirus targeting the Rb pathway produces anti-glioma effect in vivo. *Oncogene*, 2000. 19 (1): 2-12

[70] Dmitriev, I, et al., Ectodomain of coxsackievirus and adenovirus receptor genetically fused to epidermal growth factor mediates adenovirus targeting to epidermal growth factor receptor-positive cells. *J Virol*, 2000. 74 (15): 6875-84

[71] Zhang, J, Frolov, I and Russell, SJ, Gene therapy for malignant glioma using Sindbis vectors expressing a fusogenic membrane glycoprotein. *J Gene Med*, 2004. 6 (10): 1082-91

[72] Rainov, NG and Ren, H, Clinical trials with retrovirus mediated gene therapy--what have we learned? *J Neurooncol*, 2003. 65 (3): 227-36

[73] Vile, RG and Russell, SJ, Retroviruses as vectors. *Br Med Bull*, 1995. 51 (1): 12-30

[74] McConnell, MJ and Imperiale, MJ, Biology of adenovirus and its use as a vector for gene therapy. *Hum Gene Ther*, 2004. 15 (11): 1022-33

[75] Sonabend, AM, et al., Oncolytic adenoviral therapy for glioblastoma multiforme. *Neurosurg Focus*, 2006. 20 (4): E19

[76] Sandmair, AM, et al., Thymidine kinase gene therapy for human malignant glioma, using replication-deficient retroviruses or adenoviruses. *Hum Gene Ther*, 2000. 11 (16): 2197-205

[77] Lichtenstein, DL and Wold, WS, Experimental infections of humans with wild-type adenoviruses and with replication-competent adenovirus vectors: replication, safety, and transmission. *Cancer Gene Ther*, 2004. 11 (12): 819-29

[78] Fueyo, J, et al., Preclinical characterization of the antiglioma activity of a tropism-enhanced adenovirus targeted to the retinoblastoma pathway. *J Natl Cancer Inst*, 2003. 95 (9): 652-60

[79] Vandier, D, et al., Inhibition of glioma cells in vitro and in vivo using a recombinant adenoviral vector containing an astrocyte-specific promoter. *Cancer Gene Ther*, 2000. 7 (8): 1120-6

[80] Shinoura, N, et al., Adenovirus-mediated transfer of bax with caspase-8 controlled by myelin basic protein promoter exerts an enhanced cytotoxic effect in gliomas. *Cancer Gene Ther*, 2000. 7 (5): 739-48

[81] Parr, MJ, et al., Tumor-selective transgene expression in vivo mediated by an E2F-responsive adenoviral vector. *Nat Med*, 1997. 3 (10): 1145-9

[82] Ichikawa, T and Chiocca, EA, Comparative analyses of transgene delivery and expression in tumors inoculated with a replication-conditional or -defective viral vector. *Cancer Res*, 2001. 61 (14): 5336-9

[83] Markovitz, NS, Baunoch, D and Roizman, B, The range and distribution of murine central nervous system cells infected with the gamma(1)34.5- mutant of herpes simplex virus 1. *J Virol*, 1997. 71 (7): 5560-9

[84] Chung, RY, Saeki, Y and Chiocca, EA, B-myb promoter retargeting of herpes simplex virus gamma34.5 gene-mediated virulence toward tumor and cycling cells. *J Virol*, 1999. 73 (9): 7556-64

[85] Glorioso, JC and Fink, DJ, Herpes vector-mediated gene transfer in treatment of diseases of the nervous system. *Annu Rev Microbiol*, 2004. 58 253-71

[86] Shah, AC, et al., Oncolytic viruses: clinical applications as vectors for the treatment of malignant gliomas. *J Neurooncol*, 2003. 65 (3): 203-26
[87] Bischoff, JR, et al., An adenovirus mutant that replicates selectively in p53-deficient human tumor cells. *Science*, 1996. 274 (5286): 373-6
[88] Khuri, FR, et al., a controlled trial of intratumoral ONYX-015, a selectively-replicating adenovirus, in combination with cisplatin and 5-fluorouracil in patients with recurrent head and neck cancer. *Nat Med*, 2000. 6 (8): 879-85
[89] Heise, C, et al., ONYX-015, an E1B gene-attenuated adenovirus, causes tumor-specific cytolysis and antitumoral efficacy that can be augmented by standard chemotherapeutic agents. *Nat Med*, 1997. 3 (6): 639-45
[90] Kohno, S, et al., Midkine promoter-based conditionally replicative adenovirus for malignant glioma therapy. *Oncol Rep*, 2004. 12 (1): 73-8
[91] Lin, E and Nemunaitis, J, Oncolytic viral therapies. *Cancer Gene Ther*, 2004. 11 (10): 643-64
[92] Flint, J and Shenk, T, Viral transactivating proteins. *Annu Rev Genet*, 1997. 31 177-212
[93] Grand, RJ, et al., Human cells arrest in S phase in response to adenovirus 12 E1A. *Virology*, 1998. 244 (2): 330-42
[94] Ramachandra, M, et al., Re-engineering adenovirus regulatory pathways to enhance oncolytic specificity and efficacy. *Nat Biotechnol*, 2001. 19 (11): 1035-41
[95] Hall, AR, et al., p53-dependent cell death/apoptosis is required for a productive adenovirus infection. *Nat Med*, 1998. 4 (9): 1068-72
[96] Habib, NA, et al., Assessment of growth inhibition and morphological changes in in vitro and in vivo hepatocellular carcinoma models post treatment with dl1520 adenovirus. *Cancer Gene Ther*, 2002. 9 (5): 414-20
[97] O'Shea, CC, et al., Heat shock phenocopies E1B-55K late functions and selectively sensitizes refractory tumor cells to ONYX-015 oncolytic viral therapy. *Cancer Cell*, 2005. 8 (1): 61-74
[98] O'Shea, CC, et al., Late viral RNA export, rather than p53 inactivation, determines ONYX-015 tumor selectivity. *Cancer Cell*, 2004. 6 (6): 611-23
[99] Parato, KA, et al., Recent progress in the battle between oncolytic viruses and tumours. *Nat Rev Cancer*, 2005. 5 (12): 965-76
[100] Hamel, W, Westphal, M and Shepard, HM, Loss in expression of the retinoblastoma gene product in human gliomas is associated with advanced disease. *J Neurooncol*, 1993. 16 (2): 159-65
[101] Ueki, K, et al., CDKN2/p16 or RB alterations occur in the majority of glioblastomas and are inversely correlated. *Cancer Res*, 1996. 56 (1): 150-3
[102] Kratzer, F, et al., The adenovirus type 5 E1B-55K oncoprotein is a highly active shuttle protein and shuttling is independent of E4orf6, p53 and Mdm2. *Oncogene*, 2000. 19 (7): 850-7
[103] Harada, JN and Berk, AJ, p53-Independent and -dependent requirements for E1B-55K in adenovirus type 5 replication. *J Virol*, 1999. 73 (7): 5333-44
[104] Braithwaite, AW and Russell, IA, Induction of cell death by adenoviruses. *Apoptosis*, 2001. 6 (5): 359-70

[105] Tollefson, AE, et al., The adenovirus death protein (E3-11.6K) is required at very late stages of infection for efficient cell lysis and release of adenovirus from infected cells. *J Virol*, 1996. 70 (4): 2296-306

[106] Bergelson, JM, et al., Isolation of a common receptor for Coxsackie B viruses and adenoviruses 2 and 5. *Science*, 1997. 275 (5304): 1320-3

[107] Tomko, RP, Xu, R and Philipson, L, HCAR and MCAR: the human and mouse cellular receptors for subgroup C adenoviruses and group B coxsackieviruses. *Proc Natl Acad Sci U S A*, 1997. 94 (7): 3352-6

[108] Asaoka, K, et al., Dependence of efficient adenoviral gene delivery in malignant glioma cells on the expression levels of the Coxsackievirus and adenovirus receptor. *J Neurosurg*, 2000. 92 (6): 1002-8

[109] Grill, J, et al., Combined targeting of adenoviruses to integrins and epidermal growth factor receptors increases gene transfer into primary glioma cells and spheroids. *Clin Cancer Res*, 2001. 7 (3): 641-50

[110] Li, D, et al., Variability of adenovirus receptor density influences gene transfer efficiency and therapeutic response in head and neck cancer. *Clin Cancer Res*, 1999. 5 (12): 4175-81

[111] Hemmi, S, et al., The presence of human coxsackievirus and adenovirus receptor is associated with efficient adenovirus-mediated transgene expression in human melanoma cell cultures. *Hum Gene Ther*, 1998. 9 (16): 2363-73

[112] Li, Y, et al., Loss of adenoviral receptor expression in human bladder cancer cells: a potential impact on the efficacy of gene therapy. *Cancer Res*, 1999. 59 (2): 325-30

[113] Okegawa, T, et al., The dual impact of coxsackie and adenovirus receptor expression on human prostate cancer gene therapy. *Cancer Res*, 2000. 60 (18): 5031-6

[114] Uhm, JH, Gladson, CL and Rao, JS, The role of integrins in the malignant phenotype of gliomas. *Front Biosci*, 1999. 4 D188-99

[115] Bello, L, et al., IS20I, a specific alphavbeta3 integrin inhibitor, reduces glioma growth in vivo. *Neurosurgery,* 2003. 52 (1): 177-85; discussion 85-6

[116] Kawakami, M, et al., Analysis of interleukin-13 receptor alpha2 expression in human pediatric brain tumors. *Cancer*, 2004. 101 (5): 1036-42

[117] Kawakami, M, et al., Mutation and functional analysis of IL-13 receptors in human malignant glioma cells. *Oncol Res*, 2001. 12 (11-12): 459-67

[118] Mintz, A, et al., IL-13Ralpha2 is a glioma-restricted receptor for interleukin-13. *Neoplasia*, 2002. 4 (5): 388-99

[119] Saikali, S, et al., Expression of nine tumour antigens in a series of human glioblastoma multiforme: interest of EGFRvIII, IL-13Ralpha2, gp100 and TRP-2 for immunotherapy. *J Neurooncol*, 2007. 81 (2): 139-48

[120] Ulasov, IV, et al., Novel recombinant adenoviral vector that targets the interleukin-13 receptor alpha2 chain permits effective gene transfer to malignant glioma. *Hum Gene Ther*, 2007. 18 (2): 118-29

[121] Wong, AJ, et al., Increased expression of the epidermal growth factor receptor gene in malignant gliomas is invariably associated with gene amplification. *Proc Natl Acad Sci U S A*, 1987. 84 (19): 6899-903

[122] Ekstrand, AJ, et al., Genes for epidermal growth factor receptor, transforming growth factor alpha, and epidermal growth factor and their expression in human gliomas in vivo. *Cancer Res*, 1991. 51 (8): 2164-72

[123] Libermann, TA, et al., Amplification, enhanced expression and possible rearrangement of EGF receptor gene in primary human brain tumours of glial origin. *Nature*, 1985. 313 (5998): 144-7

[124] Hu, P, et al., Interaction of phosphatidylinositol 3-kinase-associated p85 with epidermal growth factor and platelet-derived growth factor receptors. *Mol Cell Biol*, 1992. 12 (3): 981-90

[125] Li, E, et al., Adenovirus endocytosis via alpha(v) integrins requires phosphoinositide-3-OH kinase. *J Virol*, 1998. 72 (3): 2055-61

[126] Graulich, W, et al., Cell type specificity of the human endoglin promoter. *Gene*, 1999. 227 (1): 55-62

[127] Dahlstrand, J, Collins, VP and Lendahl, U, Expression of the class VI intermediate filament nestin in human central nervous system tumors. *Cancer Res*, 1992. 52 (19): 5334-41

[128] Guha, A, et al., Expression of PDGF and PDGF receptors in human astrocytoma operation specimens supports the existence of an autocrine loop. *Int J Cancer*, 1995. 60 (2): 168-73

[129] Boyd, M, et al., Expression in UVW glioma cells of the noradrenaline transporter gene, driven by the telomerase RNA promoter, induces active uptake of [131I]MIBG and clonogenic cell kill. *Oncogene*, 2001. 20 (53): 7804-8

[130] Shai, R, et al., Gene expression profiling identifies molecular subtypes of gliomas. *Oncogene*, 2003. 22 (31): 4918-23

[131] Mischel, PS, et al., Identification of molecular subtypes of glioblastoma by gene expression profiling. *Oncogene*, 2003. 22 (15): 2361-73

[132] Kim, NW, et al., Specific association of human telomerase activity with immortal cells and cancer. *Science*, 1994. 266 (5193): 2011-5

[133] Le, S, et al., Telomerase activity in human gliomas. *Neurosurgery*, 1998. 42 (5): 1120-4; discussion 24-5

[134] DeMasters, BK, et al., Differential telomerase expression in human primary intracranial tumors. *Am J Clin Pathol*, 1997. 107 (5): 548-54

[135] Langford, LA, et al., Telomerase activity in human brain tumours. *Lancet*, 1995. 346 (8985): 1267-8

[136] Harada, K, et al., Telomerase activity in primary and secondary glioblastomas multiforme as a novel molecular tumor marker. *J Neurosurg*, 2000. 93 (4): 618-25

[137] Collins, VP and James, CD, Gene and chromosomal alterations associated with the development of human gliomas. *Faseb J*, 1993. 7 (10): 926-30

[138] Miyauchi, M, et al., Frequent expression of midkine gene in esophageal cancer suggests a potential usage of its promoter for suicide gene therapy. *Jpn J Cancer Res*, 1999. 90 (4): 469-75

[139] Furnari, FB, Huang, HJ and Cavenee, WK, Genetics and malignant progression of human brain tumours. *Cancer Surv*, 1995. 25 233-75

[140] Cortez, N, et al., Primary astrocytes retrovirally transduced with a tyrosine hydroxylase transgene driven by a glial-specific promoter elicit behavioral recovery in experimental parkinsonism. *J Neurosci Res*, 2000. 59 (1): 39-46

[141] Segovia, J, Vergara, P and Brenner, M, Astrocyte-specific expression of tyrosine hydroxylase after intracerebral gene transfer induces behavioral recovery in experimental parkinsonism. *Gene Ther*, 1998. 5 (12): 1650-5

[142] Miyao, Y, et al., Usefulness of a mouse myelin basic protein promoter for gene therapy of malignant glioma: myelin basic protein promoter is strongly active in human malignant glioma cells. *Jpn J Cancer Res*, 1997. 88 (7): 678-86

[143] Miyao, Y, et al., Selective expression of foreign genes in glioma cells: use of the mouse myelin basic protein gene promoter to direct toxic gene expression. *J Neurosci Res*, 1993. 36 (4): 472-9

[144] Nettelbeck, DM, Jerome, V and Muller, R, Gene therapy: designer promoters for tumour targeting. *Trends Genet*, 2000. 16 (4): 174-81

[145] Feng, J, et al., The RNA component of human telomerase. *Science*, 1995. 269 (5228): 1236-41

[146] Meyerson, M, Telomerase enzyme activation and human cell immortalization. *Toxicol Lett*, 1998. 102-103 41-5

[147] Ito, H, et al., Autophagic cell death of malignant glioma cells induced by a conditionally replicating adenovirus. *J Natl Cancer Inst*, 2006. 98 (9): 625-36

[148] Srinivasula, SM, et al., Generation of constitutively active recombinant caspases-3 and -6 by rearrangement of their subunits. *J Biol Chem*, 1998. 273 (17): 10107-11

[149] Komata, T, et al., Treatment of malignant glioma cells with the transfer of constitutively active caspase-6 using the human telomerase catalytic subunit (human telomerase reverse transcriptase) gene promoter. *Cancer Res*, 2001. 61 (15): 5796-802

[150] Yu, L, et al., Midkine promoter-driven suicide gene expression and -mediated adenovirus replication produced cytotoxic effects to immortalised and tumour cells. *Eur J Cancer*, 2004. 40 (11): 1787-94

[151] Yu, L, et al., Midkine promoter can mediate transcriptional activation of a fused suicide gene in a broader range of human breast cancer compared with c-erbB-2 promoter. *Oncology*, 2004. 66 (2): 143-9

[152] Tomizawa, M, et al., A promoter region of the midkine gene that is frequently expressed in human hepatocellular carcinoma can activate a suicide gene as effectively as the alpha-fetoprotein promoter. *Br J Cancer*, 2003. 89 (6): 1086-90

[153] Yu, L, et al., Cell growth- and P53-dependent transcriptional activity of the midkine promoter confers suicide gene expression in tumor cells. *Oncol Rep*, 2003. 10 (5): 1301-5

[154] Sakiyama, S, et al., Utilization of the promoter region of the midkine gene as a tool to drive therapeutic genes in a tumor specific manner. *Adv Enzyme Regul*, 2003. 43 57-66

[155] Adachi, Y, et al., Midkine promoter-based adenoviral vector gene delivery for pediatric solid tumors. *Cancer Res*, 2000. 60 (16): 4305-10

[156] Yang, L, et al., Tumor-specific gene expression using the survivin promoter is further increased by hypoxia. *Gene Ther*, 2004. 11 (15): 1215-23

[157] Kleinschmidt-DeMasters, BK, et al., Survivin in glioblastomas. Protein and messenger RNA expression and comparison with telomerase levels. *Arch Pathol Lab Med*, 2003. 127 (7): 826-33

[158] Kajiwara, Y, et al., Expression of survivin in astrocytic tumors: correlation with malignant grade and prognosis. *Cancer*, 2003. 97 (4): 1077-83

[159] Das, A, et al., Expression of survivin in primary glioblastomas. *J Cancer Res Clin Oncol*, 2002. 128 (6): 302-6

[160] Chen, JS, et al., Cancer-specific activation of the survivin promoter and its potential use in gene therapy. *Cancer Gene Ther*, 2004. 11 (11): 740-7

[161] Ulasov, IV, et al., Evaluation of Promoter Candidates for Transcriptional Targeting of Glioma Gene Therapy. *Cancer Biology and Therapy* 2007. Accepted for Publication.

In: New Gene Therapy and Cancer Research
Editor: Wilma B. Gustafsson, pp. 227-248

ISBN: 978-1-60021-969-6

Chapter VII

NONVIRAL CANCER VACCINES: FROM FREE ANTIGENS TO ENGINEERED CELLS

M. J. Herrero[1], R. Botella[2], R. Algás[3], F. Marco[4], S. Lledó[5] and S. F. Aliño[1,6]

[1]Unidad de Terapia Génica, Departmento de Farmacología, Facultad de Medicina, Universidad de Valencia, Spain;
[2]Servicio de Dermatología, Instituto Valenciano de Oncología (IVO), Valencia, Spain;
[3]Servicio de Radioterapia, Hospital Clínico Universitario, Valencia, Spain;
[4]ASAC Pharmaceutical International, Alicante, Spain;
[5]Servicio de Cirugía, Hospital clínico Universitario, Valencia, Spain;
[6]Unidad de Farmacología Clínica, Hospital Universitario La Fe, Valencia, Spain.

ABSTRACT

In the present work we have developed several models of cancer vaccines, employing a murine melanoma and nonviral procedures for gene transfer. Many efforts have been made in relation to cancer vaccines, attempting to elucidate the best way to induce correct activation of the immune system in order to achieve proper antitumor response. Engineered cells seem to be the most successful approach, since they better reproduce the processes that occur in real patients, including events that today still escape our understanding. However, purified antigens represent an easier approach in terms of their preparation, reproducibility and facility to become a commercial medicine. This is why they continue to center attention, though their results are still not particularly satisfactory. In an attempt to establish the best approach for stimulating the immune response and also securing the simplest treatment, we have tested different preventive vaccination models such as: a) purified antigens from irradiated B16 melanoma tumor cells (Tumor Membrane Proteins, TMP); b) such antigens encapsulated in liposomes; c) lipopolyplexes formed by cationic liposomes bearing antigens plus the cationic polymer polyethyleneimine (PEI), carrying DNA; d) freshly transfected and irradiated B16 cells, producing cytokines; and e) a very reduced number of transfected cells, selected by means of magnetic bead procedures. The results obtained show different rates of tumor growth inhibition - performance improving when adjusting the combinations of plasmid bearing the cytokine gene and TMP antigens in the lipopolyplexes. The best inhibition (total) was obtained with freshly transfected (not selected) cells, which allowed us to perform further experiments consisting of a vaccine with only the truly transfected (cytokine-producing) cells. On this occasion, reducing the cell number to only 20% that of the prior doses, we achieved about 80% of tumor growth inhibition. All these results encourage the conduction of further studies of this kind, with the purpose of increasing accuracy and optimizing cancer vaccine procedures.

Introduction

Genetically modified tumor cells have been shown to be very efficient in various models of antitumor vaccines [1,2,3]. Still, the main problem with these models is the great difficulty of obtaining tumor cells from patients and that moreover must be kept in culture, amplified to a larger number, transfected and then returned to the same patient. This is not easy, even when employing other proposed methods - not only with tumor cells, but also with syngenic or allogenic cells [4,5]. All these efforts in the field of cancer vaccine research have converged on the idea that the best results are obtained vaccinating not only with the tumor antigens, but also with the genes that the immune system itself would use to achieve a good response: the cytokine genes. However, the functioning of the immune system is very complex, and combining these two components has not always been successful [6,7], leading to immune suppression or even anergy. Our group has also made efforts to elucidate the correct time order to supply the two signals [8]. At present, the most effective way of administering these two components is the introduction of cells, or a neoplastic nature or otherwise, that produce the cytokine themselves [8,9,10]. In this context, many studies have achieved promising results, and clinical trials have been set up [11,12]. To understand what kind of antigens work best and how they awaken a truly effective response, we also wanted to work with tumor cell antigens instead of whole cells - since they offer the advantage of being easier to prepare and standardize as commercial medicines [13]. In this sense, we have worked in a murine model of melanoma, using the two above mentioned components to develop an antitumor vaccine, antigens and cytokine genes, adopting two different approaches: purified antigens or cells. As antigens, we have used irradiated whole tumor cells (murine melanoma B16 cells) or an extract of their hydrophilic membrane antigens (tumor membrane proteins, TMP). As cytokines, we have used the m-GMCSF encoding gene (Granulocytes and Macrophages Colony Stimulating Factor), which has largely demonstrated great usefulness as an antitumor tool [1,4,6,10]. However, in later experiments, our tumor cells have also been transfected with the m-B7.2 encoding gene.

The first set of experiments is based on TMP encapsulated in liposomes or lipopolyplexes, and there we have explored the best liposome type and formulation, and the quantity of TMP and quantity of GM-CSF suitable for achieving an antitumor response.

Liposomes and lipopolyplexes also have a long trajectory in the field of vaccines, and have been shown to be good adjuvants in many different settings [14-17].

Nevertheless, being aware of the more solid results obtained with whole cells instead of purified antigens, in the second set of experiments we have worked with freshly transfected B16 cells, producing GM-CSF and B7.2.

B7.2 (also called CD86) is a costimulatory molecule of the immune system, naturally expressed only at the surface of professional Antigen Presenting Cells (APCs). This molecule has been widely employed in different antitumor approaches [18-24], as it enhances the immune response by participating in the activation of T cells: after the first signal of antigen recognition in the APC, the major histocompatibility complex (MHC) molecules present the antigenic peptides to the TCR (T Cell Receptor); however, only if the second signal (costimulation) is also present, will the T cells correctly begin sustained cell proliferation, effector or memory cell generation, and the prevention of anergy or apoptosis. It is in relation to this second signal where B7.2 plays its role by positively stimulating T cells through CD28. Our aim in employing B7.2 has been to increase the T cell response against the transfected B16 cells, but we have also taken advantage of such transfection to select and purify only the truly transfected cells from a total population of freshly transfected cells and to perform a vaccination experiment with a very reduced cell number - again attempting to define the minimum number of cells required to secure good results, and thus start with "easier to prepare" cell vaccines.

Materials and Methods

Plasmids

p2F m-gmcsf, p2F m-B7.2, p2F m-gmcsf + m-B7.2 and p2F Ø, were derived from the pVITRO2 base plasmid (Invivogen, France), with the *m-gmcsf* gene, *m-B7.2*, *m-gmcsf* plus *m-B7.2* genes or the empty plasmid, respectively. pVITRO2 allows the coexpression of two genes and contains two human ferritin composite promoters, FerH (heavy chain) and FerL (light chain), combined to the SV40 and CMV enhancers respectively, and the resistance gene to Hygromycin. To eliminate the iron regulation, their 5'UTRs have been replaced by the 5'UTR of the mouse and chimpanzee EF1α genes.

All plasmids were amplified in *Escherichia coli* DH5α, in selective LB broth (Pronadisa, Spain) and extracted with the Qiagen Giga Endofree kit (Izasa SA, Spain), quantified by spectrophotometry and tested by electrophoresis to confirm their integrity and purity.

TMP Obtainment

The mixture of hydrophilic membrane proteins from B16 cells was performed following a protocol based on the work of Bordier work [25]. Briefly, after detaching and counting the irradiated cells, their pellet is resuspended in 1 ml of extraction buffer for every 10 million cells, containing Tris 10 mM, $MgCl_2$ 2 mM, Triton X-114 0.5% (Sigma, Spain) and phenylmethylsulfonylfluoride (PMSF) 0.1 mM (Sigma, Spain), pH 7.2. The mixture is incubated in ice for 45 min., shaking gently every 10 min. Then, centrifugation is carried out at 5300 rpm, 4°C, for 15 min. The supernatant is recovered and 750 μl placed above 250 μl of centrifuge buffer (sucrose 10% in extraction buffer) in microcentrifuge tubes. After incubating 3 min. at 37°C, it is centrifuged again for 5 min. at 2100 rpm. Supernatant (750 μl) is recovered and Triton X-114 added to a final concentration of 0.5% before placing the tube in ice again over 250 μl of centrifuge buffer. After incubating for 3 min. more at 37°C and centrifuging for 5 min. more at 2100 rpm, two different phases are obtained in the microcentrifuge tube: the upper one contains the hydrophilic proteins, that will be kept in aliquots at -20°C until use.

The proteins are quantified with the CBQCA protein quantitation kit (Molecular Probes-Invitrogen, Spain), following the manufacturer's instructions.

Liposomes and Lipopolyplexes

Three different types of liposome production were tested: Multilamellar Vesicles (MLV), Dehydration-Rehydration Vesicles (DRV), and Freeze-Thawed Multilamellar Vesicles (MLV-FT), proceeding according to the literature for manufacture [26,27]. Also, four different lipidic compositions were evaluated, employing Phosphatidylcholine (PC), Sphingomyelin (SM), Cholesterol (CH) and Dicetylphosphate (DP), all from Sigma (Spain), being PC:CH and SM:CH at 6:4 molar ratio and PC:CH:DP and SM:CH:DP at 5:4:1. All were formed in Milli Q water. The liposomes chosen for lipopolyplex formation were PC:CH:DP (5:4:1), which were later coupled with PEI 25 KDa (polyethyleneimine, Sigma, Spain) linked to the plasmid in use, at a ratio of 1.41:1, PEI:DNA (polyplex, also made in Milli Q) [27,28]. To test the quantity of protein encapsulated in each type of liposome, the CBQCA protein quantitation kit (Molecular Probes-Invitrogen, Spain) was employed, following the manufacturer's instructions.

Cells and Transfection Procedures

B16 murine melanoma cells have been used in all of the experiments. These cells are syngenic with the animals used for vaccination, i.e., C57BL/6 mice (Harlan, France). B16 cells were also used as source of antigen for vaccination, either as whole cells or employed to obtain an extract of their membrane proteins (TMP). To inoculate the tumors in vaccinated and control groups of mice, 10^5 freshly detached B16 cells were injected in their usual simple culture medium into the left leg of the animals, while the vaccines were injected subcutaneously into the right leg.

B16 cells are adherent cells that are grown in flasks with DMEM (Dulbecco's modified Eagle's medium) (Sigma, Spain), supplemented with 10% heat inactivated fetal bovine serum (FBS) (Biomedia, France), Penicillin (100 U/ml) and Streptomycin (100 μg/ml). They are cultured in a humidified incubator with 5% CO_2 at 37°C, and are detached from the flasks with Trypsin-EDTA. When whole cells are used for vaccinating, they are irradiated with a 150 Gy dose, after being detached from their flasks, and are later frozen in FBS with 5% DMSO to be kept at -80 or -150°C until use.

The cells were transfected by means of a chemical procedure based on PEI 25 KDa (polyethyleneimine. Sigma, Spain) polyplexes with 20 μg/ml p2F plasmids, as previously described [8,26]. The transfection percentage with this method lies between 20-40% of total cells (data not shown), as observed using the reporter EGFP gene. Cells were transfected when more than 80% confluence was reached in their flasks, irradiated 72 hours post-transfection with 150 Gy, and then frozen in DMSO 5% in FBS and kept at -80 or -150°C until use.

Determination of m-GMCSF Production

The GM-CSF production of the transfected B16 cells is determined by Enzyme Linked Immunosorbent Assay (ELISA), performed on supernatant samples of the culture media taken 72 hours post-transfection and prior to cell detachment and irradiation, having changed the media every 24 hours. The BD OptEIA ELISA kit for m-GMCSF (Pharmingen, BD Biosciences, Spain) was used. The time-point of 72 hours was chosen on the basis of prior experimental results, assessed to study cytokine production over time, and using the referred transfection conditions [8,10,26], in order to achieve adequate production according to the literature [4].

Determination of m-B7.2 production

Flow cytometry was performed to confirm the presence of m-B7.2 in the surface of the transfected cells. At 72 h post-transfection, cells were harvested and pelleted in aliquots of 500,000 cells, washed and incubated in ice for at least 30 min. in 200 μl PBS-FBS (2.5%) - Azide (0.01%) solution of primary antibody (1 μg/million cells): Biotin-conjugated rat anti-mouse CD86 monoclonal antibody (Pharmingen, BD, Spain). Then, cells were washed twice in 1 ml PBS-Azide and incubated in ice and dark with the secondary antibody (0.5 μg/million cells): Streptavidin-Fluorescein Isothiocyanate conjugate (FITC) (Pharmingen, BD, Spain).

Finally, cells were washed twice and finally resuspended in 500 μl PBS to be passed through the cytometer (Coulter Epics, XL; Beckman Coulter, Spain) and for analysis of the fluorescence in the populations, in order to discriminate the truly transfected cells. To avoid taking autofluorescence or nonspecific binding as positive results, several controls were tested. The groups were: a) non-transfected wild type B16 cells, without any antibody; b) non-transfected wild type B16 cells incubated with both antibodies; c) B16-p2F m-gmcsf + m-B7.2 transfected cells, without any antibody; d) B16-p2F m-gmcsf + m-B7.2 transfected cells, incubated only with primary antibody; e) B16-p2F m-gmcsf + m-B7.2 transfected cells, incubated only with secondary antibody; and finally f) B16-p2F m-gmcsf + m-B7.2 transfected cells, incubated with both primary and secondary antibody.

Selection and Purification of Transfected Cells

This process is carried out by means of the Automacs device for magnetic cell separation (Miltenyi Biotec, Spain), according to the manufacturer's instructions and employing the Automacs columns. At 72 h post-transfection, cells are harvested and incubated with the first antibody, in PBS, under the same conditions as in the flow cytometry experiments; the Streptavidin Microbeads protocol is then followed (Miltenyi Biotec, Spain), and transfected cells are separated and purified employing the "Posseld 2" program. Lastly, cells are counted and frozen until the time of the vaccination experiments.

Preventive Vaccination Procedures

C57BL/6 mice (8-10 weeks old) kept under standard laboratory conditions were housed 5 mice per cage. All the experiments were approved by the Biological Research Committee of the University of Valencia (Spain). In all cases, mice were vaccinated (right leg) with a single dose per week, in weeks -3, -1 and +1 (days –21, -7 and +7), with respect to tumor injection (day 0) in the form of 10^5 wild type B16 cells in the left leg.

For experiments with liposomes and lipopolyplexes, 100 µl of liposomes or lipopolyplexes in Milli Q water were injected at each dose, the treatment groups for the liposomes containing TMP vaccine being: a) 10 µg of TMP alone; b) PC:CH liposomes containing 10 µg of TMP; c) SM:CH liposomes containing 10 µg of TMP; and d) Control group (100 µl saline solution). For the lipopolyplexes vaccine, the complexes were prepared with 10 or 50 µg of p2F *m-gmcsf* plasmid (GM10 or GM50) and 2 or 20 µg of TMP (TMP2 or TMP20), being GM10/TMP2, GM10/TMP20, GM50/TMP2, GM50/TMP20.

For experiments with freshly transfected B16 cells (non-selected), cells were thawed and counted for $2x10^5$ B16 cells (previously transfected, irradiated and frozen) per dose (groups p2F∅, B7.2, GM, GM+B7.2/200) per mouse, in 100 µl DMEM. For p2F m-gmcsf + m-B7.2 treatment, two different cell doses were studied: one with the usual cell dose ($2x10^5$), GM+B7.2/200; and another with cells sufficient to reach the same GM-CSF production as in the GM group, according to previous ELISA experiments of GM-CSF production (data not shown), i.e., group GM+B7.2/500. In the B16* group, $2x10^5$ wild type irradiated B16cells (150 Gy) were injected in 100µl DMEM, while in the Control group only 100 µl DMEM was injected, at every three vaccination dose.

For experiments with transfected and selected B16 cells (beads selection), we chose a vaccine dose that represented only the truly transfected cells of the "non-selected cells vaccine". Thus, we had to vaccine only with 20% of the previous doses, since in this case all of the employed cells would be transfected cells. Our two groups were: Control (100 µl DMEM) and GM+B7.2/40, employing only 40,000 selected cells per mouse, per dose, in 100 µl DMEM.

In all vaccination experiments, blood samples were taken from all the animals, pooling blood from the animals from the same group at each time-point. The samples were taken on days –22 (before any manipulation of the animals, serving as base level or control in each group), -1 (the day before tumor implantation, day 0, with two vaccination doses already performed), and +15 (one week after the third and last dose was administered). Plasma was obtained by centrifugation at 3000 rpm for 5 min. and kept at –20°C until use.

Tumor Growth Measurement, Survival and Statistical Analysis

Tumor growth in mice was monitored visually and measured with a caliper in two dimensions, A, the long diameter and B, the short diameter. Tumor volume was calculated with the formula $V = (AxB^2)/2$, and expressed in mm^3. Total or partial survival was achieved in some of the treated groups; animals were collected at their death date to construct the survival curves. To statistically compare the results of the different treatment groups, a two-tailed ANOVA was used, with Bonferroni post hoc testing (95% confidence interval, 95%CI), expressing statistically significant differences on the basis of $P<0.05$, $P<0.01$ and $P<0.001$.

Specific anti-TMP IgG ELISA

Measurement of IgG and IgG subclass antibodies to TMP was performed in serum samples by specific ELISA, as previously described [13]. Plates were coated by overnight incubation of TMP at 0.8 μg/ml in carbonate buffer, pH 9.6. The next day, plates were neutralized with 1% BSA solution before addition of serum samples. For analysis, sera were diluted in dilution buffer (PBS-BSA 1%-Tween 20 0.1%) at 1/1000 for total IgG and IgG1 subclass and at 1/100 for IgG2a. Bound antibodies were detected with goat antisera to total IgG (Biocheck, USA) at 1/10000 or mouse IgG subclasses at 1/1000 (Sigma, Mouse monoclonal isotyping reagents, Spain), followed by 1/5000 dilution of biotinylated rabbit antiserum to goat IgG (Sigma, Spain) and streptavidin coupled to horseradish peroxidase (Sigma, Spain). Plates were developed with a mixture of orthophenylenediamine (OPD, Sigma, Spain) and hydrogen peroxide (Fluka, Spain), and read at 492 nm. All samples were assayed in duplicate, allowing the estimation of mean OD value and standard deviation.

RESULTS

Efficacy of Protein Encapsulation in Liposomes

The different procedures of liposome preparation revealed a very different ability for encapsulating BSA Protein (Bovine Serum Albumin), as seen in Figure 1-A. The freeze and thaw cycles performed during the formation of MLV-FT liposomes enable these vesicles to entrap nearly 90% of the protein present in the medium. These results made us continue with this kind of liposomes, as our purpose was to use them simply as a delivery vehicle for our tumor antigens (TMP), so the more effective the better, in the sense that we would be able to deliver more antigen with less lipid.

As we wanted to simultaneously transport proteic antigens (TMP) and DNA encoding cytokine genes (GM-CSF) in two independent compartments, we prepared a lipopolyplex complex in which TMP were encapsulated in anionic liposomes, whereas DNA was prepared as a PEI/DNA polyplex. For this reason, we were interested in obtaining good encapsulation of TMP in anionic liposomes - in our case liposomes containing the anionic DP lipid. In Figure 1-B, the best encapsulation percentages are achieved with PC:CH, for the simple formulations, and are equivalent in PC:CH:DP and SM:CH:DP. The best encapsulation was achieved when liposomes incorporated 10% DP, which is why we used the more classical PC:CH:DP liposomes for the following lipopolyplex experiments.

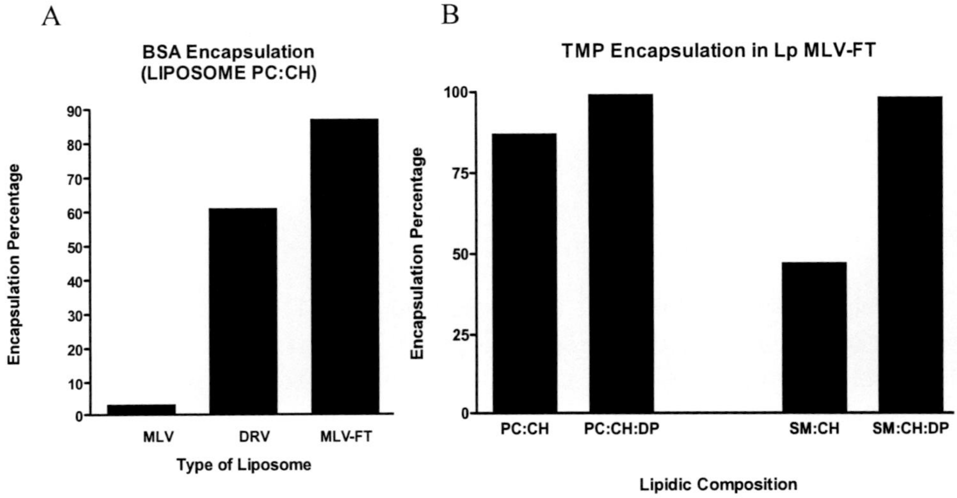

Figure 1. A- BSA protein encapsulation in liposomes. Ability for encapsulating BSA protein in different procedures of liposome preparation: Multilamellar Vesicles (MLV), Dehydration-Rehydration Vesicles (DRV) and Freeze-Thawed Multilamellar Vesicles (MLV-FT). B- TMP encapsulation in Lp MLV-FT. Percentage of TMP encapsulation in MLV-FT liposomes with different lipidic compositions: Phosphatidylcholine (PC), Sphingomyelin (SM), Cholesterol (CH) and Dicetylphosphate (DP).

Liposomes and Lipopolyplexes Vaccine

With the aim of evaluating the efficacy of TMP vaccines employing liposomes or lipopolyplexes as carriers, C57BL/6 mice (n=5 per group) were vaccinated in the right leg at a single dose per week, on weeks -3, -1 and +1 (days –21, -7 and +7), with respect to tumor injection (day 0) with 10^5 wild type B16 cells in left leg. Liposomes or lipopolyplexes (100 μl) were injected at each dose in the following groups: a) 10 μg of TMP alone; b) PC:CH liposomes containing 10 μg of TMP; c) SM:CH liposomes containing 10 μg of TMP; and d) Control group (100 μl saline solution), as seen in Figure 2. For the lipopolyplexes vaccine, in Figure 3, complexes made of 10 or 50 μg of p2F *m-gmcsf* plasmid (GM10 or GM50) and 2 or 20 μg of TMP (TMP2 or TMP20) were employed, according to the following groups: a) GM10/TMP2, b) GM10/TMP20, c) GM50/TMP2, and d) GM50/TMP20. Tumor growth was monitored in mice, measuring the long diameter (A) and the short diameter (B) with calipers.

The tumor volume was calculated with the formula $V= (AxB^2)/2$, and expressed in mm^3. Statistical tests were performed by two-way ANOVA and Bonferroni post hoc testing. In Figure 2, "a" represents a statistically significant difference of $P<0.05$ regarding the TMP Lp SM group; "b" the same, but regarding the Control group; and "c" is $P<0.01$ compared also with the Control group. Tumor growth is inhibited (40-50%) with statistically significant differences on day +22 after tumor implantation (Day 0), when comparing TMP 10 µg or TMP Lp PC versus TMP Lp SM or Control, and no differences were found within the two couples. These results led us to continue working with PC liposomes.

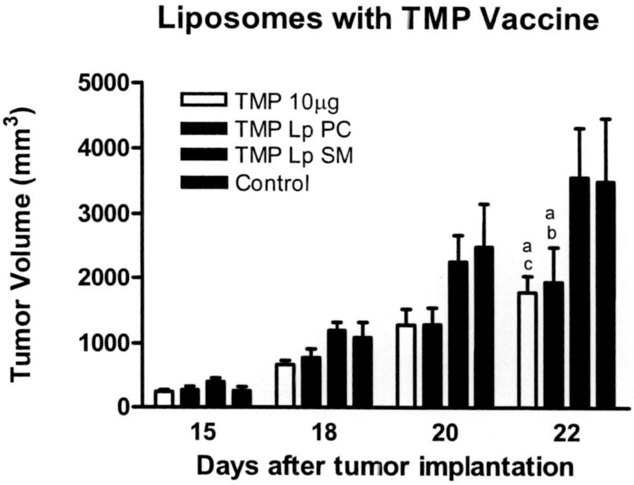

Figure 2. Liposomes with TMP vaccine. C57BL/6 mice (n=5 per group) were vaccinated in the right leg on days –21, -7 and +7 with respect to tumor injection on day 0 (10^5 wild type B16 cells) in the left leg. Treatments: a) 10 µg of TMP alone; b) PC:CH liposomes containing 10 µg of TMP; c) SM:CH liposomes containing 10 µg of TMP; d) Control group (100 µl saline solution). Tumor volume was calculated from $V = (AxB^2)/2$, where A is the long diameter and B the short diameter, with volume expression in mm^3. Statistical tests were performed by two-way ANOVA and Bonferroni post hoc testing. Statistically significant difference of $P<0.05$ regarding TMP Lp SM group = a, b is the same but regarding Control group, and c is $P<0.01$ likewise versus the Control group.

In Figure 3, "a, b, c, d" represent a statistically significant difference of $P<0.001$ comparing GM10/TMP20 with each following group in the figure, respectively. The figure shows statistically significant differences in tumor growth inhibition on days +20 and +23, regarding tumor implantation, achieved only by group GM10/TMP20 (40-50%) when compared with all other treatments, and reaching the maximum degree of significance. The other groups did not show any difference between each other. Thus, the best combination in this experiment was vaccinating with a lipopolyplex that contained the lowest DNA and the highest antigen quantities.

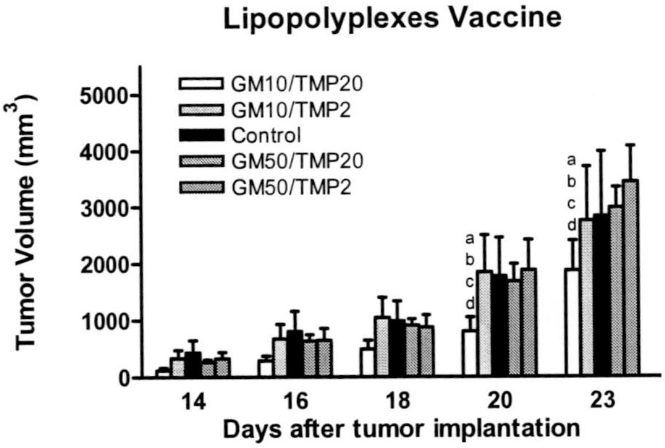

Figure 3. Lipopolyplexes vaccine. The same vaccination pattern as in Fig. 2 was followed, but treatments were lipopolyplexes prepared with 10 or 50 μg of p2F *m-gmcsf* plasmid: PEI polyplexes (GM10 or GM50) linked with 2 or 20 μg of TMP (TMP2 or TMP20) in PC:CH:DP liposomes, being GM10/TMP2, GM10/TMP20, GM50/TMP2, GM50/TMP20. Volume formula and statistical analysis were the same as in Fig. 2. Statistically significant difference of $P<0.001$ comparing GM10/TMP20 with each following group in the figure is represented by a, b, c and d, respectively.

Although similar growth inhibition was achieved in liposomes and lipopolyplex vaccines, differences were observed in the survival results. While in the Liposome Vaccine experiment we did not observe any differential survival between treated and control groups (data not shown), better survival results were observed in the Lipopolyplex Vaccine experiment (Figures 4-A and B). In Fig. 4-A, the groups with the lower DNA doses are represented, both of them achieving longer survival periods than the control group. According to the results of tumor growth inhibition, the longest survival was reached with 10 DNA μg of GM-CSF, while the groups treated with higher than 50 μg DNA doses (Figure 4-B) performed worse than the control group.

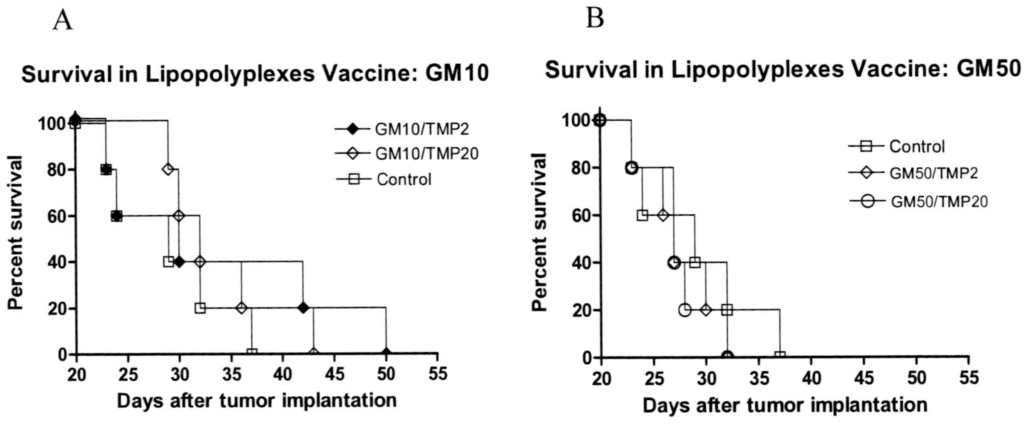

Figure 4. Survival in lipopolyplexes vaccine. Animal death dates were collected to construct survival curves. A- Results of Control and groups treated with lipopolyplexes containing 10 μg p2F *m-gmcsf*. B- Results of Control and groups treated with lipopolyplexes containing 50 μg p2F *m-gmcsf*.

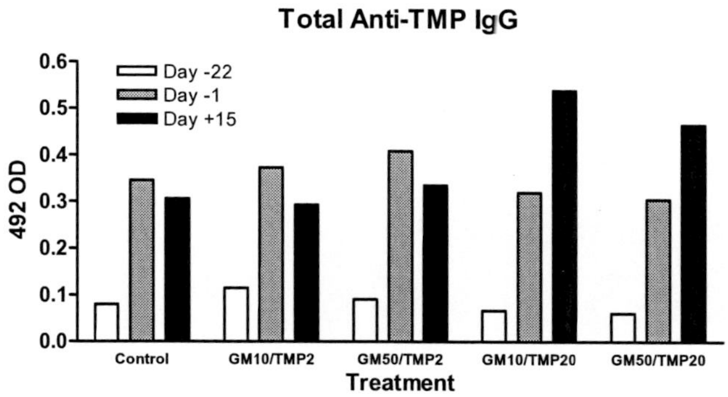

Figure 5. Total Anti-TMP IgG in lipopolyplex vaccine. Blood samples were taken from all the animals on days -22, -1 and +15, pooling the blood of the animals from the same group at each time-point, with respect to the tumor transplant day (day 0). Plasma was obtained by blood centrifugation at 3000 rpm during 5 min. Specific anti-TMP IgG were measured in plasma by ELISA: Plates were coated by overnight incubation of TMP at 0.8 μg/ml in carbonate buffer, pH 9.6. The next day, plates were neutralized with 1% BSA solution before addition of serum samples. For analysis, sera were diluted in dilution buffer (PBS-BSA 1%-Tween 20 0.1%) at 1/1000 for total IgG and IgG1 subclass and at 1/100 for IgG2a. Bound antibodies were detected with goat antisera to total IgG (Biocheck, USA) at 1/10000 or mouse IgG subclasses at 1/1000 (Sigma, mouse monoclonal isotyping reagents, Spain), followed by 1/5000 dilution of biotinylated rabbit antiserum to goat IgG (Sigma, Spain) and streptavidin coupled to horseradish peroxidase (Sigma, Spain). Plates were developed with a mixture of orthophenylenediamine (OPD, Sigma, Spain) and hydrogen peroxide (Fluka, Spain), and read at 492 nm. All samples were assayed in duplicate, allowing the estimation of mean OD value and standard deviation.

Blood samples were taken from all the animals during the experiment, pooling blood from the animals from the same group at each time-point, with respect to the tumor transplant day (day 0). The samples were taken on days –22 (before any manipulation of the animals, which serves as base level or control in each group), day -1 and day +15. The total anti-TMP IgG found by ELISA in the vaccinated mice and control group is shown in Figure 5. The measurements were made in duplicate, and means and standard deviations (SD) were calculated and represented, although SD is inappreciable, since it was less than 5% of the mean value, which also happened in the rest of the vaccine experiments in this work. In this figure, the treatments with higher antigen doses (20 μg TMP) show the maximum IgG response on day +15, whereas the two groups with the lower TMP dose (2 μg), show their maximums on day -1, and these levels are always lower than those recorded for the other two groups. In order to know the immunoglobulin switch induced by vaccination, specific subtypes IgG1 and IgG2a were also studied, and the results were summarized in Figures 6-A and B, respectively. The same pattern as for total IgG is observed, with more relevant differences between the two TMP conditions in IgG1. On the other hand, optimal responses in IgG2a are achieved when 20 μg TMP and 10 μg DNA GM-CSF were employed, since higher DNA doses did not offer any advantages. Also, GM50/TMP2 increased IgG2a response, but mainly limited to day-1.

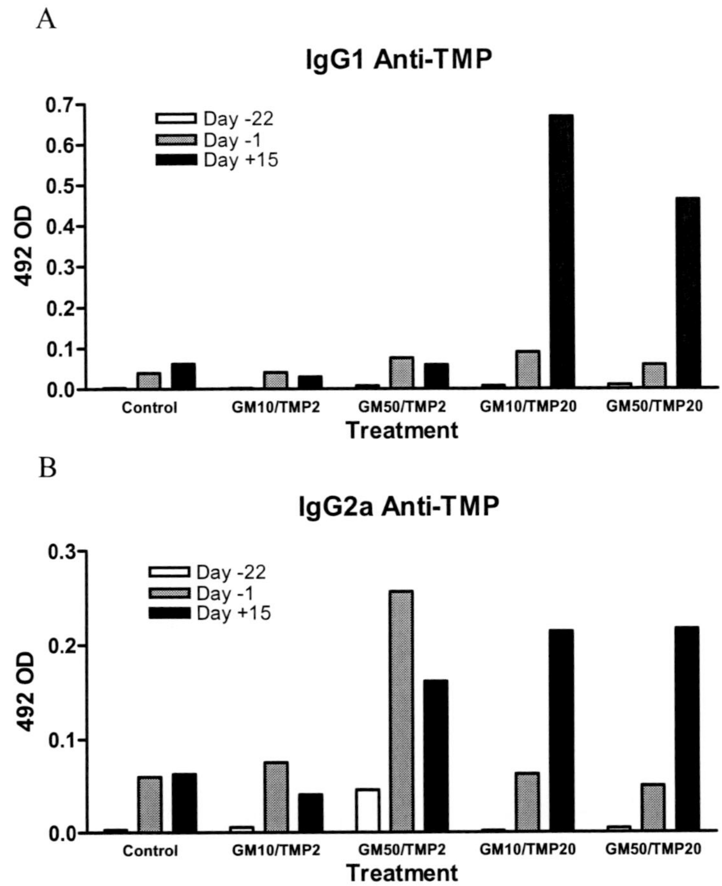

Figure 6. Specific anti-TMP IgG subclasses in lipopolyplexes vaccine. The same protocol as described in Fig. 5 was used, this time for IgG1 subclass (A) and IgG2a subclass (B).

Determination of m-B7.2 Production

The efficiency of m-B7.2 expression on B16 cell surface 72 h after transfection was evaluated by flow cytometry. The results are summarized in Figure 7, which plots counts versus F1 Log, and where we can identify specific surface expression of m-B7.2 in the right peak of the figure, whereas the middle and left peaks correspond to the transfected and non-transfected control cells, respectively. The intersection area between the middle peak and the right peak represents the proportion of transfected cells that are also fluorescent, i.e., the cells that express m-B7.2 at their surface. This area is approximately 20-40% of the right peak, which was our expected transfection efficacy, according to our previous experiments (data not shown).

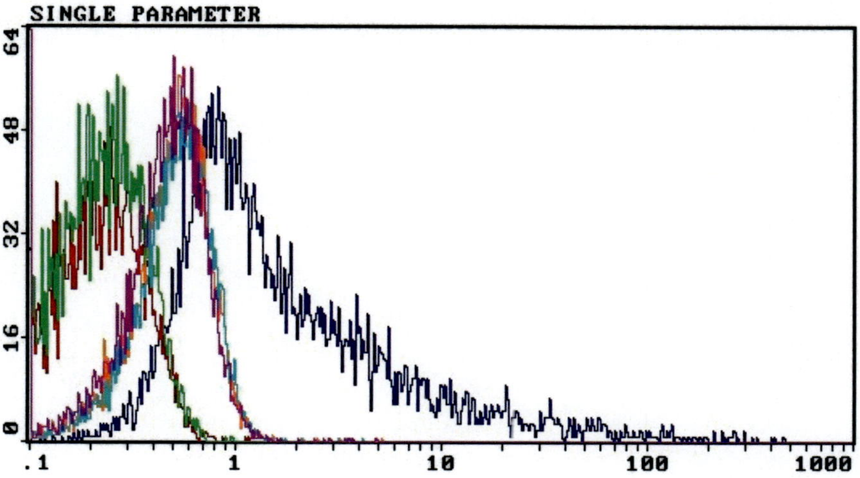

Figure 7. Flow cytometry of p2F m-gmcsf+mB7.2 transfected B16 cells. Groups of B16 cells were passed through the cytometer: a) non-transfected wild type B16 cells, without antibodies; and b) non-transfected wild type B16 cells incubated with both antibodies, both corresponding to the left peaks. Corresponding to the middle peak: c) B16-p2F m-gmcsf + m-B7.2 transfected cells, without antibodies, d) B16-p2F m-gmcsf + m-B7.2 transfected cells, only with primary antibody, e) B16-p2F m-gmcsf + m-B7.2 transfected cells, only with secondary antibody. Finally, f) B16-p2F m-gmcsf + m-B7.2 transfected cells, with both primary and secondary antibody, corresponding to the right peak. The figure plots counts versus FL1 log.

Cell Vaccine Employing Non-Selected Freshly Transfected Cells

The aim of this experiment was to evaluate the efficacy of the antitumor vaccine with genetically engineered tumor cells, expressing cytokines such as mGM-CSF and mB7.2. Thus, $2x10^5$ B16 cells previously transfected (p2F∅, B7.2, GM, GM+B7.2/200), irradiated (150 Gy) and frozen, were injected on days -21, -7 and +15 with 100 μl DMEM. For p2F m-gmcsf + m-B7.2 treatments, two different cell doses were studied: one with the usual cell dose ($2x10^5$), GM+B7.2/200; and another with cells sufficient to reach the same GM-CSF production as in the GM group, according to the ELISA experiments of GM-CSF production (data not shown), i.e., group GM+B7.2/500 ($5x10^5$ cells). In the B16* group, $2x10^5$ irradiated wild type B16 cells (150 Gy) were injected, and in the Control group, only DMEM was injected for each dose. The best results (Figure 8) were obtained employing GM+B7.2/200 and GM alone groups, since no tumor development was observed (marked with arrows in the figure) in any of the animals with those treatments 23 days after tumor implantation, when animals from other groups had started to die. In the figure,"a" corresponds to the maximum statistically significant difference, P= 0.001, and "b" represents P= 0.01, both versus the Control group. The survival curves of these groups are shown in Figure 9, and were consistent with the tumor inhibition results. In group GM, 100% mice survival was observed more than three months after tumor transplant. The GM+B7.2/200, GM+B7.2/500 and B7.2 groups achieved 80, 40 and 20% survival, respectively. Groups B16* and p2F Ø failed to increase survival versus the control group.

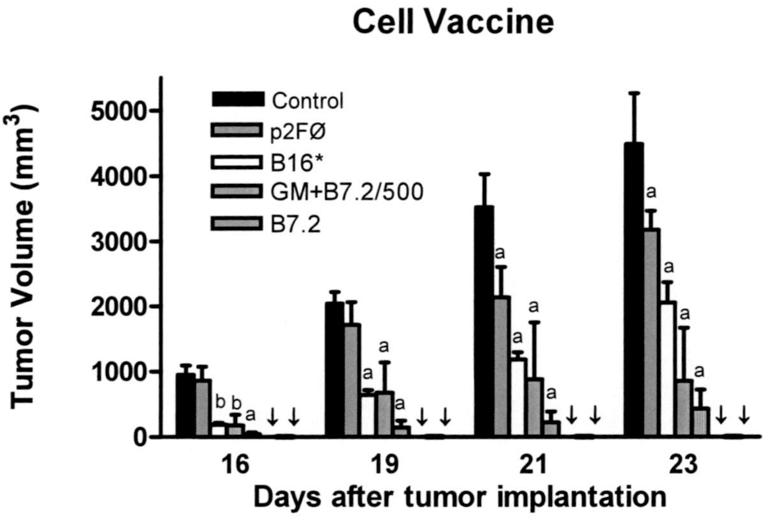

Figure 8. Cell vaccine. The freshly transfected (non-selected) cell vaccine followed the same pattern as in Fig. 2. Treatment groups were $2x10^5$ B16 cells (previously transfected, irradiated and frozen, then thawed and counted) per dose (groups p2F∅, B7.2, GM, GM+B7.2/200) per mouse, in 100μl DMEM. For p2F m-gmcsf + m-B7.2 treatment, two different cell doses were studied: one with the usual cell dose ($2x10^5$), GM+B7.2/200; and the other with cells sufficient to reach the same GM-CSF production as in group GM, i.e., GM+B7.2/500. In the B16* group, $2x10^5$ wild type irradiated B16 cells (150 Gy) were injected in 100 μl DMEM, while in the Control group only 100 μl DMEM, at every three vaccination dose. Arrows show the position in the figure of groups GM, GM+B7.2/200, which developed no tumors at all. The symbol "a" represents P<0.001, and "b" P<0.01, statistically significant difference versus the Control group.

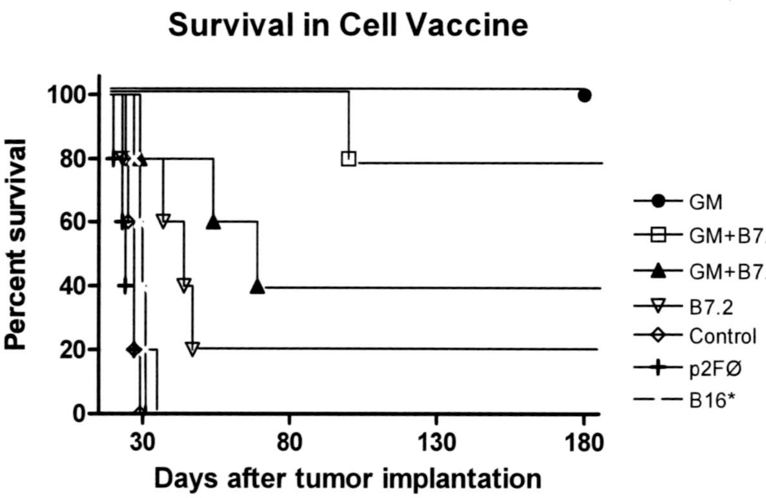

Figure 9. Survival in cell vaccine. As in Fig. 4, the figure plots the survival curves of mice from the Cell Vaccine experiment. In group GM, 100% mice survival was observed more than 3 months after tumor transplant. The GM+B7.2/200, GM+B7.2/500 and B7.2 groups achieved 80, 40 and 20% survival, respectively. The groups B16* and p2F Ø failed to increase survival versus the Control group.

Figure 10 shows the total specific IgG found in the plasma of the animals from this experiment, as explained also for Figure 5. All the groups showed the highest production on day +15, the best performance corresponding to the groups containing GM-CSF in the transfection. In addition, the study of IgG1 and IgG2a subtypes supports the same idea. GM-CSF transfection must contribute to the efficacy of the antitumor response in a significant way, while B7.2 exerts a more limited effect, and no synergistic effect was observed with GM-CSF gene.

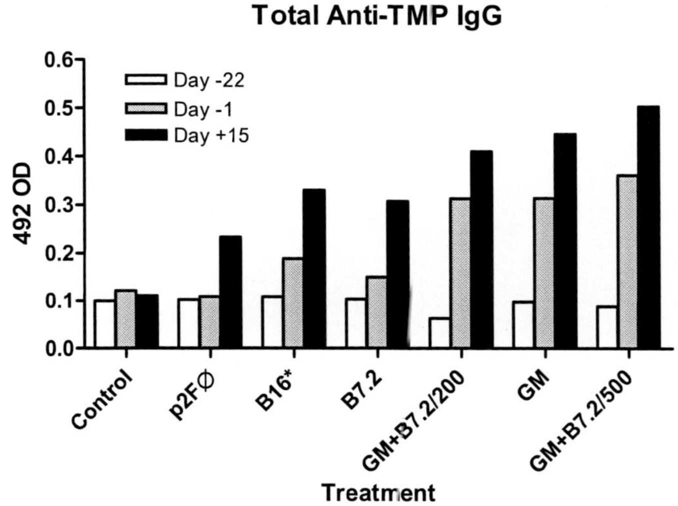

Figure 10. Total anti-TMP IgG production in cell vaccine. As in Fig. 5, this figure shows the specific anti-TMP total IgG from the different groups. Data were obtained from ELISA made with the plasma obtained on days -21, -1 and +15, with respect to tumor injection (day 0).

Expression-Selected Cell Vaccine

Since the maximal efficacy of our non-viral transfection procedure was 20-40% of the cells, we must expect that the non-transfected cells (80-60%) contribute poorly to vaccine efficacy. Therefore, we thought that our previous procedure, employing non-selected transfected cells, could be improved if only the cytokine-expressing cells, selected by magnetic beads purification, were used in the vaccine. For this purpose, we designed the experiments employing both GM-CSF and B7.2, due to their contribution to antitumor vaccine success and the B7.2 protein membrane location serving for cell magnetic selection. Thus, two groups were established: Control (100 μl DMEM) and GM+B7.2/40, employing only 40,000 selected cells per dose, in 100 μl DMEM.

A

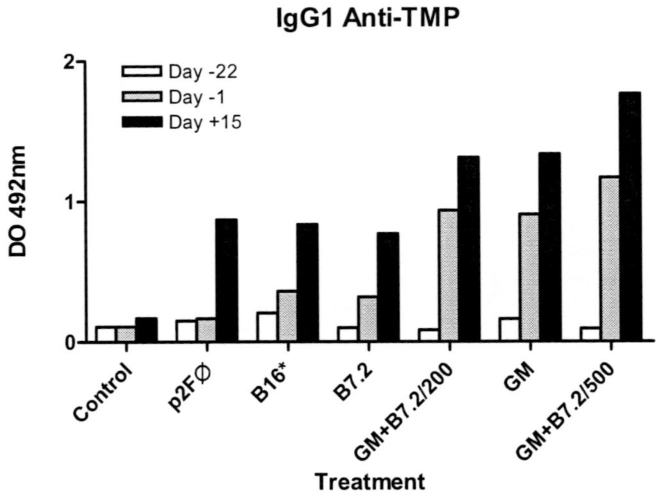

B

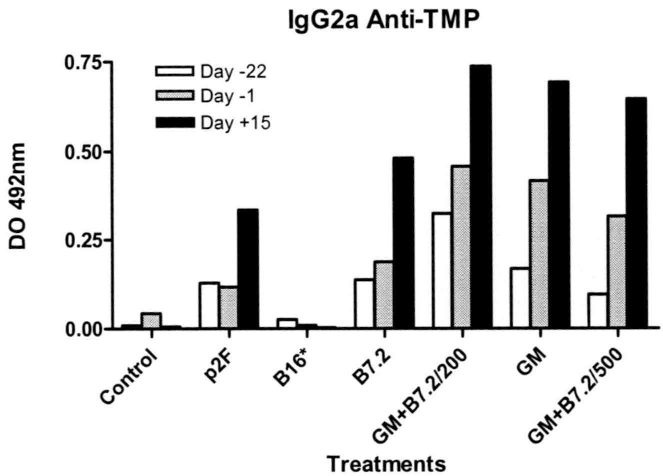

Figure 11. Specific anti-TMP IgG subclasses in cell vaccine. Following the same protocol as in Fig. 5, IgG1 analysis (A) and IgG2a (B) were performed.

The tumor growth inhibition results of the Selected Cells Vaccine are shown in Figure 12. The results on each measurement day were maximally significant (a= P<0.001), achieving reductions of more than 80% in tumor volume. These results are consistent with increased survival (Figure 13) in the GM+B7.2/40 group.

The total specific anti-TMP IgG and the IgG1 and IgG2a subtypes are shown in Figures 14-A and B, respectively. The immunoglobulin levels are again consistent with the tumor growth inhibition and survival data.

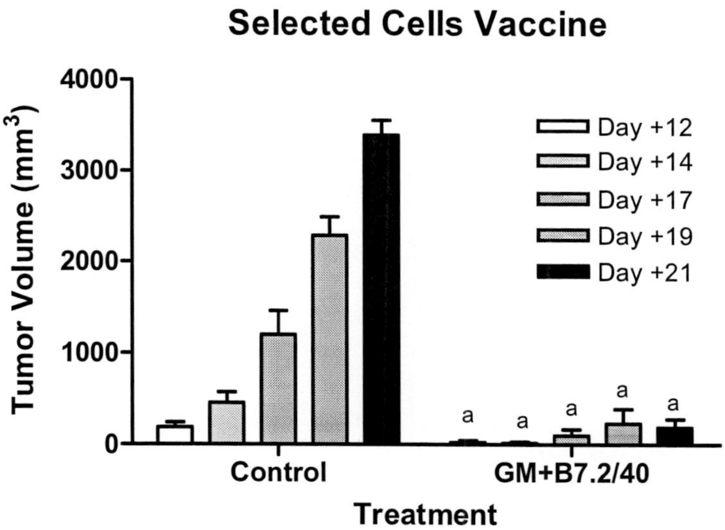

Figure 12. Selected cells vaccine. The tumor growth inhibition obtained in this vaccine is represented. Control and GM+B7.2/40 group, which is 40,000 selected by expression transfected B16 cells. The selection is made by Streptavidin microbeads, thanks to m-B7.2 surface expression. The symbol "a" represents $P<0.001$, statistically significant difference versus the Control group, where only DMEM was injected at each dose.

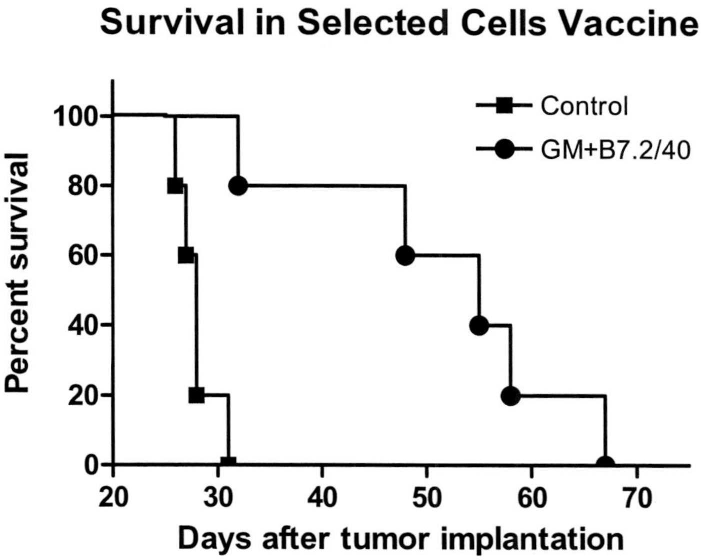

Figure 13. Survival in selected cells vaccine. As in Fig. 4, the survival curves are plotted.

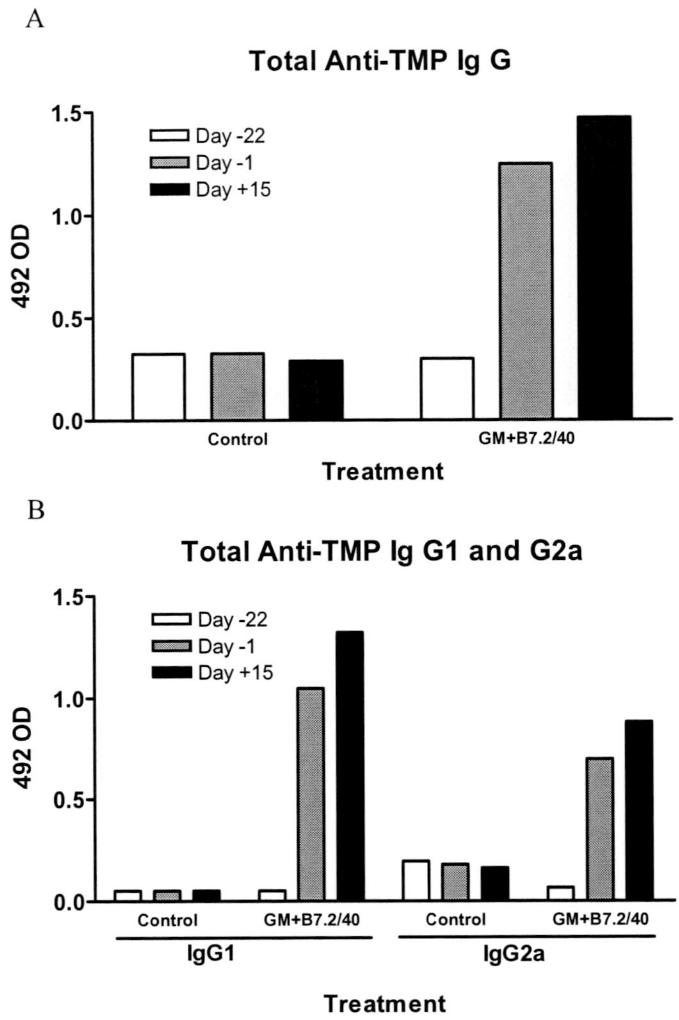

Figure 14. Specific anti-TMP IgG in selected cells vaccine. As in Fig. 5, the total IgG production (A) and the subclasses IgG1 and IgG2a (B) are represented in the graphs.

Conclusion

The aim of this work has been to try to improve the antitumor vaccine methods in order to establish the easiest and most efficient protocol. Engineered cells secreting cytokines have been widely demonstrated to be the most effective vaccines [1-7,9,11], as we have also seen [8,10,12], though we are aware of the great difficulty of working with this approach in actual clinical practice. In effect, taking cells from the patients that also must be kept in culture, amplified to a larger number, transfected and then returned to the same patient, guaranteeing sterility, no contamination, an acceptable number of cells, as well as cytokine production, is not an easy task. This is why we decided to focus effort on two different fronts. The first involved an attempt to reduce the cell number required to start a proper immune response against the tumor, thus avoiding very complex cell work in future patients. The second front focusing our effort is more difficult, because not so good results have been achieved with this kind of procedure to date [13,16], i.e., forgetting about cells and returning to the origins: vaccines made only of components supposed to be necessary, i.e., tumor antigens derived from cell membrane proteins (TMP) and plasmids containing the *gm-csf and B7.2* genes.

For the antigens approach, we studied the antitumor efficacy of several models: TMP alone, TMP encapsulated in liposomes, and finally lipopolyplexes bearing both TMP antigens and the GM-CSF cytokine gene. After choosing the best liposome type, we performed two vaccination experiments and conclude that although the tumor growth inhibitions were similar in the best groups from the three models, the best survival results were obtained with the lipopolyplexes comprising liposomes PC:CH:DP and polyplex PEI:p2F *m-gmcsf*, containing 20 μg TMP and 10 μg of the plasmid per dose. These results were also reflected in mice IgG production, not only in terms of total production but also in terms of the IgG1 and IgG2a subtypes. It should be noted that the groups with the higher TMP dose in the lipopolyplexes showed a later maximum production of IgG2a (day +15), while the groups with the lower TMP dose peaked earlier (day-1). However, this difference is apparently not correlated to survival. In contrast, high and low GM-CSF doses, which discriminated between better or worse survival results, did not have significant effect upon IgG2a plasma levels, suggesting that while IgG switching should be interesting for cell memory induction and antitumor response activation, this effect must be limited and other mechanisms must be involved in a negative regulation [7].

The best results were obtained with the cell vaccine approach on vaccinating with $2x10^5$ transfected cells, 100% and 80% survival levels were achieved in GM and GM+B7.2/200 groups, respectively. This cell vaccine also confirms the idea that higher amounts of GM-CSF production are not necessarily better [4,6,7]; on the contrary, GM+B7.2/500 induced poorer survival results than GM+B7.2/200, which had half the GM-CSF production. However, we think that synergistic effects between GM-CSF and B7.2 must exist, due to the good survival response promoted by the GM+B7.2/200 group. Again, the GM-CSF transfected cell groups showed the highest IgG productions. In this vaccine, a good correlation was observed between IgG response and survival, mainly in relation to the IgG2a subtype. Finally, from all these experiments, we must consider that in some cases the humoral response may not show a good correlation to survival, probably due to other phenomena such as regulatory T cell immune suppression.

Since the survival results suggest that cell vaccines achieve significant antitumor effects, we made additional efforts to improve the efficacy of the procedure by reducing the cell number required for each vaccine dose. In this respect, we knew that only 20-40% of the cells that we had employed in cell vaccination were transfected, and for this reason we designed new vaccine experiments employing only the cytokine-expressing cells. Thus, we made use of the B7.2 surface membrane expression strategy because it has been shown in our experiments and in the literature [18-24] to be helpful and even synergistic with GM-CSF in some cases. Moreover, its location in the cell could help us select the cells expressing the protein on their membranes, i.e., only the transfected cells. The aim of the experiment was to determine whether only the transfected cells (20% of $2x10^5$ = 40,000 cells) were able to mediate the same successful results as those obtained in nonselected-cell vaccines. The selected cells vaccine showed a very significant tumor growth reduction employing only

40,000 cells, and this reduction correlated to a longer survival and good IgG response of the treated mice. Although the results were not as good as those with the non-selected cells vaccine, no conclusions can be drawn before a dose-dependent study is made. It remains to be elucidated how synergistic effects between antigens, GM-CSF and costimulatory B7.2 molecules cooperate in the generation of efficient antitumor response or toxicity. We cannot exclude a lack of net antigen contribution due to the reduction in cell number or, contrarily, an excess in GM-CSF production which could result in a loss of vaccine efficacy. These experiments will focus our future attention, and will contribute to clarify the exact need of each component in a cell vaccine that could become suitable for use in clinical practice.

ACKNOWLEDGEMENTS

This work has been partially supported by the *Ministerio de Educación y Ciencia* SAF 2004-08161 and SAF 2007-64492 and the *Generalitat Valenciana* GVACOMP 2006-217.

REFERENCES

[1] Dunussi-Joannopoulos K, Dranoff G, Weinstein HJ, Ferrara JLM, Bierer BE, Croop JM. Gene immunotherapy in murine acute myeloid leukemia: granulocyte-macrophage colony-stimulating factor tumor cell vaccines elicit more potent antitumor immunity compared with B7 family and other cytokine vaccines. *Blood*, 1998, Vol 91, No 1, 222-230.

[2] Mastrangelo MJ & Lattime EC. Virotherapy clinical trials for regionale disease: *in situ* immune modulation using recombinant poxvirus vectors. *Cancer Gene Therapy*, 2002, 9, 1013-1021.

[3] Se-Heon K, Carew JF, Kooby DA, Shields J, Entwisle C, Patel S, Shah JP, Fong Y. *Cancer Gene Therapy*, 2000, Vol 7, No 9, 1279-1285.

[4] Borrello I & Pardoll D. *Cytokine and Growth Factor Reviews*, 2002, 13, 185-193.

[5] Jaffee EM, Abrams R, Cameron J et al. A phase I clinical trial of lethally irradiated allogeneic pancreatic tumor cells transfected with the GM-CSF gene for the treatment of pancreatic adenocarcinoma. *Human Gene Therapy*, 1998, 9, 1951-1971.

[6] Serafini P, Carbley R, Noonan KA, Tan G, Bronte V, Borrello I. High-dose granulocyte-macrophage colony-stimulating factor-producing vaccines impair the immune response through the recruitment of myeloid suppressor cells. *Cancer Research*, 2004, 64, 6337-6343.

[7] Rodríguez-Lecompte JC, Kruth S et al. Cell-based cancer gene therapy: breaking tolerante or inducing autoimmunity? *Anim Health Res Rev.*, 2004, Dec; 5(2), 227-234.

[8] Herrero MJ, Botella R, Dasí F, Algás R, Sánchez M, Aliño SF. Antigens and cytokine genesin antitumor vaccines: the importance of teh temporal delivery sequence in antitumor signals. *Ann. N.Y. Acad. Sci.*, 2006, 1091, 412-424.

[9] Shi FS, Weber S, Gan J, Rakhmilevich A, Mahvi DM. Granulocyte-macrophage colony-stimulating factor (GM-CSF) secreted by cDNA-transfected tumor cells induces a more

potent antitumor response than exogenous GM-CSF. *Cancer Gene Therapy*, 1999, Vol 6, 81-88.

[10]Moret-Tatay I, Diaz J, Marco FM, Crespo A, Aliño SF. Complete tumor prevention by engineered tumor cell vaccines employing nonviral vactors. *Cancer Gene therapy*, 2003, 10, 887-897.

[11]Wiley, J and sons, Ltd. Gene Therapy Clinical Trials Worldwide. 2007. Available from: www.wiley.co.uk/genmed/clinical

[12]Moret-Tatay I, Sanmartín I, Marco FM, Díaz J, Aliño SF. Nonviral therapeutic cell vaccine mediates potent antitumor effects. *Vaccine*. 2006, 24, 3937-3945.

[13]Aliño SF, Lejarreta M et al. Antimetastatic effect of immunization with liposome-encapsualted tumor cell-membrane proteins obtained from experimental tumors. *Immunopharmacology and immunotoxicology*, 1995, 17 (3), 419-436.

[14]Guillem VM, Tormo M, et al. Targeted oligonucleotide delivery in human lymphoma cell lines using a polyethileneimine based immunopolyplex. *Journal of controlled release*, 2002, 83, 133-146.

[15]Guillem VM, Tormo M, et al. Polyethyleneimine-based immunopolyplex for targeted gene transfer in human lymphoma cell lines. *The Journal of Gene Medicine*, 2002, 4, 170-182.

[16]Massó O, Aliño SF et al. Specific serological response by active immunization with GD3-bearing liposomes. *The Journal of Pharmacology and Experimental Therapeutics*, 1996, 278(3), 1114-1120.

[17]Garcia L, Bunuales M, Duzgunes N, Tros de Ilarduya C. Serum-resistant lipopolyplexes for gene delivery to liver tumor cells. *Eur J Pharm Biopharm*, 2007.

[18]Zajac P, Oertli W at al. Phase I/II Clinical trial of a nonreplicative vaccinia virus expressing multiple HLA-A0201-restricted tumor-associated epitopoes and costimulatory molecules in metastatic melanoma patients. *Human Gene Therapy*, 2003, 14, 1497-1510.

[19]Chong H, Todryk S et al. Tumor cell expression of B7 costimulatory molecules and interleukin-12 or granulocyte-macrophage colony-stimulating factor induces a local antitumor response and may generate systemis protective immunity. 1998, *Gene Therapy*, 5, 223-232.

[20]Pizzoferrato E. B7-2 expression above a threshold elicits anti-tumor immunity as effective as interleukin-12 and prolongs survival in murine B-cell lymphoma. *Int J Cancer*, 2004, 110, 61-69.

[21]Kim k-Y, Kang M-A, Nam M-J. Enhancement of natural killer cell-mediated cytotoxicity by coexpression of GM-CSF/B70 in hepatoma. *Cancer Letters*, 2001, 166, 33-40.

[22]Grosenbach DW, Barrientos JC, et al. Synergy of vaccine strategies to amplify antigen-specific immune responses and antitumor effects. *Cancer Research*, 2001, 61, 4497-4505.

[23]Parney IF, Farr-Jones MA et al. Human autologous in vitro models of glioma immunogene therapy using B7-2, GM-CSF and IL-12. *Can J Neurol Sci*, 2002, 29(3), 267-275.

[24]Mukherjee S, Nelson D, et al. The immune anti-tumor effects of GM-CSF and B7-1 gene transfection are enhanced by surgical debulking of tumor. *Cancer Gene Therapy*, 2001, 8, 580-588.

[25]Bordier C. Phase separation of integral membrane proteins in Triton X-114 solution. *J Biol Chem.* 1981, 25, 1604-1607.

[26]Guillem VM & Aliño SF. Transfection pathways of nonspecific and targeted PEI-polyplexes. *Gene Therapy and Molecular Biology*, 2004, Vol 8, 369-384.

[27]Walde P & Ichikawa S. Enzymes inside lipid vesicles: preparation, reactivity and applications. *Biomolecular Engineering*, 2001, 18, 143-177.

[28]Moret I, Peris JE, Guillem VM, Benet M, Revert F, Dasí F, Crespo A, Aliño SF. Stability of PEI-DNA and DOTAP-DNA complexes: effect of alkaline pH, heparin and serum. *Journal of controlled Release,* 2001, 76, 169-181.

In: New Gene Therapy and Cancer Research
Editor: Wilma B. Gustafsson, pp. 249-278
ISBN: 978-1-60021-969-6

Chapter VIII

Biodegradable Poly (β- Amino Ester) Derivatives for Gene and siRNA Delivery

Dhananjay Jere[1], Rhohidas Arote[1], Myung-Haing Cho[2] and Chong-Su Cho[1,*]

[1]School of Agricultural Biotechnology, Seoul National University, Seoul 151-921, South Korea;

[2]College of Veterninary Medicine, Seoul National University, Seoul 151-742, South Korea.

Abstract

The availability of human genome sequence has revolutionalized the ability of medical science to manipulate genes either by inducing or silencing specific gene expression which modulates many grave diseases and disorders including cancer. Vectors are being developed based on the capacity of polymers or lipids to mediate appropriate interactions with the cellular environment or to interface with specific cellular processes. Number of novel delivery strategies has been proposed to improve the efficiency of *in vivo* plasmid DNA or siRNA tansfection. However, only few of these strategies have been shown to enhance the expression of injected plasmid DNA or siRNA. Non-viral delivery methods, especially ones that focus on the use of biodegradable synthetic polymers represent the persistent future of polynucleotide based therapy. This chapter describes recent success of poly (β-amino ester)s (PAE)s as non-viral vectors and highlights their future in the development of polynucleotide based cancer therapy. Among non-viral vectors, PAEs received high attention owing to their safety and high transfection efficiency *in vitro* and *in vivo*. Ease of synthesis and efficient manipulation of physicochemical properties have made PAEs polymer of choice for gene

* Correspondence concerning this article should be addressed to: Chong-Su Cho, chocs@plaza.snu.ac.kr; Tel: +82 2 880 4636; Fax: +82 2 875 2494.

delivery studies. Purpose of this chapter is to provide novel insight with respect to this type of gene delivery system. It primarily reports the chemical structure of frequently studied PAE backbones along with the classification on the basis of their chemical nature. Secondly, the influence on transfection by polymer backbones is described. Thirdly, important properties such as surface properties, molecular weight, dissociation and degradation, structural chemistry and charge density of polyplexes are considered. Fourthly, chapter highlights potential of PAEs in the siRNA delivery for cancer therapy and finally, chapter gives a very brief look at success of PAEs *in vivo* gene and siRNA delivery.

Keywords: Cancer; Non-viral vectors; Poly (amino ester); Gene delivery; siRNA delivery.

1. Introduction

The human genome project has substantially increased our knowledge of the molecular mechanisms of cancer during the last decade and raised the hope of cancer gene therapy. Gene therapy may be defined as the expression of a gene that has been introduced into a target cell or a target tissue to alter an existing function or to introduce a new function in order to cure a patient from a specific disease or genetic disorder. Innate or acquired genetic defects are responsible for number of disorders such as Alzheimer, hemophilia, cystic fibrosis (mucovisidosis), adenosine-deaminase (ADA) deficit and also cancer [1]. Gene delivery has been studied extensively to overcome theses genetic problems by genetic manipulations. Along with gene delivery, discovery of RNA based silencing has given new vision to cancer therapy [2] and further boosted nucleotide based therapeutic research [3,4]. RNA interference (RNAi) is a process, whereby the introduction of short double-stranded RNA (shRNA or siRNA) (21-23 nucleotides) in the cells causes sequence specific degradation of homologous mRNA which results in specific gene silencing. Although siRNA delivery or gene delivery has an enormous therapeutic potential, lack of safe and efficient vector system has limited their clinical success.

Viral and non-viral vectors systems have been studied for gene and siRNA delivery. Viral vectors have an older history than non-viral vectors for transfection studies. Although systematic *in-vitro* transfection studies were initiated in late 1950, some of the earliest experiments scientifically performed more than 78 years back. Griffith, for example, had proved the transformation of pneumococcus bacteria from nonpathogenic to pathogenic phenotype in 1928 [1]. Alexander et al. showed that purified poliovirus RNA was infectious in HeLa cells in 1958 [5]. Further Holland et al. originated the concept of nonviral transfer and they proved that a hypertonic saline solution (1M NaCl) could enhance infectivity of the purified RNA by about 100-folds [6]. This has given birth to the concept that living virus particles are not required to produce infectious replicating virus and this was subsequently confirmed and extended by using improved methods for polynucleotide delivery [7]. The concept of gene therapy for human genetic diseases was introduced in 1972 by Friedmann [8] and the idea rapidly immerged as a field with immense potential. The discovery of cationic synthetic vectors has brought revolution in the field of gene delivery research. Currently, many non-viral cationic lipid based vectors are under clinical investigation along with viral vectors. Above all, cationic polymeric vectors are rapidly immerging over viral and lipid based vectors owing to their better safety and ease of modification [9]. Ideal gene delivery vector should be biodegradable, nontoxic, non-immunogenic, and stable during storage. It should be target-specific, and should be able to navigate series of extra- and intracellular barriers in order to deliver the gene to the required cells. In past decade, numerous papers have been published describing the barriers to effective delivery [10-13]. Viruses are naturally evolved vectors and highly efficient in crossing all cellular barriers to deliver loaded genetic material. Viral vectors are made by replacing part of viral genome with therapeutic genetic material [14]. Viral vectors can be classified as:

a) Retrovirus: It is a Eukaryotic virus. It uses viral enzymes to copy its genome into DNA and integrate into host chromosome. Long term gene expression can be achieved with this vector, but only in cycling cells [15].
b) Adenovirus: Adenovirus contains large DNA genome. Unlike retrovirus, it can infect both dividing and non-dividing cells. However, gene expression lasts for only short time as adenoviral genome is not integrated into the host DNA [16].
c) Adeno-Associated Virus: It is a small nonpathogenic DNA virus. It can only produce progenies in the presence of a helper virus, such as adeno or herpes virus. Both dividing and non-dividing cells can be infected; however, low viral titer is a major limitation [17].
d) Other viral vectors: Herpes simplex virus (HSV) [18], vaccinia virus [19], baculo virus [20] , measles virus [21], polio virus [22], and bacteriophage [23] are additional examples of viral vectors.

Although, till now, viral vectors are efficient gene delivery systems and have been tried in the majority of clinical trials, there have been a number of problems with their application in human gene therapy, the major disadvantages of viral delivery include:

- Generation of immune responses to expressed viral proteins that subsequently kill the target cells required to produce the therapeutic gene product.
- Random integration of some viral vectors into the host chromosome.
- Clearance of viral vectors delivered systemically.
- Difficulties in engineering viral envelopes or capsids to achieve specific delivery to cells other than those with natural tropism for the virus.
- Potential recombination of the viral vector with DNA sequences in the host chromosome that generates a replication-competent, infectious virus.
- Inability to administer certain viral vectors more than once.
- High costs for producing large amounts of high-titer viral stocks for use in the clinic.
- Limited size of the nucleic acid that can be packaged and used for viral gene therapy.

Actual death occurred during the clinical trial and also reports of leukemia development due to viral vector based therapy have questioned the safety of viral vectors. These safety issues of viral vectors have given birth to alternative non-viral vector systems. Non-viral vectors were designed on the potential of synthetic systems to bind and condense the genetic material effectively. Non-viral vectors have received glorious success in gene delivery, *in vitro* as well as *in vivo*. Non-viral vector systems can be classified as:

a) Naked DNA: Intratumoral injection of the naked DNA can induce transgene expression at a level that is high enough to elicit therapeutic response [24,25].
b) Gene gun: Shooting DNA into cells can be carried out by using a physical method such as bioballistic bombardment or gene gun after exposing tissue surgically [26].
c) Liposome/DNA complex or Lipoplex: Because of charge interaction, a complex can be easily formed between cationic liposomes and anionic DNA [27]. Several different kinds of cationic lipids, including quaternary ammonium detergents, cationic derivatives of cholesterol and diacyl glycerol, and lipid derivatives of polyamines, have been developed.
d) Polymer/DNA complex or Polyplex: Polymeric materials have found wide use in gene delivery applications [28]. Several examples include poly(lysine), polyethylenimine (PEI), poly(amido amine) dendrimers. These polymers generally serve as gene carriers through either electrostatic complexation or physical entrapment for the intracellular delivery of preloaded genetic material.
e) Liposome/Polymer/DNA complex or Lipopolyplex: Incorporation of polylysine into lipoplex to form ternary complexes leads to a tight condensation of DNA [29]. Similarly attachment of PEG on liposomes leads to reduced aggregation and nuclease degradation [30,31].

The safety of non-viral vectors over viral vectors has enlightened the development of synthetic vector systems for gene delivery. Although, presently cationic lipid based vectors are more successful commercially, cationic polymeric vectors are gaining popularity because of their ease of modification and biocompatibility.

2. Cationic Polymers for Gene Delivery

Cationic polymers are promising non-viral vectors with many unique advantages for efficient gene delivery. They have been widely investigated as transfection vectors due to the facility with which they condense and protect negatively charged DNA. Cationic polymers are cheap and easily available commercially. They can be specifically tailored for proposed application with desirable physicochemical or physiological properties such as degradation under certain conditions or cell-specific targeting. A wide variety of cationic polymers have been characterized for their transfection potential (Figure 1). Many natural polymers, such as protein [32] peptides [33], chitosan [34-36] spermine [37,38] chitosan-graft-polyethylenimine [39], urocanic acid-modified chitosan [40,41] and synthetic polymers such as polyethylenimine [42,43], poly(L-lysine) [44], poly(L-histidine)-graft-poly(L-lysine) [45,46], poly(amino ester) [47], polyanhydrides [48], poly(amido amines) [49,50] are extensively studied as vectors for gene delivery. All these polymers contain positively-charged amino groups which govern transfection efficiency of these polymers.

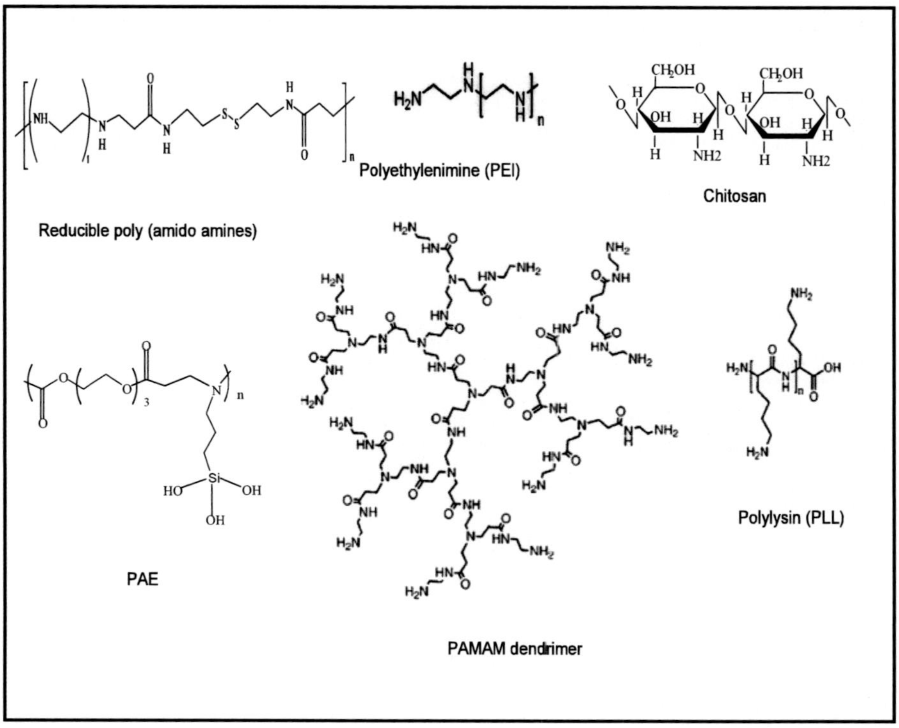

Figure 1. Structure of cationic polymers used for gene delivery.

As cells more efficiently take up compact particles via adsorptive endocytosis, cationic polymers should form a compact complex with anionic DNA through charge interaction. Extensive studies on structure and properties of polyamine/DNA complex have shown that the complex is largely toroidal in shape [51-53]. DNA stoichiometrically binds to polyamine and is governed by structure of polyamine [54]. For an effective binding, all of the positive charges must interact simultaneously and the position of these charges plays an important role in optimal interaction [55]. It is also reported that about 90% of the phosphates must be neutralized for a complete compaction [55]. The extent of compaction between the polycation and DNA depends on the charge ratio [56]. In case of polyamines (where protonation of amine groups depends on pH), the charge ratio is defined as the N/P i.e. ratio of number of nitrogen atoms from polycation to phosphate groups from DNA. At low N/P ratios, the complexes are large and electrically neutral; however, at high N/P ratios polyplexes are compact and positively charged. Excess of positive charge is essential that interacts with proteoglycans of the cell surface and enhances cellular binding to assist complex uptake. However, very high positive charge may increase uptake levels until the high concentration of polymer results in toxicity and cell death [56]. Also complexes made with an excess of cationic polymer have been shown to be heterogeneous mixture of polymer-DNA particles and free polymer. This suggests that an equilibrium state can be achieved for the condensation of these complexes. Although these separated complexes had reduced gene transfer activity in serum free conditions, they exhibited less toxicity, and demonstrated better activity in serum supplemented medium [56]. Thus, amount of binding is positively correlated with increasing cationic charge ratio [56]. The computed cation to anion ratio can be compared to the actual charge exhibited by the polyplex by measuring particle surface charge, or zeta potential. The zeta potential usually transits from negative to positive between 1:1 and 2:1 theoretical net charge. Slight variation in the transition point may occur based on the ionic concentration of the medium, the pH of the medium and actual pKa's of the amines [56]. A number of physical techniques have been developed to characterize the condensation of polycation-DNA complexes, including; size or shape (electrophoretic mobility on agarose gels, electron or atomic force microscopy and laser light scattering), charge (electrophoretic mobility and zeta potential), conformation and condensation (circular dichroism, ethidium bromide exclusion and centrifugation).

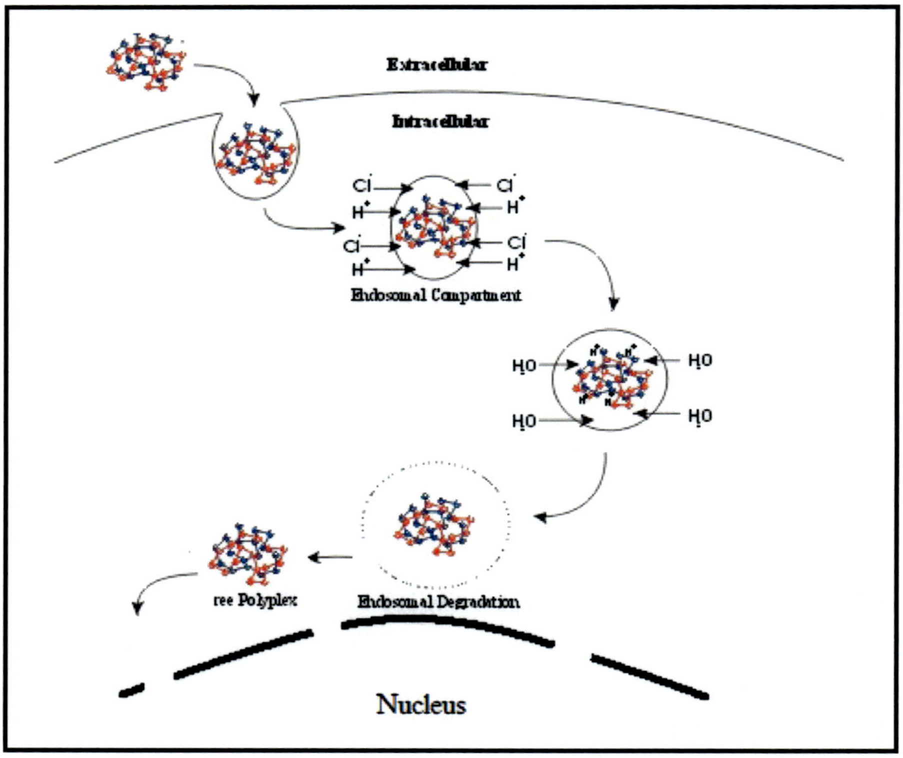

Figure 2. Proton sponge hypothesis.

Although size, shape, charge, conformation and condensation are important parameters in designing good non-viral vectors, the endosome lysis and release of DNA into cytosol as major limiting steps need to be studied carefully. Along with DNA condensation and endocytosis, amine groups are also essential to release complex by endosome lysis. Endosome lysis occurs due to the high buffering capacity of amine groups at physiological pH. These groups reduce the acidification of the endosome, increase Cl^- influx and subsequently lead to the osmotic swelling and rupture of endosomal membrane, known as 'proton sponge effect' (Figure 2) [57]. Although, cationic charge on polyamine is sufficient to condense DNA and promote its endocytosis, it is not adequate to achieve good transfection. Sonawane et. al. studied proton sponge effect for buffering and non-buffering polyamines. They reported that cationic polyamines with fixed non-titrable charges have poor ability of endosomal escape and hence, are less efficient in transfection than polyamines with titrable charges [58]. Thus, cationic polymers like PEI, PAMAM dendrimers having titrable amines are good transfection vectors. Although PEI and PAMAM dendrimers have good transfection efficiency, they are toxic to the cells due to the absence of biodegradable linkage. Recently many polymeric systems such as poly(β-amino ester) (PAE) [47], reducible poly(amido ethylenimine) [59-62] and reducible poly(amido amines) [63,64] are designed to take advantages of special intracellular environment to release DNA or siRNA. These polymers get easily degrade in cell cytoplasm into small fragments which can be easily removed from the cells. Reducible polymers have disulphide linkages which can be easily broken under reducing cytosolic environment while polyesters can be easily hydrolyzed in cytosol to form nontoxic metabolites. Among different types of polyesters, PAEs have been extensively investigated for their gene delivery ability. This chapter will further emphasize on characterization and success of PAEs in gene and siRNA delivery.

3. Characteristics of PAEs

3.1. Synthesis of PAEs

Poly(β-amino ester) (PAE) is a class of biodegradable polymers having ester linkages in their backbone and titrable amines at β-carbon atom. PAEs are mainly synthesized by Michael addition reaction, particularly, via the conjugate addition of either primary or secondary aliphatic amines to α, β-unsaturated carbonyl compounds to produce the β-amino derivatives [65]. Usually, these conjugate addition reactions are carried out either without solvent or in anhydrous organic solvents to minimize hydrolytic degradation during synthesis. This straight forward synthetic procedure makes it feasible to synthesize a variety of different PAE structures from a diverse pool of commercially available monomers [66]. Also commercial scale up of optimized PAE will be easy and accurate. Thus, easy and economical synthetic procedure and beneficial structural properties like juxtaposition of amines and esters within the backbone have increased the importance of PAEs in gene and siRNA delivery. Although PAEs have these beneficial properties, number of parameters need to be studied carefully for their successful applications as biodegradable gene and siRNA carriers.

3.2. Degradation and Cytotoxicity

PAEs are biodegradable due to the rapid hydrolysis of ester linkages under physiological conditions. Hydrolysis of PAE produces small non-toxic molecules bis(β-amino acids) and diols which can be easily removed by the cells. As PAEs are synthesized by Michael addition reaction, it is possible that the degradation could occur via retro-Michael reaction to regenerate acrylate monomers. As acrylates are DNA alkylating agents, degradation by this pathway will be potentially harmful and toxic to the cells. However, Lynn et al. confirmed the absence of this degradation pathway under physiological conditions [47]. Also, degradation of PAEs depends on the nature of PAE and pH of the system. Park et al. synthesized linear PAEs from three different molecular weight poly(ethylene glycol) diacrylate (PEGDA) and low molecular weight linear polyethylenimine (PEI) (Figure 3) [67]. They observed that the molecular weights of the synthesized PAEs were maintained relatively constant at about 4000 after 72 h regardless of molecular weight of PEGDA. However, different half-lives were observed depending on the molecular weight of PEGDA [67]. PAE composed of PEGDA 575 exhibited a half-life of 8 h, while those of 25 h for PAEs with PEGDA 700, based on the remaining molecular weight of the copolymers (Figure 4A). This rapid degradation in case of linear PAEs is plausible as even few cleavages may reduce chain length rapidly with quick drop in molecular weight. In contrast, branched PAEs from polycaprolactone (PCL) and branched PEI exhibited half-life 4.5-5 days [68] (Figure 4B). This higher half-life with branched PAEs is due to more stable polymeric structure as few cleavages do not change chain length or molecular weight drastically. Hence, stability of polyplex is higher with branched PAEs over that of linear PAEs [69]. Although linear PAE degrades rapidly than branched PAE at pH 7.4, its degradation is reduced at lower endosomal pH 5.1 [47], while degradation of branched PAE is relatively constant at both pH [70]. Moderate or slight degradation of PAE in polyplex has no significant effect on DNA condensation and protection [70]. Moreover, complexation with plasmid DNA is effective in reducing degradation rate of PAEs [47]. Intracellular degradation of PAE is responsible for its low toxicity; however, it is not the only factor governing the safety of PAEs. Safety of PAE was also significantly affected by the end group chemistry which is governed by monomer concentrations [71]. PAEs synthesized with excess of diacrylate monomer resulted in acrylate terminated PAEs which were found to be toxic to the cells [72]. It is plausible that the increase in diacrylate monomer increases hydrophobicity of the polymer and hence making it toxic to the cells. It should be noted that these studies are preliminary indicator of biocompatibility of PAEs and additional work must be done to more firmly establish the safety of PAE as gene delivery agents *in vivo*. Subsequent work with broader range of polymers has suggested that cytotoxicity is a function of polymer structure and self-assembled polymer-DNA complexes formed from certain polymers may be more toxic than the free, uncomplexed polymers themselves [73,74]. This observation highlights the importance of evaluating new polymers such as these over the full range of conditions in the context of gene and siRNA delivery.

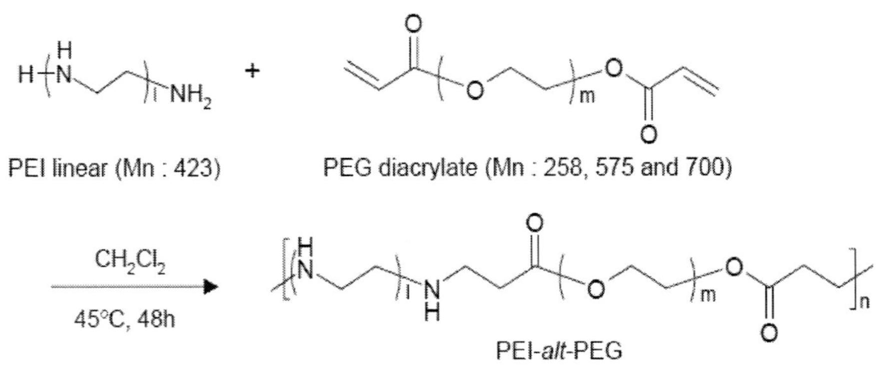

Figure 3. Synthesis of linear PAE composed of PEI and PEG [67].

3.3. Plasmid DNA Binding, Condensation and Protection

For successful DNA delivery to the cells, a cationic polymer must be able to self-assembled with DNA through electrostatic interactions and condensed it into positively charged nanometer-scale polymer-DNA conjugates [75]. Moreover, complex should protect DNA from degradation in cytosol by DNase enzymes for its successful transfection. Among variety of techniques popular to study these characteristics, agarose gel electrophoresis is most commonly used to study DNA binding, retention and protection. Both, linear PAEs from PEI-PEGDA [67], Spermine-PEGDA [76] and branched PAE from PCLDA-PEI [68], were able to interact electrostatically with pDNA and retard the migration of DNA on an agarose gel. As shown in Figure 5A, for the self-assembly of polymer Spermine-PEGDA with pCMV-Luc, DNA migration is completely retarded at DNA:polymer ratio above 1: 10 (w/w) [76]. PAEs from PEGDA-PEI [67] and PCLDA-PEI [68] have also effectively inhibited the migration of plasmid DNA at N/P ratio above 11.7 and 5, respectively. Also, these polymers effectively protected DNA from DNase enzyme as observed with DNase protection assay (Figure 5B) [67,68]. Dynamic light scattering and zeta potential analysis demonstrated that these PAEs can condense pDNA into small, positively charged polymer-DNA complexes less than 200 nm in diameter under physiological conditions [67,68]. Atomic force microscopy (AFM) further confirmed the morphology of complexes. Figures 6A, 6B, 6C and 6D show representative particle sizes and zeta potential profiles for complexes formed using linear PAE from PEGDA-PEI and branched PAE from PCLDA-PEI at different N/P ratios [67,68].

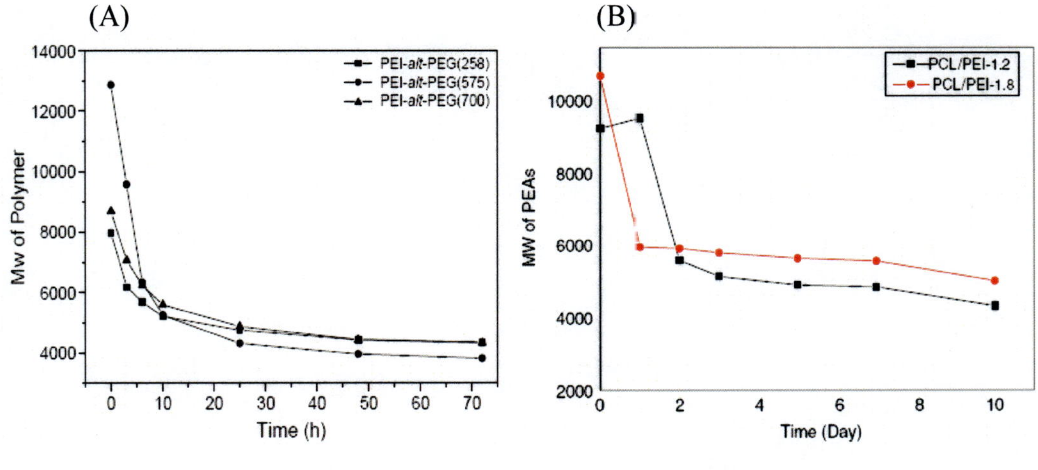

Figure 4. Degradation profile for (A) linear PAE [67], (B) branched PAE [68].

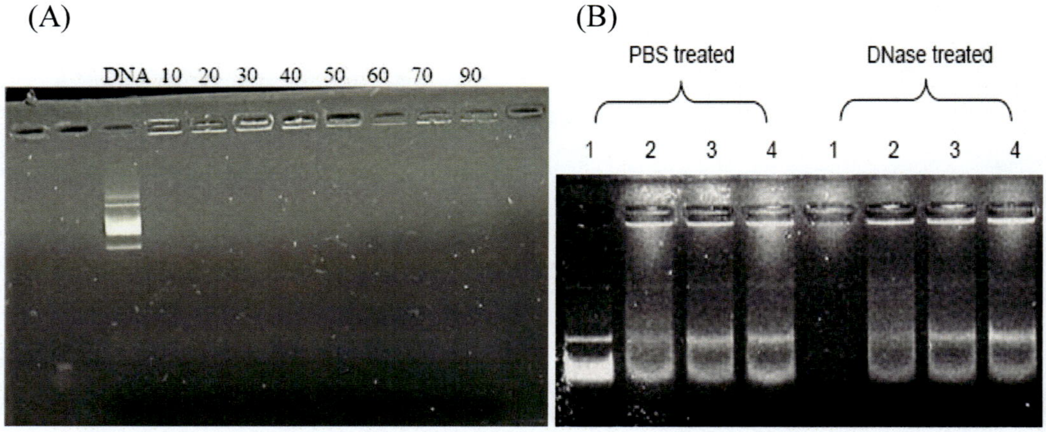

Figure 5. Gel electrophoretic determination for (A) DNA condensation and binding ability of PAEs [76]. (B) Protection of plasmid DNA from DNase by PAEs [67].

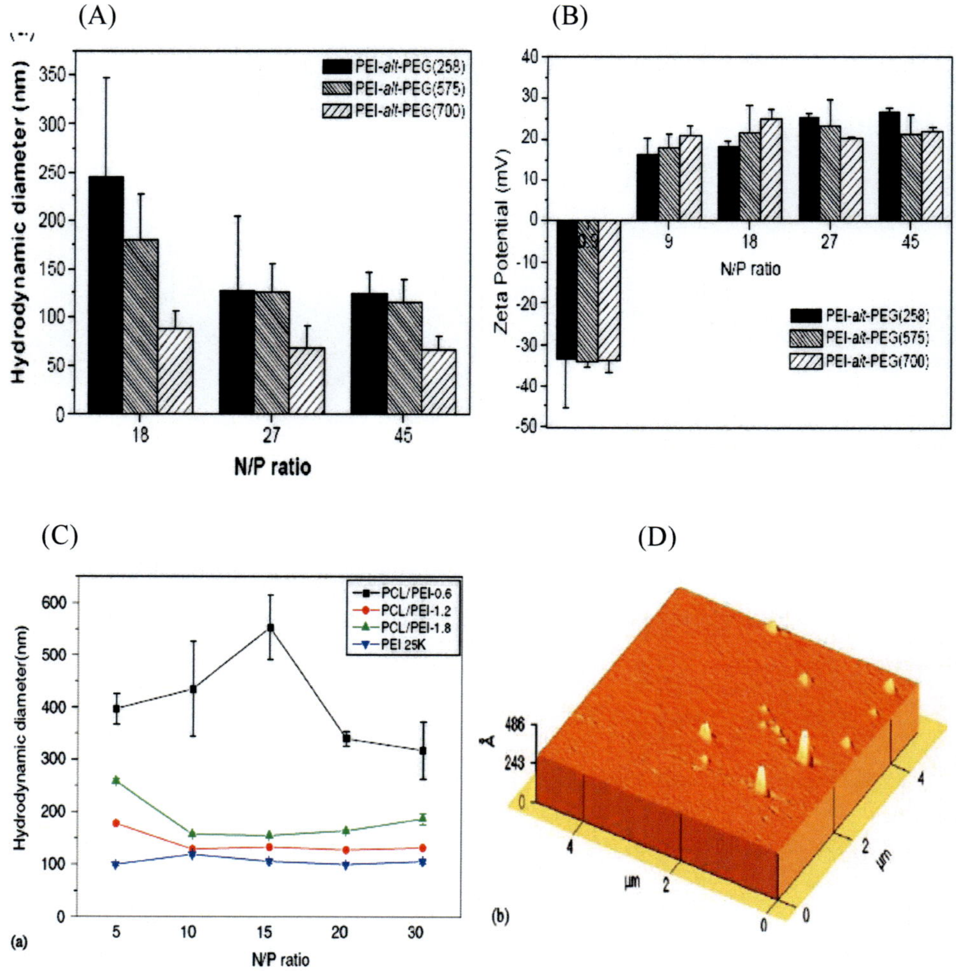

Figure 6. Particle sizes (A) and zeta potential (B) of linear PAE/DNA complexes [67]; Particle sizes (C) and AFM imgae (D)of branched PAE/DNA complexes [68].

4. CLASSIFICATION OF PAEs

PAEs exhibit variety of structural differences, primarily governed by the nature and concentration of monomers and secondly by reaction conditions. They are mainly different in their back bone structure which is either linear or branched. These linear and branched PAEs have different physicochemical properties and gene delivery efficiencies.

4.1. Linear PAEs

Linear PAEs have gained remarkable success in gene delivery. They are synthesized by conjugate addition of small molecular weight linear amines over diacrylate monomers. The final structure and molecular weight of these PAEs are predominantly governed by nature of amine groups in monomer, reaction conditions and monomer concentration. When PAEs were synthesized from polyamine monomers, nature of amine groups should be considered carefully. Lynn et al. reported that difunctional secondary amine monomers are more efficient in synthesis of linear PAEs [47]. Addition of the secondary amines to the diacrylate moieties results into tertiary amines which do not participate in subsequent addition reactions, that otherwise leads to polymer branching or cross linking. In other hand, difunctional primary amines may form extensively branched PAE if reaction conditions are not controlled explicitly [47]. Liu et al. used trifunctional amine monomers with primary and secondary amines for the stepwise synthesis of PAEs from linear to branch types by carefully monitoring reaction conditions [77] (Figure 7). Also during parallel PAE synthesis, Anderson et al. observed that reaction conditions play an important role. Optimum temperature and solvent are necessary for homogenous and complete reaction [71]. Although maximizing monomer concentration in reaction mixture is desirable to obtain high molecular weight PAE, it leads to insoluble gel formation in many cases [71,76]. Use of solvent may favor the homogenous and complete reaction; however, selection, optimization and removal of solvent are critical. Moreover, different solvents have significant effect on yield and performance of final PAEs [76]. As higher concentration of monomers favors intermolecular addition over intramolecular cycliazation, hence optimum solvent is essential. Concentration of monomers is deciding factor in end-terminal chemistry of PAEs. End-terminal chemistry significantly affects gene delivery efficiency of PAEs. Depending on the ratio of monomers used during synthesis, PAE can be made to have either amine or acrylate terminated chains. Akinc et al. observed that PAEs synthesized with amine monomers in excess have better transfection efficiency than acrylate monomers in excess [72] (Figure 8). Excess of amine monomer results into amine terminated polymer which effectively binds with cell membrane and promotes its uptake whereas acrylate terminated polymer has poor cellular entry and hence low transfection efficiency [72]. Along with nature and concentration of amine monomers, nature and molecular weight of diacrylate monomers are also important in determining transfection efficiency of PAEs. As diacrylates are mainly hydrophobic, they help in optimizing hydrophilic-lipophilic balance of PAEs. They reduce particle aggregation by reducing surface charges and also promote hydrophobic interactions with the cells. Moreover, hydrophobic units in polymeric carriers may assist dissociation of polymer/DNA complexes in order to release DNA which otherwise strongly bound with ionic interactions between cationic units and DNA phosphates. Although hydrophobic interactions reduce particle aggregation *in vivo*, use of lyoprotectants may be beneficial to prevent particle aggregation during lyophilization [78]. Molecular weight of diacrylate monomers also has significant effect on transfection efficiency. Park et al. noticed significant decrease in the transfection efficiency of PAEs with increase in molecular weight of PEGDA due to increased charge masking [67] (Figure 9). Screening of PAE library by Anderson et al. revealed that the transfection potential was proportional to the molecular weight of polymer [71]. PAEs with molecular weight smaller than 10 KDa have poor transfection potential [71]. They also discovered three linear PAEs having excellent transfection efficiency and safety [66,71]. These PAEs were synthesized from low molecular weight amino alcohols, namely, aminobutanol and aminopentanol having primary amine and alcohol groups. Accordingly, they suggested the importance of hydroxyl groups in transfection efficiency of PAEs, however, exact role of hydroxyl moieties in transfection is unclear [66]. Similar study on mini-library of γ-aminopropyl triethoxysilane (APES) based linear PAEs by Jere et al. revealed that the transfection efficiency and safety of PAE are highly dependent on monomer concentrations [79]. Even marginal changes in APES concentration showed drastic effects on transfection and safety of these PAEs [79]. In co-ordinance with finding of Akinc et al., they observed that amine terminated PAEs exhibited better transfection efficiency than acrylate terminated polymers. These polymers also contain alcohol-functionalized side chains after hydrolysis of ethoxysilane groups and are functionally similar to hydroxyl functionalized polymers identified by Langer group (Figure 10). Moreover, these PAEs exhibited good transfection efficiency even in the presence of serum.

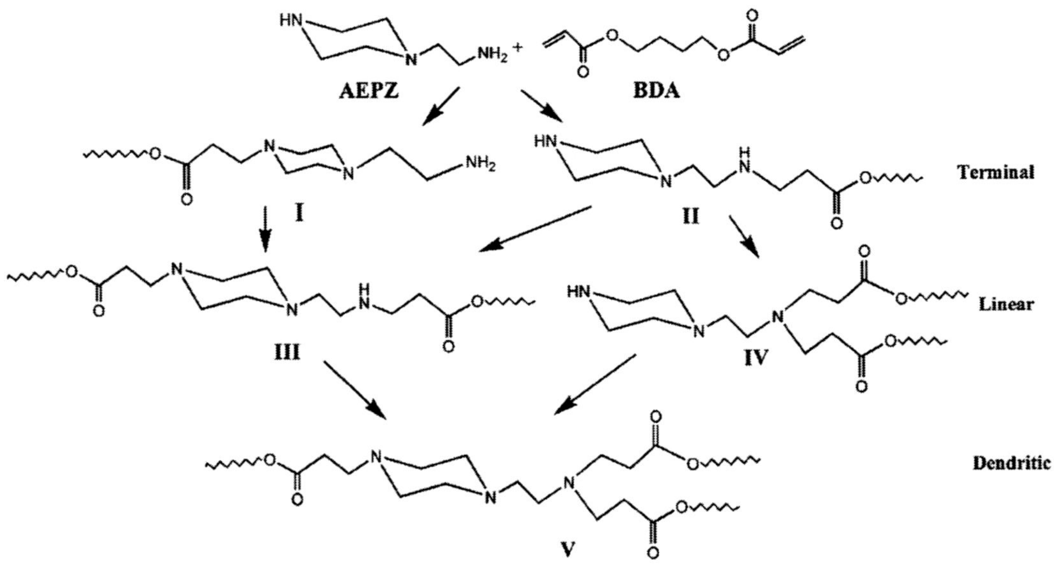

Figure 7. Synthesis of linear to branch PAEs by using trifunctional amines [77].

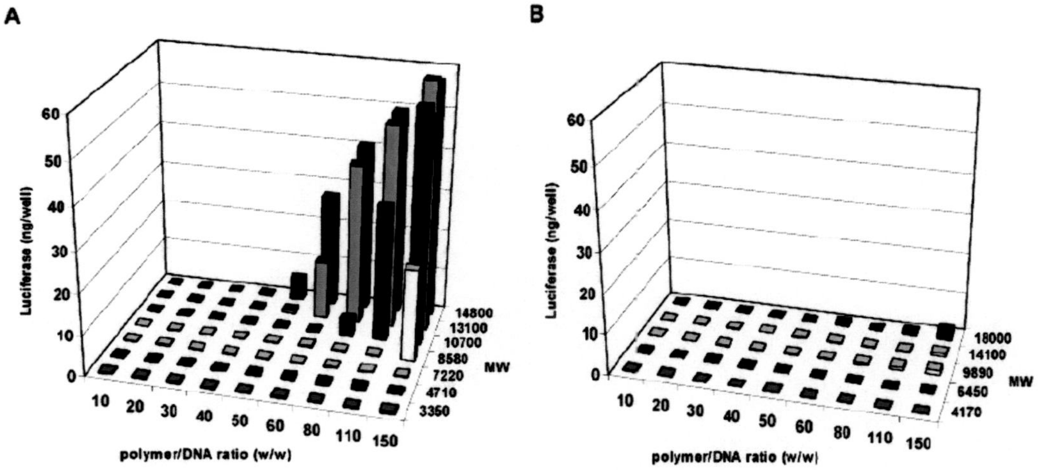

Figure 8. Transfection efficiency of PAEs depends on molecular weight [72].

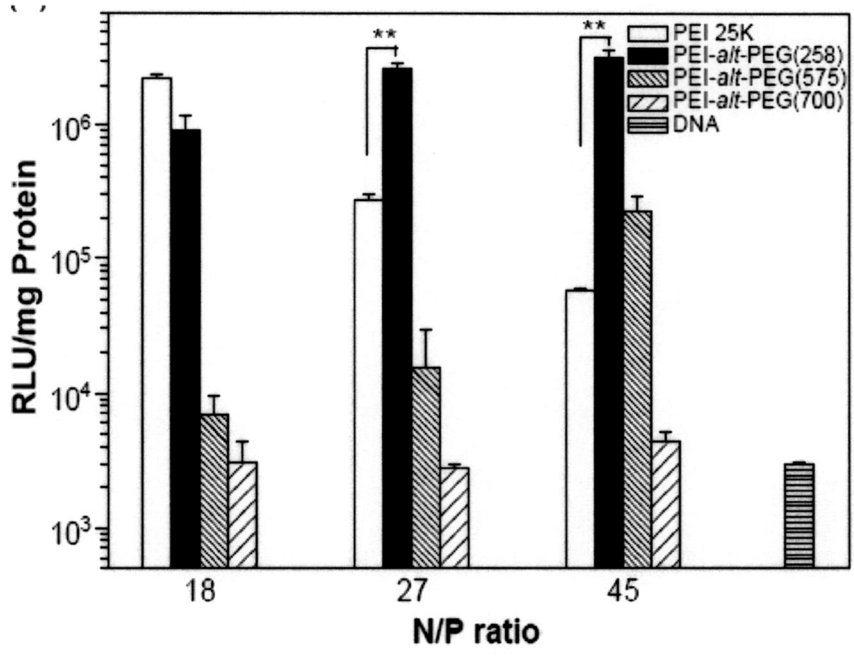

Figure 9. Decrease in transfection efficiency of PAEs with increase in molecular weight. of PEG [67].

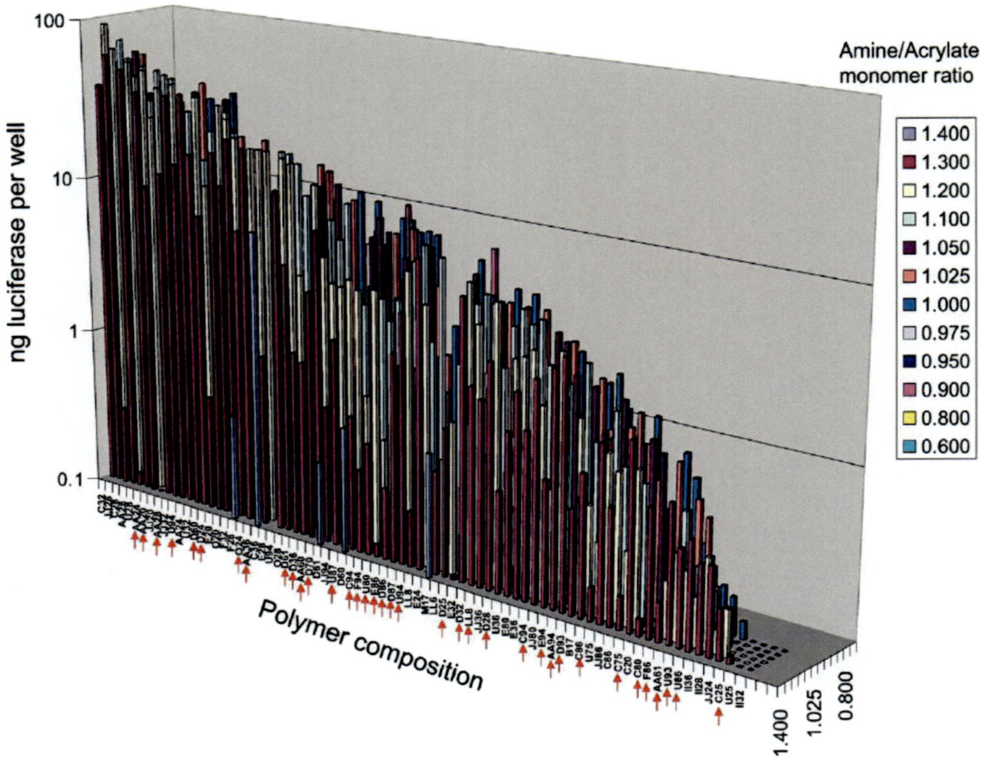

Figure 10. Transfection efficiency of PAE library [71].

4.2. Branched PAEs

Unlike linear PAEs, branched ones need more detail investigation for optimal mole ratio of monomers. Similar fashioned study of cross linked PAE was performed by Kim et al [80]. Biodegradable cross linked poly (β-amino ester) (CLPAE) was synthesized by Michael addition of pentaerythritol triacrylate and N,N-dimethyl-ethylenediamine and was further modified with aminohexanoic acid and lysine for gene delivery system. The CLPAEs showed residual unreacted acrylate groups at reaction mole ratio of 1 after confirmation by ^{1}HNMR whereas peaks of acrylate groups had vanished completely at mole ratio 2. It was also found that these CLPAE degraded more slowly than linear type polyesters and controled the release of DNA [80]. Meanwhile Liu et al. reported a mechanism of synthesis of PAEs from trifunctional amine monomers and 1,4-butanediol dicarylate (BDA) (Figure 7). Michael addition reaction was carried out with 1-(2-amino ethyl) piperazine (AEPZ) to which BDA solution was slowly added in equimolar concentrations at 45°C for 72 h using chloroform as a solvent. The polymerization of AEPZ with diacrylates was reported but hyperbranched PAEs with primary, secondary and tertiary amines were supposed to be formed based on unsolidified experimental evidence, suggesting that secondary amines are more reactive than primary ones in case of trifunctional cyclic amines [77]. To support this mechanism of polymerization with trifunctional amine and diacrylates, they reported that the reactivity sequence of three types of amines was 2° amine (original) > 1° amine >> 2° amine (formed).

It was also supported that reactivity of 1° amines in all trifunctional amines can be considered to be similar. Also stearic hindrance directs the reactivity of 2° amines including 2° amines (formed) among all the amines [81]. Same group further synthesized protonated hyperbranched PAEs and characterized for their gene delivery ability (Figure 11). It was found that all these hyperbranched PAEs degraded in a controlled manner within 40-45 days and it was speculated that this phenomenon may be due to the lesser water accessibility of the ester groups in hyperbranched structures. Furthermore, these hyperbranched PAEs revealed 80% cell viability even at 250μg/ml concentration and significant transfection efficiency in various cell lines compared with PEI 25K [82].

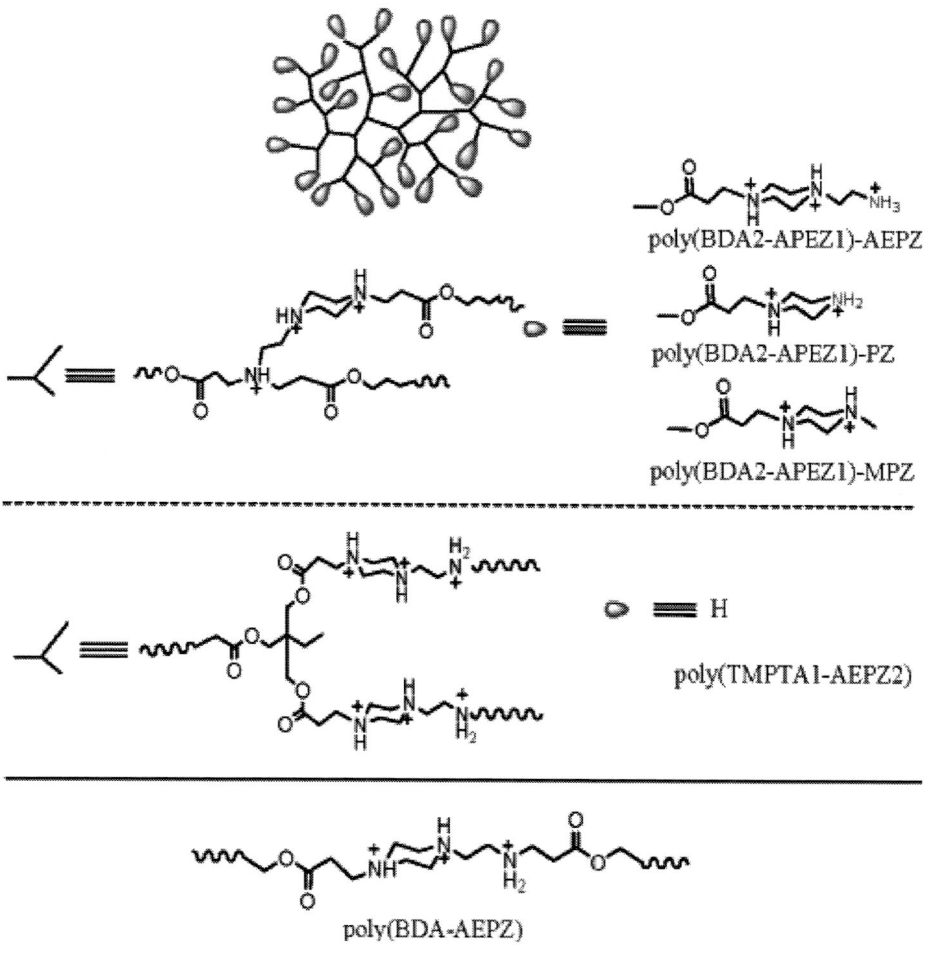

Figure 11. Structure of linear and hyperbranched PAE obtained via Michael addition polymerization of trifunctional amines with diacrylates and triacrylates [82].

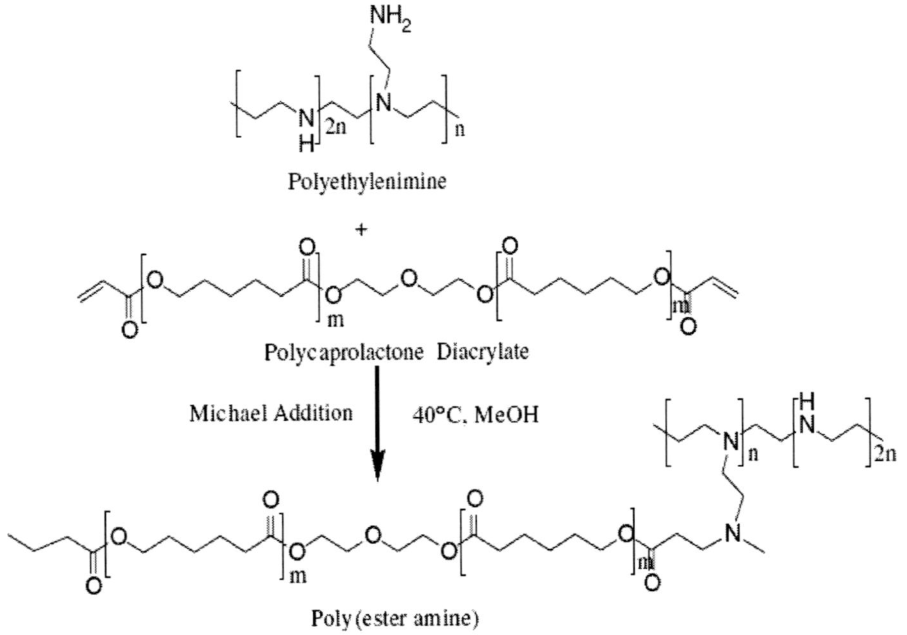

Figure 12. Synthetic scheme of PAEs from polycaprolactone and low molecular weight PEI [68].

A large library of PAEs was synthesized by Michael addition and identified by various promising candidates with remarkable in vitro and in vivo gene transfection efficiency with low cytotoxicity [71]. Similar fashioned synthesis of PAE was carried out by Forrest et al. under the label of degradable polyethylenimines and these degradable polymers mediated gene expression 2 to 16 fold more efficiently and reduced toxicity than commercially available PEI 25K [70]. Recently Arote et al. synthesized branch PAE by Michael addition, based on hydrophobic PCL and low molecular weight PEI. The branched PAE depicted at least 70-80% cell viability even at higher N/P ratios when measured in three different cell lines as shown in Figure 13A. Interestingly the transfection efficiency was found to be 15-25 folds higher than PEI 25K as a control in vitro (Figure 13B). It was simply an indication of application of ester linkage which supports the easy degradation leaving non-toxic building blocks, thereby increased transfection efficiency and reduced cytotoxicity. The PAE showed controlled degradation with the half life of 4-4.5 days [68]. Large library of PAEs reported by Langer group showed that majority of these linear PAEs were unable to condense DNA, probably owing to the fact that these linear PAEs contain merely tertiary amino group located in the stearically crowded environment [71]. In order to overcome these problems, Kim et al. recently reported another degradable branched PAE based on poloxamer diacrylate and low molecular weight PEI. These hyper branched PAEs can be easily synthesized by Michael type addition reaction between poloxamer diacrylate and low molecular weight PEI. These hyper branched PAEs showed slow degradation at physiological conditions which was greatly dependent on hydrophilicity of poloxamer and revealed around 80% cell viability along with good transfection efficiency [83].

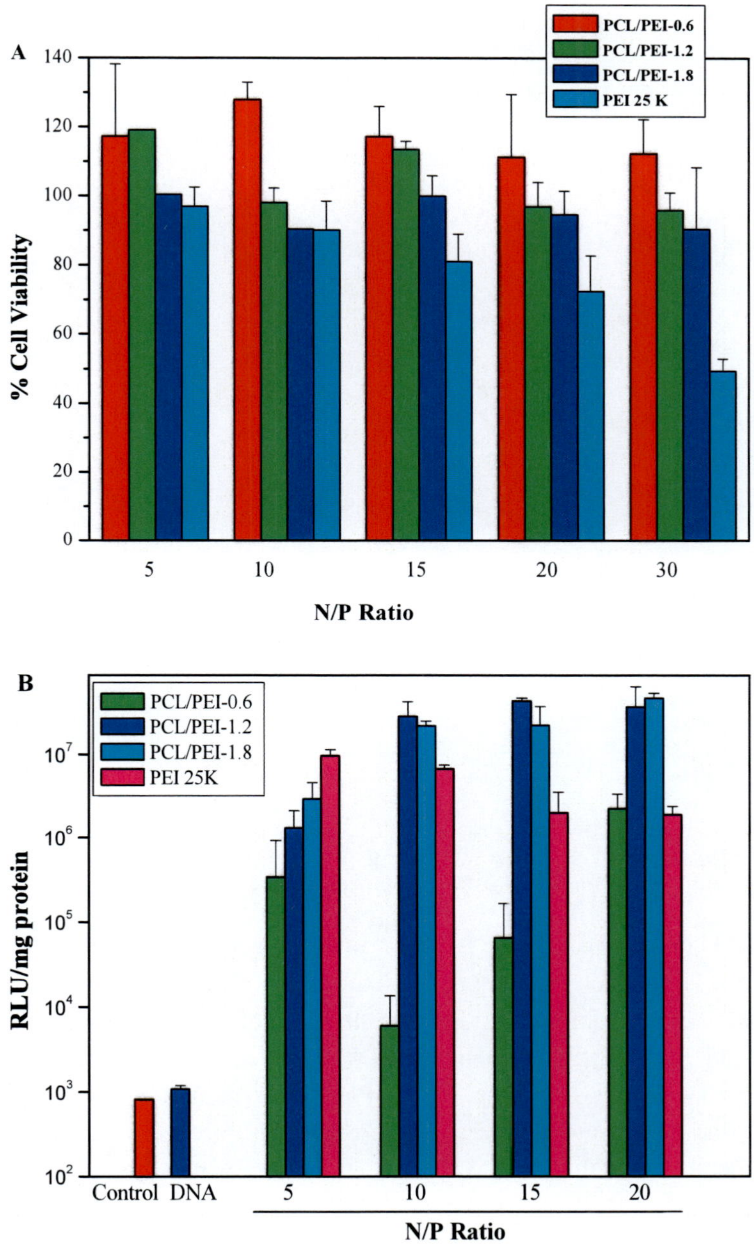

Figure 13. Cell viability (A) and transfection efficiency (B) of PAE's on HeLa cell line measured by MTS and Luciferase assay respectively [68].

4.3. Ligand Modified PAEs

Target-specific gene delivery is another important requirement for any gene delivery vector. Efforts are being done to develop degradable PAEs using various ligands for targeted delivery. New PAEs using primary amine monomer, 2-(pyridyldithio)-ethylamine (PDA) has been synthesized speculating that pyridyldithio groups in these side chains display fast and selective reactivity with thiols without alteration of charge density of the polymer backbone as shown in Figure 14. This property of PDA based PAEs further led to the conjugation of cell targeting peptides or ligands for targeted and site specific delivery.

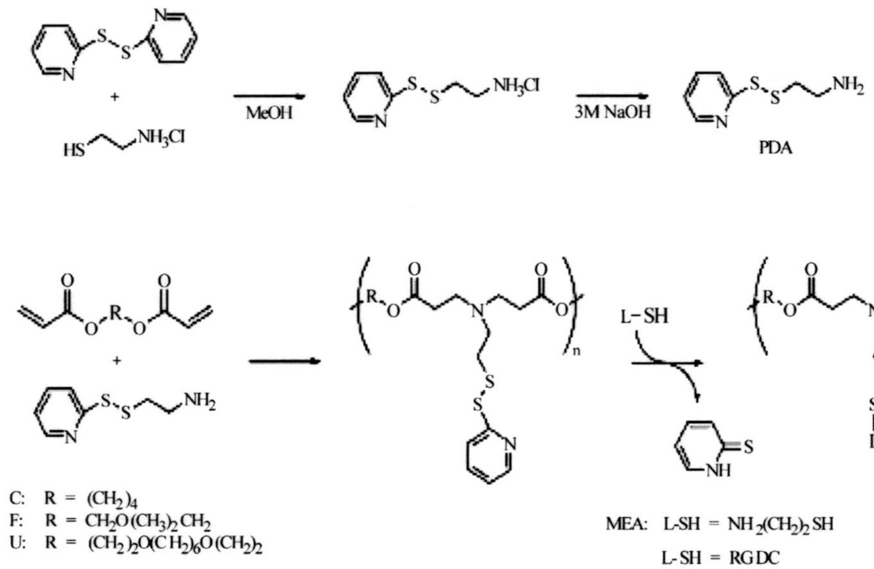

Figure 14. Synthesis scheme of amine monomer, 2-(pyridyldithio)-ethylamine hydrochloride from mercaptoethylamine hydrochloride and 2,2'-dipyridyl sulfide [84].

Mercaptoethylamine (MEA) and RGDC peptide attachment as a ligand to PDA-PAEs revealed potential application as a targeted delivery system [84]. It was found that both these polymers condensed DNA into nanosized particles with effective diameters around 100 nm. This MEA based PAE is capable of delivering DNA without exogenous endosomal buffering agent like poly (4-hydroxy-L-proline ester) (PHP ester) and poly [α-(4 amino butyl)-L-glycolic acid] (PAGA) reported by Lim et al. [85,86]. MEA based PAEs have an advantage that it has response to glutathione. It was reported that MEA based polymer delivery system is relatively stable in the extra cellular space but responsive to intracellular conditions in which partial unpacking is triggered. Significant increase in transfection efficiency by MEA based PAE was found over PAE when tested on human hepatocellular carcinoma cell lines. It could be the advantage of side chain reactivity. All three polymers with MEA substitution showed elevated transfection levels and low cytotoxicity [84].

Arote et al. coupled folic acid moiety for folate receptor targeting to PAE backbone using poly (ethylene glycol) as a linker. At initial stage, folate conjugated PAE revealed folate receptor mediated endocytosis and elevated levels of luciferase expression in three different, folate receptor cancer cell lines (A549, KB and NCI-H226), suggestion of the application of specific ligand modified PAE [87].

5. *In Vivo* Results of PAEs

For clinical feasibility of gene delivery, the vector system should be efficient and safe. Moreover, for in vivo success of non-viral gene delivery vector, additional challenges such as stability of vector system in proteins and serum, avoidance of reticuloendothelial system, protection from various nucleases and specificity to target the cell population should be successfully faced. To address these challenges various groups reported their success using PAE *in vivo*. Little et al. reported the encapsulation of plasmid DNA within hybrid PLGA/PAE microparticles and demonstrated the resulting enhancement in intracellular delivery compared with encapsulation by PLGA alone [88]. The hypothesis is that the incorporation of biodegradable, pH sensitive PAE in conventional PLGA microparticle formulations would increase the gene delivery capacity by facilitating intracellular release of plasmid payload upon phagosomal acidification. These microspheres fabricated from PAE, rapidly released the contents when exposed to acidic endosomal pH. The immunogenic efficacy of PAE containing microparticle formulations was compared by vaccinating B6 mice (five per group) with plasmid (pCMV-SIY) containing microparticles, naked DNA and empty microparticles. As shown in Figure 15, results showed that formulations composed of 15% and 25% PAE with pCMV-SIY, distinctly reduced the average growth rate of the tumor expressing SIY.

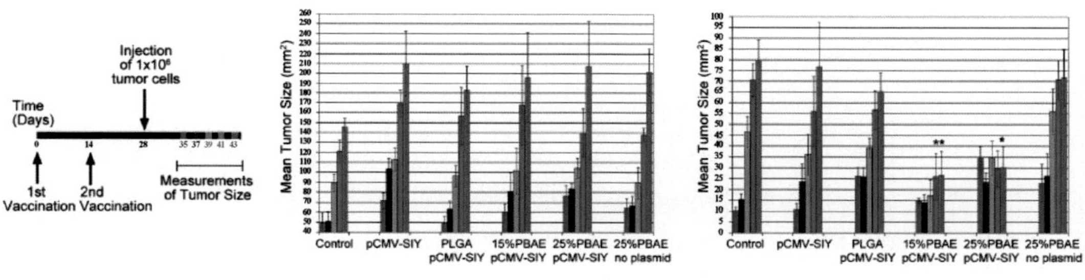

Figure 15. *In vivo* tumor rejection in B6 mice after treatment with genetic vaccine formulations. Mice were vaccinated and challenged by using the schedule shown in *Left*, and mean tumor size was measured by using a caliper in 2D 7 (blue), 9 (red), 11 (orange), 13 (green), and 15 (pink) days after s.c. injection of 3 x 10^6 normal EL4 thymoma cells (*Center*) or EL4 cells that are transfected with SIY and express it on their surface (*Right*). Standard error bars are shown for comparison. * indicates one mouse in which the tumor expressing SIY had completely regressed by this time point [88].

In another report by Greenland et al. to enhance the plasmid DNA immunogenecity of CRL1005 formulation of poloxamer, PAE was used to further enhance the transgene expression and it was expected to potentiate immune responses more dramatically [89]. To evaluate the boosting effect of CRL1005 formulation with PAE, mice were inoculated intramuscularly with 50 µg plasmid DNA, formulated with either 100 µg of CRL1005 or 100 µg of each candidate PAE. These candidates from a family of PAEs tested were found to enhance β-galactosidase activity by 4-10 folds (Figure 16). Formulations with poly [(1,6-di (acryloxyethoxy) hexane)-co-(4-aminobutanol)] (U28) enhanced β-galactosidase activity 7 folds on repeated administration. In subsequent experiment, to determine whether the enhancement in local transgene expression with these polymer-DNA formulations would result in enhanced immunogenicity, immune responses were examined following the immunization with plasmid expressing both β-galactosidase and HIV gp120. It was found that highest frequency of β-galactosidase responses was observed in the mice inoculated with plasmid DNA adjuvanted with two PAEs. Interestingly, some inconsistencies between transfection efficiencies *in vitro* and *in vivo* were observed. Also it was found during structural analysis that PAEs from amine monomers with terminal alcohol showed increased transfection efficiency *in vitro* and *in vivo*. However, PAEs based on hydrophobic diacrylates were successful *in vitro* but less successful at enhancing transfection *in vivo*.

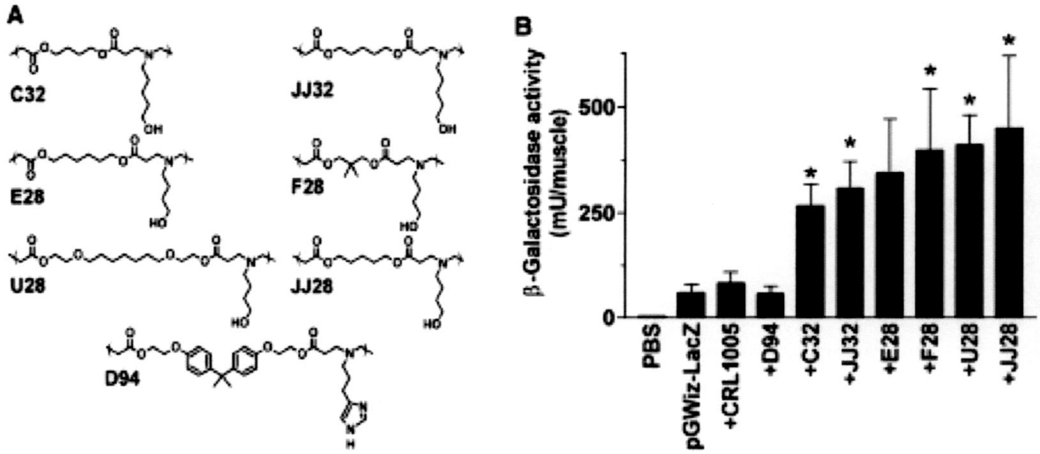

Figure 16. Formulation of plasmid DNA with selected h-amino ester polymers results in enhanced plasmid transgene expression levels. (A) Chemical structures of h-amino ester polymers selected for their effect on plasmid transgene expression in vitro. (B) Mice were inoculated with 50 μg pGWiz-LacZ and 100 μg of the indicated polymers divided between both quadriceps muscles. Seven days following inoculation, muscles were isolated (n = 10) and β-galactosidase activity was measured in homogenates as determined by FDG conversion rate. Asterisk denotes P b 0.05 for a Mann–Whitney test comparingthe β-galactosidase activity with that observed in muscles inoculated with unformulated plasmid DNA [89].

Arote et al. reported the *in vivo* success of PAEs based on PCLDA and low molecular weight PEI after aerosol administration [68]. Introduction of biodegradable ester linkages from hydrophobic PCLDA and highly cationic PEI as well as better biophysical properties tended to increase *in vivo* gene expression in lung than highly PEI 25K. Polyplexes prepared from biodegradable PCL/PEI-1.2 (1:2) and pEGFP-N_2 at charge ratio of 30 was aspirated to 13 week old female BALB/c mice. The GFP expression was determined after 2 days by confocal laser scanning microscopy. In agreement with *in vitro* results, PAEs depicted increased level of GFP expression than PEI 25 K as a control (Figure 17). Alveolar cells of lung were much compatible with PAEs than the cytotoxic PEI 25K owing to the introduction of biodegradable ester linkages.

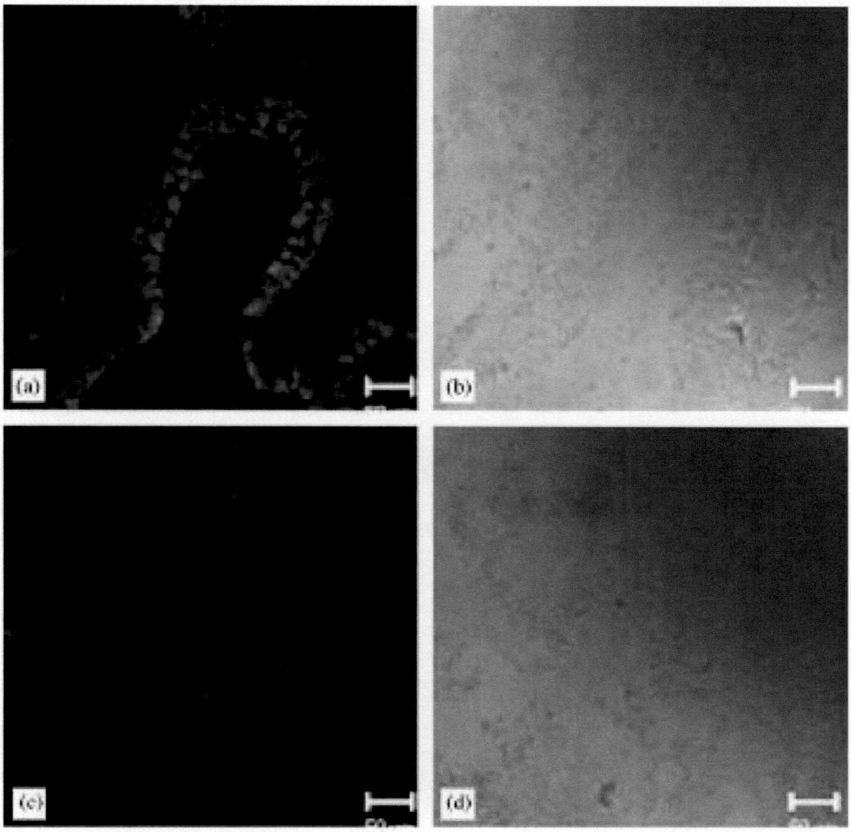

Figure 17. In vivo GFP expression analysis after aerosol administration to lung (bar = 50 μm). (a) Fluorescent microscopic image of PCL/PEI-1.2, (b) Phage contrast image of PCL/PEI-1.2, (c) Fluorescent microscopic image of PEI 25 K, (d) Phage contrast image of PEI 25 K [68].

6. siRNA Delivery by PAEs

Discovery of RNA based silencing has given new therapeutic vision to the treatment of incurable diseases and genetically associated disorders. RNA interference (RNAi) is a process, first described in the worm *Caenorhabditis elegans*, whereby the introduction of long double-stranded RNA (dsRNA) in cells results in the degradation of homologous mRNA [90,91]. Long dsRNA is processed to 21–23 bp small interfering RNA (siRNA) with 2nt 3' overhangs by the RNAseIII-like protein Dicer [92]. These cleavage products are subsequently incorporated into the RNA-induced silencing complex (RISC) [93]. Delivery of chemically synthesized siRNAs, mimicking Dicer cleavage substrates, results in sequence-specific, robust silencing of the expression of the corresponding endogenous gene [94], thus bypassing the non-specific inhibitory mechanisms elicited by longer dsRNA in mammalian cells [95]. Successful applications of RNAi in mammalian cells depend upon effective knockdown of targeted transcripts and efficient intracellular delivery of either preformed siRNAs or vector expressed siRNAs.

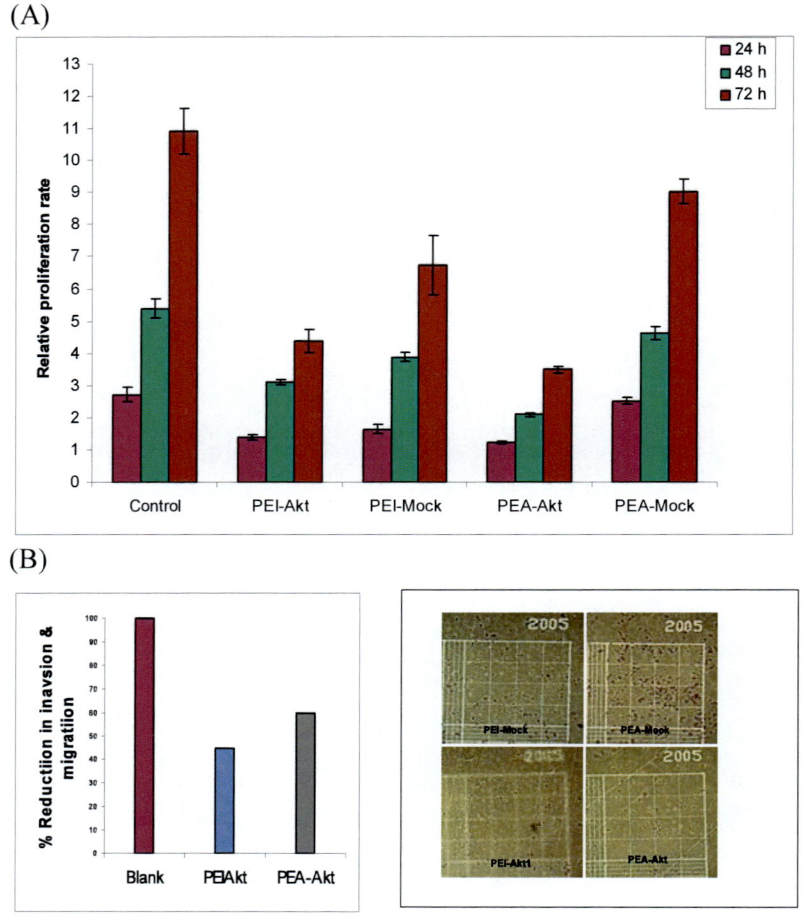

Figure 18. Akt1 siRNA treatment by using linear PAE from PEG-PEI (A) and branched PAE from PCL-PEI (B) reduces A549 cell proliferation and metastasis [97,98].

Many researchers and companies are working on developing strategies to deliver siRNAs or shRNAs to cells in culture and in tissues in various animal models. In some organisms like C. elegans, the presence of RNAdependent RNA polymerase allows for the amplification of siRNAs, and potentially even passes it on through the germ line, resulting in a long-lived, stable gene silencing. However, mammalian cells do not possess this mechanism, and, thereby, gene silencing is only seen for a few days after treatment with siRNA or shRNA. Plasmid-based expression systems have been developed for the stable expression of siRNAs in most of the other cell types [2,96]. Viral vectors like retrovirus-, adenovirus- and lentivirus-based vectors have been quite successful in obtaining efficient and longer gene silencing effects using RNAi. However, biosafety is the major concern which again makes non-viral vectors as an inevitable option in RNAi based therapeutics. PAEs are already successful in gene delivery; in above sections, we have given plethora of references proving safety and efficiency of PAEs in gene delivery. In this part we will highlight potential of PAEs in siRNA based gene silencing studies. Also the state of siRNA delivery using PAEs in vitro and in vivo will be explained even though reported research in this area is limited at this moment. Already efforts have been initiated to explore PAEs in siRNA based studies which may explore new era in cancer therapeutics. Jere et al. delivered synthetic and vector based siRNAs by using linear and branched type of PAEs composed of PEGDA-PEI and PCLDA-PEI, respectively. Both PAEs successfully delivered synthetic as well as vector based siRNAs. Delivery of therapeutic Akt1 siRNA expressing vector by these PAEs have been achieved with remarkable success in non-small cell lung carcinoma cells. This treatment has effectively altered and to some extent reversed cancer cell properties *in-vitro*. The results also showed high silencing when PAE used as a carrier over PEI 25K. Treatment of Akt1 siRNA with linear PAE has reduced proliferation of A549 cells more than two folds when compared with PEI 25K (Figure 18A) [97]. Also reduction in invasion, migration and malignancy was high when PAE used as a carrier to prove its superiority over prototype cationic polymer PEI 25K (Figure 18B). Branched PAEs also exhibited superiority over PEI 25K in similar type of studies [98]. Both these reports highlighted the potential of linear and branched PAEs in siRNA based cancer studies [97,98]. Furthermore, aerosol delivery of PAE/Akt1 siRNA nanoparticles by Xu et al. in K-*ras* null mice offered a non-invasive way in siRNA based therapy for lung cancer. This treatment significantly suppressed tumor numbers as well as adenoma and hyperplasia in mice as shown in Figure 19. Aerosol delivered PAE/Akt1 siRNA complexes efficiently suppressed lung cancer progression through regulating proteins important for Akt-related signals, and cell cycle regulation [99].

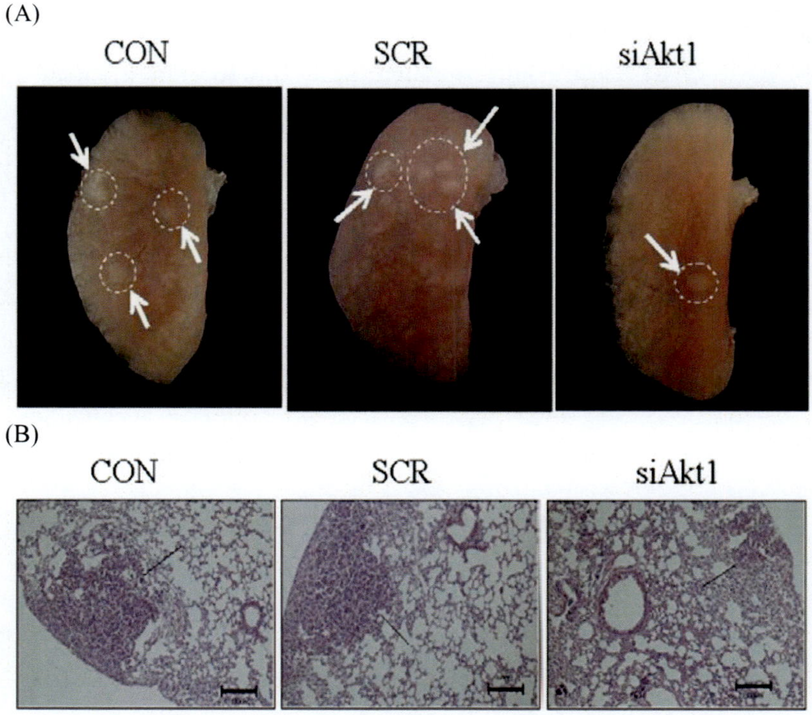

Figure 19. Tumor pathology of lungs in K-*ras* null mice. (A) K-*ras* null mice lungs showing numerous visible lesions (arrows and dotted circles). (B) Histological characteristics of K-*ras* null mice lungs. Arrows indicate the adenocarcinoma in the lungs of K-*ras* null mice. CON, control; SCR, scrambled control; siAkt1, Akt1 siRNA. X100, Scale bar represents 100 μm [99].

7. Summary and Future Prospective

PAEs comprise a class of degradable cationic polymers with many desirable properties in the perspective of gene and siRNA delivery. Their synthesis is straightforward and economical. Variety of structural variants can be generated from a broad array of commercially available monomers. PAEs can be either linear or branched that mainly depends on the nature of amine monomer and on reaction conditions. The branched PAEs are more stable than linear ones; however, linear PAEs with tertiary amine and alcohol functionalities have higher transfection efficiency than branched ones. Linear as well as branched PAEs have been proved efficient *in vitro* and *in vivo*. Moreover, PAEs demonstrated high potential in siRNA based non-invasive cancer therapies. Overall PAEs are non-viral vectors with high potential in gene and siRNA based therapies, however, important steps for the continued development and optimization of PAEs include improving serum stability and reducing plasma clearance, improving target specificity and maximizing tumor specific uptake, and finally optimizing it for controlled release applications.

8. Acknowledgement

We would like to acknowledge Korea Science and Engineering Foundation (KOSEF) (ROI-2005-000-10087-0) for providing funding. D. J and R. A. are supported by Korea Research Foundation (KRF) scholarship.

9. References

[1] Wagner LHM-CHE. *Nonviral Vectors for Gene Delivery*. International ed: Academic Press 1999.

[2] Devi GR. siRNA-based approaches in cancer therapy. *Cancer Gene Ther*. 2006 Sep;13(9):819-29.

[3] Dallas A, Vlassov AV. RNAi: a novel antisense technology and its therapeutic potential. *Med Sci Monit*. 2006 Apr;12(4):RA67-74.

[4] Leung RK, Whittaker PA. RNA interference: from gene silencing to gene-specific therapeutics. *Pharmacol Ther*. 2005 Aug;107(2):222-39.

[5] Alexander H. E. KG, Sprunt K., Van Damme. Infectivity of ribonucleic acid of poliovirus on HeLa cell monolayers. *Journal of Experimental Medicine*. 1958;108:493-506.

[6] Holland J. J. and Syverton J. T. The Mammalian cell-virus relationship. III. Poliovirus production by non-primate cells exposed to poliovirus ribonucleic acid. *Proceedings of the Society for Experimental Biology and Medicine*. 1959;100(1959):843-5.

[7] Graham F.L. A new technique for the assay of infectivity of human adenovirus 5 DNA. *Virology*. 1973;52:456-67.

[8] Friedmann T, Roblin R. Gene therapy for human genetic disease? *Science* (New York, NY. 1972 Mar 3;175(25):949-55.

[9] De Smedt SC, Demeester J, Hennink WE. Cationic polymer based gene delivery systems. *Pharm Res*. 2000 Feb;17(2):113-26.

[10]Roth CM, Sundaram S. Engineering synthetic vectors for improved DNA delivery: insights from intracellular pathways. *Annu Rev Biomed Eng*. 2004;6:397-426.

[11]Nishikawa M, Huang L. Nonviral vectors in the new millennium: delivery barriers in gene transfer. *Human gene therapy*. 2001 May 20;12(8):861-70.

[12]Lechardeur D, Lukacs GL. Nucleocytoplasmic transport of plasmid DNA: a perilous journey from the cytoplasm to the nucleus. *Human gene therapy*. 2006 Sep;17(9):882-9.

[13]Godbey WT, Mikos AG. Recent progress in gene delivery using non-viral transfer complexes. *J Control Release*. 2001 May 14;72(1-3):115-25.

[14]Kootstra NA, Verma IM. Gene therapy with viral vectors. *Annual review of pharmacology and toxicology*. 2003;43:413-39.

[15]Anderson WF. Human Gene Therapy. Science (New York, NY. 1992;256(5058):808-13.

[16]Grunhaus AaH, M. S. Adenoviruses as cloning vectors. *Seminars in Virology*. 1992;3:237-52.

[17]Muzyczka N. Use of adeno-associated virus as a general transduction vector for mammalian cells. *Current topics in microbiology and immunology*. 1992;158:97-129.

[18]Vlazny DA, Frenkel N. Replication of herpes simplex virus DNA: localization of replication recognition signals within defective virus genomes. *Proc Natl Acad Sci U S A*. 1981 Feb;78(2):742-6.

[19]Lyerly HK, DiMaio JM. Gene delivery systems in surgery. *Arch Surg*. 1993 Nov;128(11):1197-206.

[20]Kim YK, Park IK, Jiang HL, Choi JY, Je YH, Jin H, et al. Regulation of transduction efficiency by pegylation of baculovirus vector in vitro and in vivo. *Journal of biotechnology*. 2006 Aug 20;125(1):104-9.

[21]Fooks AR, Schadeck E, Liebert UG, Dowsett AB, Rima BK, Steward M, et al. High-level expression of the measles virus nucleocapsid protein by using a replication-deficient adenovirus vector: induction of an MHC-1-restricted CTL response and protection in a murine model. *Virology*. 1995 Jul 10;210(2):456-65.

[22]Yang WX, Terasaki T, Shiroki K, Ohka S, Aoki J, Tanabe S, et al. Efficient delivery of circulating poliovirus to the central nervous system independently of poliovirus receptor. *Virology*. 1997 Mar 17;229(2):421-8.

[23]Monaci P, Urbanelli L, Fontana L. Phage as gene delivery vectors. *Curr Opin Mol Ther*. 2001 Apr;3(2):159-69.

[24]Jiao S, Williams P, Berg RK, Hodgeman BA, Liu L, Repetto G, et al. Direct gene transfer into nonhuman primate myofibers in vivo. *Human gene therapy*. 1992 Feb;3(1):21-33.

[25]Wolff JA, Budker V. The mechanism of naked DNA uptake and expression. *Advances in genetics*. 2005;54:3-20.

[26]Yang NS, Burkholder J, Roberts B, Martinell B, McCabe D. In vivo and in vitro gene transfer to mammalian somatic cells by particle bombardment. *Proc Natl Acad Sci U S A*. 1990 Dec;87(24):9568-72.

[27]Gershon H, Ghirlando R, Guttman SB, Minsky A. Mode of formation and structural features of DNA-cationic liposome complexes used for transfection. *Biochemistry*. 1993 Jul 20;32(28):7143-51.

[28]Zhou XH, Klibanov AL, Huang L. Lipophilic polylysines mediate efficient DNA transfection in mammalian cells. *Biochimica et biophysica acta*. 1991 May 31;1065(1):8-14.

[29]Gao X, Huang L. Potentiation of cationic liposome-mediated gene delivery by polycations. *Biochemistry*. 1996 Jan 23;35(3):1027-36.

[30]Shi F, Wasungu L, Nomden A, Stuart MC, Polushkin E, Engberts JB, et al. Interference of poly(ethylene glycol)-lipid analogues with cationic-lipid-mediated delivery of oligonucleotides; role of lipid exchangeability and non-lamellar transitions. *Biochem J*. 2002 Aug 15;366(Pt 1):333-41.

[31]Martin-Herranz A, Ahmad A, Evans HM, Ewert K, Schulze U, Safinya CR. Surface functionalized cationic lipid-DNA complexes for gene delivery: PEGylated lamellar complexes exhibit distinct DNA-DNA interaction regimes. *Biophys J*. 2004 Feb;86(2):1160-8.

[32]Ding ZM, Cristiano RJ, Roth JA, Takacs B, Kuo MT. Malarial circumsporozoite protein is a novel gene delivery vehicle to primary hepatocyte cultures and cultured cells. *J Biol Chem*. 1995 Feb 24;270(8):3667-76.

[33]Murphy JE, Uno T, Hamer JD, Cohen FE, Dwarki V, Zuckermann RN. A combinatorial approach to the discovery of efficient cationic peptoid reagents for gene delivery. *Proc Natl Acad Sci U S A*. 1998 Feb 17;95(4):1517-22.

[34]Erbacher P, Zou S, Bettinger T, Steffan AM, Remy JS. Chitosan-based vector/DNA complexes for gene delivery: biophysical characteristics and transfection ability. *Pharm Res*. 1998 Sep;15(9):1332-9.

[35]Lee KY, Kwon IC, Kim YH, Jo WH, Jeong SY. Preparation of chitosan self-aggregates as a gene delivery system. *J Control Release*. 1998 Feb 12;51(2-3):213-20.

[36]Gao S, Chen J, Xu X, Ding Z, Yang YH, Hua Z, et al. Galactosylated low molecular weight chitosan as DNA carrier for hepatocyte-targeting. *Int J Pharm*. 2003 Apr 14;255(1-2):57-68.

[37]Kim TW, Chung H, Kwon IC, Sung HC, Shin BC, Jeong SY. Polycations enhance emulsion-mediated in vitro and in vivo transfection. *Int J Pharm*. 2005 May 13;295(1-2):35-45.

[38]Hardy JG, Kostiainen MA, Smith DK, Gabrielson NP, Pack DW. Dendrons with spermine surface groups as potential building blocks for nonviral vectors in gene therapy. *Bioconjug Chem*. 2006 Jan-Feb;17(1):172-8.

[39]Jiang HL, Kim YK, Arote R, Nah JW, Cho MH, Choi YJ, et al. Chitosan-graft-polyethylenimine as a gene carrier. *J Control Release*. 2007 Feb 12;117(2):273-80.

[40]Jin H, Kim TH, Hwang SK, Chang SH, Kim HW, Anderson HK, et al. Aerosol delivery of urocanic acid-modified chitosan/programmed cell death 4 complex regulated apoptosis, cell cycle, and angiogenesis in lungs of K-ras null mice. *Molecular cancer therapeutics*. 2006 Apr;5(4):1041-9.

[41]Kim TH, Ihm JE, Choi YJ, Nah JW, Cho CS. Efficient gene delivery by urocanic acid-modified chitosan. *J Control Release*. 2003 Dec 12;93(3):389-402.

[42]Boussif O, Lezoualc'h F, Zanta MA, Mergny MD, Scherman D, Demeneix B, et al. A versatile vector for gene and oligonucleotide transfer into cells in culture and in vivo: polyethylenimine. *Proc Natl Acad Sci U S A*. 1995 Aug 1;92(16):7297-301.

[43]Lemkine GF, Demeneix BA. Polyethylenimines for in vivo gene delivery. *Curr Opin Mol Ther*. 2001 Apr;3(2):178-82.

[44]Martinez-Fong D, Mullersman JE, Purchio AF, Armendariz-Borunda J, Martinez-Hernandez A. Nonenzymatic glycosylation of poly-L-lysine: a new tool for targeted gene delivery. *Hepatology* (Baltimore, Md. 1994 Dec;20(6):1602-8.

[45]Benns JM, Choi JS, Mahato RI, Park JS, Kim SW. pH-sensitive cationic polymer gene delivery vehicle: N-Ac-poly(L-histidine)-graft-poly(L-lysine) comb shaped polymer. *Bioconjug Chem*. 2000 Sep-Oct;11(5):637-45.

[46]Fajac I, Allo JC, Souil E, Merten M, Pichon C, Figarella C, et al. Histidylated polylysine as a synthetic vector for gene transfer into immortalized cystic fibrosis airway surface and airway gland serous cells. *The journal of gene medicine*. 2000 Sep-Oct;2(5):368-78.

[47]Langer DMLaR. Degradable Poly(β-amino esters): Synthesis, Characterization, and Self-Assembly with Plasmid DNA *J Am Chem Soc*. 2000;122:10761- 8.

[48]Quick DJ, Macdonald KK, Anseth KS. Delivering DNA from photocrosslinked, surface eroding polyanhydrides. *J Control Release*. 2004 Jun 18;97(2):333-43.

[49]Bielinska A, Kukowska-Latallo JF, Johnson J, Tomalia DA, Baker JR, Jr. Regulation of in vitro gene expression using antisense oligonucleotides or antisense expression plasmids transfected using starburst PAMAM dendrimers. *Nucleic acids research*. 1996 Jun 1;24(11):2176-82.

[50]Yoo H, Sazani P, Juliano RL. PAMAM dendrimers as delivery agents for antisense oligonucleotides. *Pharm Res*. 1999 Dec;16(12):1799-804.

[51]Hud NV, Vilfan ID. Toroidal DNA condensates: unraveling the fine structure and the role of nucleation in determining size. *Annual review of biophysics and biomolecular structure*. 2005;34:295-318.

[52]Mahato RI, Takakura Y, Hashida M. Nonviral vectors for in vivo gene delivery: physicochemical and pharmacokinetic considerations. *Critical reviews in therapeutic drug carrier systems*. 1997;14(2):133-72.

[53]Liu G, Molas M, Grossmann GA, Pasumarthy M, Perales JC, Cooper MJ, et al. Biological properties of poly-L-lysine-DNA complexes generated by cooperative binding of the polycation. *J Biol Chem*. 2001 Sep 14;276(37):34379-87.

[54]Balasundaram D, Tyagi AK. Polyamine--DNA nexus: structural ramifications and biological implications. *Molecular and cellular biochemistry*. 1991 Feb 2;100(2):129-40.

[55]Smirnov IV, Dimitrov SI, Makarov VL. Polyamine-DNA interactions. Condensation of chromatin and naked DNA. *Journal of biomolecular structure & dynamics*. 1988 Apr;5(5):1149-61.

[56]Alain Rolland SS, ed. *Pharmaceutical Gene Delivery System*: Marcel Dekker, Inc. 2003.

[57]Sonawane ND, Thiagarajah JR, Verkman AS. Chloride concentration in endosomes measured using a ratioable fluorescent Cl- indicator: evidence for chloride accumulation during acidification. *J Biol Chem*. 2002 Feb 15;277(7):5506-13.

[58]Sonawane ND, Szoka FC, Jr., Verkman AS. Chloride accumulation and swelling in endosomes enhances DNA transfer by polyamine-DNA polyplexes. *J Biol Chem.* 2003 Nov 7;278(45):44826-31.

[59]Christensen LV, Chang CW, Kim WJ, Kim SW, Zhong Z, Lin C, et al. Reducible poly(amido ethylenimine)s designed for triggered intracellular gene delivery. *Bioconjug Chem.* 2006 Sep-Oct;17(5):1233-40.

[60]Lee Y, Mo H, Koo H, Park JY, Cho MY, Jin GW, et al. Visualization of the degradation of a disulfide polymer, linear poly(ethylenimine sulfide), for gene delivery. *Bioconjug Chem.* 2007 Jan-Feb;18(1):13-8.

[61]Carlisle RC, Etrych T, Briggs SS, Preece JA, Ulbrich K, Seymour LW. Polymer-coated polyethylenimine/DNA complexes designed for triggered activation by intracellular reduction. *The journal of gene medicine.* 2004 Mar;6(3):337-44.

[62]Christensen LV, Chang CW, Yockman JW, Conners R, Jackson H, Zhong Z, et al. Reducible poly(amido ethylenediamine) for hypoxia-inducible VEGF delivery. *J Control Release.* 2007 Apr 2;118(2):254-61.

[63]Lin C, Zhong Z, Lok MC, Jiang X, Hennink WE, Feijen J, et al. Linear poly(amido amine)s with secondary and tertiary amino groups and variable amounts of disulfide linkages: synthesis and in vitro gene transfer properties. *J Control Release.* 2006 Nov 28;116(2):130-7.

[64]Hoon Jeong J, Christensen LV, Yockman JW, Zhong Z, Engbersen JF, Jong Kim W, et al. Reducible poly(amido ethylenimine) directed to enhance RNA interference. *Biomaterials.* 2007 Apr;28(10):1912-7.

[65]Brian D. Mather KV, Kevin M. Miller , Timothy E. Long Michael addition reactions in macromolecular design for emerging technologies. *Progress in Polymer Science.* 2006;31:487-531.

[66]Anderson DG, Lynn DM, Langer R. Semi-automated synthesis and screening of a large library of degradable cationic polymers for gene delivery. *Angew Chem Int Ed Engl.* 2003 Jul 14;42(27):3153-8.

[67]Park MR, Han KO, Han IK, Cho MH, Nah JW, Choi YJ, et al. Degradable polyethylenimine-alt-poly(ethylene glycol) copolymers as novel gene carriers. *J Control Release.* 2005 Jul 20;105(3):367-80.

[68]Arote R, Kim TH, Kim YK, Hwang SK, Jiang HL, Song HH, et al. A biodegradable poly(ester amine) based on polycaprolactone and polyethylenimine as a gene carrier. *Biomaterials.* 2007 Feb;28(4):735-44.

[69]Lim YB, Kim SM, Suh H, Park JS. Biodegradable, endosome disruptive, and cationic network-type polymer as a highly efficient and nontoxic gene delivery carrier. *Bioconjug Chem.* 2002 Sep-Oct;13(5):952-7.

[70]Forrest ML, Koerber JT, Pack DW. A degradable polyethylenimine derivative with low toxicity for highly efficient gene delivery. *Bioconjug Chem.* 2003 Sep-Oct;14(5):934-40.

[71]Anderson DG, Akinc A, Hossain N, Langer R. Structure/property studies of polymeric gene delivery using a library of poly(beta-amino esters). *Mol Ther.* 2005 Mar;11(3):426-34.

[72]Akinc A, Anderson DG, Lynn DM, Langer R. Synthesis of poly(beta-amino ester)s optimized for highly effective gene delivery. *Bioconjug Chem.* 2003 Sep-Oct;14(5):979-88.

[73]Lynn DM, Anderson DG, Putnam D, Langer R. Accelerated discovery of synthetic transfection vectors: parallel synthesis and screening of a degradable polymer library. *J Am Chem Soc.* 2001 Aug 22;123(33):8155-6.

[74]Akinc A, Lynn DM, Anderson DG, Langer R. Parallel synthesis and biophysical characterization of a degradable polymer library for gene delivery. *J Am Chem Soc.* 2003 May 7;125(18):5316-23.

[75]Luo D, Saltzman WM. Synthetic DNA delivery systems. *Nat Biotechnol.* 2000 Jan;18(1):33-7.

[76]Jere D J, Kim TH, Arote R, Jiang HL, Cho MH, JWN, Cho CS. A poly(β-amino ester) of spermine and poly(ethylene glycol) diacrylate as a gene carrier. *Key Engineering Materials.* 2007;342-343:425-8.

[77]Liu Y, Wu D, Ma Y, Tang G, Wang S, He C, et al. Novel poly(amino ester)s obtained from Michael addition polymerizations of trifunctional amine monomers with diacrylates: safe and efficient DNA carriers. *Chem Commun (Camb).* 2003 Oct 21(20):2630-1.

[78]Sameti M, Bohr G, Ravi Kumar MN, Kneuer C, Bakowsky U, Nacken M, et al. Stabilisation by freeze-drying of cationically modified silica nanoparticles for gene delivery. *Int J Pharm.* 2003 Nov 6;266(1-2):51-60.

[79]Jere D. J. Yoo MK, Arote R, Kim T. H, Cho M. H, Nah J. W, Choi Y. J, Cho C. S. Poly (amino ester) composed of poly (ethylene glycol) and aminosilane Prepared by combinatorial chemistry as a gene carrier. *Unpublished data.*

[80]Kim TI, Seo HJ, Choi JS, Yoon JK, Baek JU, Kim K, et al. Synthesis of biodegradable cross-linked poly(beta-amino ester) for gene delivery and its modification, inducing enhanced transfection efficiency and stepwise degradation. *Bioconjug Chem.* 2005 Sep-Oct;16(5):1140-8.

[81]Wu D C LY, He C B, Chung T S and Goh S H. Effect of chemistries of trifunctional amines on mechanism of Michael addition polymerization with diacrylates. *Macromolecules.* 2004;37:6763-70.

[82]Wu D C LY, Jiang X, He C B, Goh S H and Leong K W. Hyperbranched poly(amino etser)s with different terminal amine groups for DNA delivery. *Biomacromolecules.* 2006;7:1879-83.

[83]Kim TH, Cook SE, Arote RB, Cho MH, Nah JW, Choi YJ, et al. A degradable hyperbranched poly(ester amine) based on poloxamer diacrylate and polyethylenimine as a gene carrier. *Macromol Biosci.* 2007 May 10;7(5):611-9.

[84]Zugates GT, Anderson DG, Little SR, Lawhorn IE, Langer R. Synthesis of poly(beta-amino ester)s with thiol-reactive side chains for DNA delivery. *J Am Chem Soc.* 2006 Oct 4;128(39):12726-34.

[85]Lim Y B CYHaPJS. A self-destroying polycationic polymer: biodegradable poly(4-hydroxy-L-proline ester). *J Am Chem Soc.* 1999;121: 5633-9.

[86]Lim YB, Han SO, Kong HU, Lee Y, Park JS, Jeong B, et al. Biodegradable polyester, poly [alpha-(4-aminobutyl)-L-glycolic acid], as a non-toxic gene carrier. *Pharm Res.* 2000 Jul;17(7):811-6.

[87]Arote R et al. Folate conjugated poly (ester amine) for lung cancer therapy. *Unpublished data.*

[88]Little SR, Lynn DM, Ge Q, Anderson DG, Puram SV, Chen J, et al. Poly-beta amino ester-containing microparticles enhance the activity of nonviral genetic vaccines. *Proc Natl Acad Sci U S A*. 2004 Jun 29;101(26):9534-9.

[89]Greenland JR, Liu H, Berry D, Anderson DG, Kim WK, Irvine DJ, et al. Beta-amino ester polymers facilitate in vivo DNA transfection and adjuvant plasmid DNA immunization. *Mol Ther*. 2005 Jul;12(1):164-70.

[90]Fire A X S, Mello C.C. Potent and specific genetic interference by double-stranded RNA in Caenorhabditis elegans. *Nature*. 1998;391:806-11.

[91]Hannon G J. RNA Intereference. *Nature*. 2002;418:244-51.

[92]Bernstein E CAA, Hammond S.M. and Hannon G.J. Role for a bidentate ribonuclease in the initiation step of RNA interference. *Nature*. 2001;409:363-6.

[93]Hammond S.M BE, Beach D. and Hannon G.J. An RNA-directed nuclease mediates post-transcriptional gene silencing in Drosophila cells. *Nature*. 2000;404:293-6.

[94]Elbashir S.M HJ, Tuschl T. Duplexes of 21-nucleotide RNAs mediate RNA interference in cultured mammalian cells. *Nature*. 2001;411:494-8.

[95]Williams B R. PKR; a sentinel kinase for cellular stress. *Oncogene*. 1999;18:6112-20.

[96]Engelke D R. ; Rossi J J, ed. *RNA Interference*. USA: Elsevier 2005.

[97]Jere D. J et al. Aktl siRNA delivery for lung carcinoma using poly (ester amine). *Unpublished data.*

[98]Jere D. J et al. Biodegradable poly (ester amine) for efficient Akt1 siRNA delivery to non small cell lung carcinoma cells. *Unpublished data.*

[99]Xu C. H Jere D, Jin H, Chang S.H, Chung Y. S, Shin J. Y, Park S. J, Lee Y. H, Chae C. H, Lee K. H, Beck G. R, Cho C. S, Cho M. H. Poly(ester amine)-mediated Akt1 siRNA delivery via aerosol suppressed lung tumorigenesis in K-ras null mice. *Unpublished data.*

In: New Gene Therapy and Cancer Research
Editor: Wilma B. Gustafsson, pp. 279-292

ISBN: 978-1-60021-969-6

Chapter IX

CANCER GENE THERAPY IN LARGE ANIMALS

Liliana M. E. Finocchiaro and Gerardo C. Glikin
Unidad de Transferencia Genética, Instituto de Oncología "Ángel H. Roffo", Universidad de Buenos Aires, (1417) Buenos Aires, Argentina.

ABSTRACT

Despite the important progress obtained in the treatment of many malignancies, the need to develop new treatments to fight cancer is compelling.

Artificially created tumor models can be useful in the early stages of basic and applied research. The laboratory controlled disease, based on heterotopically grafted tumors in genetically identical small rodents that usually are young and healthy at the beginning of the trial, usually differs from human cancer in patients that spontaneously contracted the disease. Such patients are genetically heterogeneous and predominantly aged people whose immune system failed in fighting against the disease. These disparate situations can explain the failure of the translation to the field of some successful trials conducted in the laboratory. On the other hand, millions of pet dogs and cats will have cancer diagnosed every year. In many of those animals, the malignancy will look and behave as much as it would in humans, spreading to the same organs. In this context, spontaneous tumors appearing in large animals (especially companion animals) could offer a unique opportunity for both: (i) to develop new therapies for inherent pathologies and (ii) as models for human cancer biology and translational cancer therapeutics. With a potentially large population of cases for investigation, veterinary clinical trials can be completed faster and at significantly lower expense than similar human clinical trials. The successful trials could be easily translated to humans being benefited both humans and animal patients.

This review discusses the outcomes of different assayed gene therapy approaches reported by many research centers on a variety of tumors such as melanoma, soft tissue sarcoma, fibrosarcoma and osteosarcoma, as well as our own experience on spontaneous canine and equine melanoma.

The encouraging results obtained by means of these spontaneous cancer models in large animals supports not only their ready application in veterinary clinical oncology, but also as preclinical proof of concept and safety assay for forthcoming human gene therapy trials.

Introduction

Up to date most of the gene transfer experiments for cancer treatment have been mainly performed in small rodents, usually young healthy syngeneic immunocompetent mice injected heterotopically with artificially induced histocompatible murine tumors, or immunodeficient mice injected with human tumor cell lines. Meanwhile, human cancer patients that spontaneously contracted the disease are genetically heterogeneous, predominantly aged, with some degree of multifactorial immune disorder and about 2,000-fold bigger than mice. All these differences preclude precise extrapolation of safety data, and the particular pharmacokinetic distributions and routes of administration in each situation difficult the translation from basic to clinical research. This could explain the failure of some human clinical trials based on laboratory scale research.

In this context, spontaneous tumors appearing in large animals (especially companion animals) could offer a unique opportunity for both: (i) to develop new therapies for inherent pathologies and (ii) as models for human cancer biology and translational cancer therapeutics. With a potentially large population of cases for investigation, veterinary clinical trials can be completed in one fifth of the time (1-3 years) at significantly lower expense than similar human clinical trials. Vail and MacEwen [2000] and Hansen and Khanna [2004] largely reviewed the field of naturally occurring tumors in companion animals and its present and future role as models for human cancers.

Whereas nearly all the patients subjected to a variety of gene therapy methodologies were canine, some data also raised from feline and equine patients. As it is the case in human clinical trials, cancer gene therapy is largely leading the major attention, mainly by using immunostimulatory cytokine genes such as GM-CSF and IL-2. Different kinds of tumors were targeted but spontaneous melanoma, a highly aggressive tumor resistant to current therapies, was the preferred model. Both viral and no-viral vectors as well as cytokine producing transgenic cells were used to deliver gene products as cytokines, suicide genes, xenogeneic tumor antigens and pro-apoptotic genes.

Even though large animals were used in many gene therapy assays as reviewed by Casal *et al.* [2006], trials on spontaneous diseases were centered almost exclusively on cancer. We are currently focusing this review only on those papers reporting clinical data collected from client-owned patients with spontaneously arising tumors: those trials where the owners informed written consent was granted and the welfare of the patients was a main concern. At present, an increasing number of non-invasive or slightly-invasive techniques that allow *in vivo* monitoring of treatments effects are available [Vassaux and Groot-Wassink, 2003] and they could be implemented soon to optimize the efficacy of the procedures.

Amazingly cancer gene therapy clinical trials started much earlier in humans [Rosenberg *et al.*, 1990] than in companion animals [Quintin-Colonna *et al.*, 1996]. A comprehensive review on the past, present and future of gene therapy for cancer treatment, emphasizing the results obtained by human clinical trials, was recently published [Cross and Burmester, 2006].

The general trend in gene types used for veterinary cancer gene therapy clinical trials reflects what happens for humans. As updated on January 2007 by the Journal of Gene Medicine (http://www.wiley.co.uk/genmed/clinical/) 67% (total=1283) of clinical protocols were focused on cancer. Human cancer gene therapy trials (total=860) were grouped in 4 main gene types: 31% cytokines, 29% antigens, 17% tumor suppressors and 13 % suicide genes. On the other hand veterinary cancer gene therapy trials concentrated in 3 main gene types: 68% cytokines, 18% antigens, 14% suicide genes. Nevertheless, when vectors usage is analyzed, the pattern appears very different. Most of the human cancer gene therapy trials were performed with viral vectors: 29% adenovirus, 18% retrovirus and 9% poxvirus. They were followed by non viral vectors such as 16% naked plasmid and 10% lipofection. Conversely, most of the veterinary cancer gene therapy trials used non viral vectors: 31% naked plasmid, 31% lipofection and 13% gene gun. Viral vectors were represented by 17% adenovirus, 4% poxvirus and 4% retrovirus (Table 1).

Most of the veterinary gene therapy assays intended to generate an immune response able to control the minimal residual disease as well as any metastatic development. Different approaches were assayed as described below and in Table 2.

Table 1. Gene and vector types in large animal and human cancer gene therapy trials worldwide (January 2007)

GENES	LARGE ANIMALS	HUMANS*
Antigens	4	245
Cytokines	14	262
Marker	3	23
Suicide	4	108
Tumor suppressor/pro-apoptotic molecule	1	154

VECTORS	LARGE ANIMALS	HUMANS*
Adenovirus	4	245
Gene gun	3	5
Lipofection	7	84
Naked-DNA	7	134
Poxvirus	1	77
Retrovirus	1	151
TOTAL	23	854

(*) Data for human gene therapy trials were obtained from the on line site of *The Journal of Gene Medicine:* www.wiley.co.uk/genmed/clinical. Some trials combined genes and/or vectors, thus the total values can differ from the respective sums.

Table 2. Veterinary cancer gene therapy trials

#	CANINE	GENE	VECTOR	MODE	RESULTS	AUTHORS / YEAR
1	MEL	hIL-2	Irradiated hIL-2 producing xenogeneic cells made by plasmid transfection	*Ex vivo – p.t.*	(n=16) NR, 480 d. Control: 1 / Treated: 6 Median Survival: Treated: 270 d / Control: 75 d	Quintin-Colonna *et al.* 1996
2	MEL FSA OSA	hGM-CSF	Irradiated hGM-CSF producing autologous tumor cells plasmid transferred by gene gun	*Ex vivo – i.d.*	MEL (n=10) 1 CR (300 d), 1 PR (300 d), 1 NED (250 d), 1 SD (125 d) FSA (n=3) 1 PR, 1 NED (175 d)	Hogge *et al.* 1998 Chauvet *et al.* 1999
3	MGA	EcLac Z	Adenovirus	*In vivo – i.a.*	Feasibility study: successful marker expression	Chauvet *et al.* 1998
4	MEL	Enterotoxin-B + cGM-CSF	Plasmid/cationic lipid	*In vivo – i.t. / p.t. / i.l.n.*	(n=12) Median survival (stage III): Treated: 168 d / Historical surgery controls: 105 d	Dow *et al.* 1998
5	MEL	hGM-CSF	Irradiated hGM-CSF producing autologous tumor cells plasmid transferred by gene gun	*Ex vivo – i.d.*	Feasibility study: successful therapeutic gene expression and safety.	Hogge *et al.* 1999
6	MMT	rCYT-P450	Encapsulated xenogeneic human 293 made by plasmid transfection	*Ex vivo – p.t.*	Clinical trial proposal	Winiarczyk *et al.* 2002
7	CAR STS LYP	mpGHRH	Naked plasmid electroporation	*In vivo – i.m.*	At 56 d, treated (n=16) improved hematological parameters compared to control (n=19)	Draghia-Akli *et al.* 2002 Tone *et al.* 2004
8	STS	Enterotoxin-A + cIL-2	Plasmid/cationic lipid	*In vivo – i.t.*	(n=16) 3 CR, 1 PR, 1 SD (84 d). Responders survival > 540 d w/o relapse.	Thamm *et al.* 2003
9	MEL	hTyr	Naked plasmid – Jet injection	*In vivo – i.m.*	(n=9) 1 CR, 2 NED, 1 SD (14 d) / Median survival: Treated 389 d. Historical controls (stage II 150 d, stage III 60 d). Humoral antibodies detected: 3/9	Bergman *et al.* 2003 Liao *et al.* 2006
10	MEL	hFasL	Plasmid/cationic lipid	*In vivo – i.t.*	(n=5) GT: 3 TR, 1 SD / CT: 2 CR, 2 PR Survival: 168-574 d	Bianco *et al.* 2003 Modiano *et al.* 2006

Table 2. (Continued)

#	CANINE	GENE	VECTOR	MODE	RESULTS	AUTHORS / YEAR
11	MEL	hTyr / mTyr mgp75 hGM-CSF	Naked plasmid – Jet injection	*In vivo – i.m.*	Different combinations and doses. Median survival Stages II-III (n=33) w/ locoregional control: 569 d. 25/33 still alive.	Bergman *et al.* 2006
12	MEL	hgp100	Autologous Adenovirus transduced dendritic cells	*Ex vivo – s.c.*	(n=3) survival ranging 210 - 1440 d	Gyorffy *et al.* 2005
13	OSA	cIL-2	Plasmid/cationic lipid	*In vivo – i.v.*	(n=20) 84 d: 1 CR, 2 PR, 4 SD. Median survival (stage IV): Treated: 82 d / Historical untreated surgery controls: 58 d	Dow *et al.* 2005
14	MBT	nlsLacZ neo^R	Retrovirus	*In vivo – i.v.i.*	Feasibility study: successful marker expression.	Dumey *et al.* 2005
15	MEL	hgp100	Irradiated allogeneic hgp100 expressing tumor cells plasmid transferred by gene gun	*Ex vivo – i.d.*	(n=34) Median survival: Responders (CR,PR,SD) (n=12), 337 d / Non-responders (n=20), 95 d	Alexander *et al.* 2006
16	STS	hNIS	Adenovirus	*In vivo – i.t.*	Feasible and manageable toxicity.	Siddiqui *et al.* 2007
17	MEL	HSV-*tk* hIL-2 hGM-CSF	Cationic lipid-complexed Plasmid HSV-*tk* + GCV. Irradiated xenogeneic hIL-2 and hGM-CSF producing cells made by plasmid lipofection	*In vivo (SG) – i.t. / Ex vivo (CPXC) – i.t.*	Combined treatment (n=45) / Surgery controls (n=23). Median survival: 160 d / 82 d. Metastasis-free median survival: >509 d / 133 d. Combined treatment: CR=16%, PR=31%, SD=27%, PD=27%.	Finocchiaro *et al.* 2007.
18	MEL	HSV-*tk* hIL-2 hGM-CSF	Cationic lipid-complexed Plasmid HSV-*tk* + GCV. Irradiated xenogeneic hIL-2 and hGM-CSF producing cells made by plasmid lipofection	*In vivo (SG) - i.t. / Ex vivo (CPXC)+ (TV) – s.c.*	Combined treatment (n=100) / Surgery controls (n=51): Local disease-free patients: 58% / 6%. Metastasis-free patients: 78% / 43%. Median survival: >1312 d / 78 d. Metastasis-free median survival: >1312 d / 112 d.	Finocchiaro and Glikin. 2007

Table 2. (Continued)

#	FELINE	GENE	VECTOR	MODE	RESULTS	AUTHORS / YEAR
1	FSA	hIL-2	Irradiated xenogeneic hIL-2 producing cells made by plasmid transfection	*Ex vivo – i.t.*	(n=16) NR, 480 d: Control: 5 / Treated: 11 Median Survival: Control: 240 d/ Treated: >480 d	Quintin-Colonna *et al.* 1996
2	FSA	hIL-2/fIL-2	Poxviruses	*In vivo – i.t.*	(n=18) NR 365 d: Control: 7 / fIL-2: 13 / hIL-2: 11	Jourdier *et al.* 2003
3	STS	fIL-12	Adenovirus	*In vivo – i.t.*	(n=13) Feasible and manageable toxicity.	Siddiqui *et al.* 2007

#	EQUINE	GENE	VECTOR	MODE	RESULTS	AUTHORS / YEAR
1	MEL	hIL-12	Naked plasmid	*In vivo – i.t.*	(n=7) PR: 59 % reduction of injected tumors burden.	Heinzerling *et al.* 2001
2	MEL	HSV-*tk* hIL-2 hGM-CSF	Plasmid/cationic lipid for HSV-*tk*+ GCV. Irradiated xenogeneic hIL-2 and hGM-CSF producing cells made by plasmid lipofection	*In vivo (SG) - i.t. Ex vivo (CPXC)+ (TV) – s.c.*	(n=1) Case report. Reduction of injected tumors burden. Prevention of post-surgical local relapse. Survival > 600 d (alive).	Finocchiaro *et al.* Submitted

CAR, carcinoma; FSA, fibrosarcoma; LYP, lymphoma; MBT, malignant bladder tumors; MEL, melanoma; MGA, meningioma; MMT, malignant mammary tumors; OSA, osteosarcoma; STS, soft tissue sarcoma; cGM-CSF, canine granulocyte macrophage colony stimulating factor; cIL-2, canine interleukin-2; EcLacZ, *E. coli* lacZ; fIL-12, feline interleukin-12; fIL-2, feline interleukin-2; hFasL, human Fas ligand; hGM-CSF, human granulocyte macrophage colony stimulating factor; hgp100, Human glycoprotein 100; hIL-12, human interleukin-12; hIL-2, human interleukin-2; HSV-*tk*, herpes simplex thymidine kinase; hTyr, human tyrosinase; mgp75, mouse glycoprotein 75; mpGHRH, mutated porcine growth hormone releasing hormone; neo^R, neomycin resistance gene; NIS, Na^+/I^- symporter; nlsLacZ, *E. coli* lacZ with nuclear localization sequence; rcytP450, rat cytochrome P450; CR, complete response; NED, no evidence of disease; NR, no relapse; PR, partial response; SD, steady disease; CPXC, cytokine producing xenogeneic cells; d, days; GCV, ganciclovir; SG, suicide gene; TV, tumor vaccine; *i.a.*, intra-arterial; *i.d.*, intradermal; *i.l.n.*, intra-lymph node; *i.m.*, intramuscular, *i.t.*, intratumoral; *i.v.*, intravenous; *i.v.i.*, intra-vesical instillation; *p.t.*, peritumoral; *s.c.*, subcutaneous.

Canine Cancer Gene Therapy

The pioneering work of Quintin-Colonna *et al.* [1996] published about 11 years ago described an *ex vivo* genetically engineered xenogeneic cell gene therapy approach (that also could be defined as a transgenic xenogeneic cell therapy) for spontaneous canine melanoma. This highly aggressive tumor of the oral cavity, digit/footpad, and mucocutaneous junctions, appears clinically similar to aggressive human melanoma. Both diseases are chemo- and radio-resistant, do not respond well to treatment with conventional biological response modifiers and share similar metastatic phenotypes and site selectivity [Vail and MacEwen, 2000; Hansen and Khanna, 2004]. Like in human melanoma, the prognosis for canine melanoma correlates directly with tumor stage. At the time of diagnosis, the disease is often metastatic and has an extremely poor prognosis because rapid invasion of surrounding normal tissue and high likelihood of regional and distant metastasis early in the course of the disease. The high metastatic rate observed with this disease and the inefficacy of current therapies, warranted the investigation into novel therapies. In this work, the effects of repeated peritumoral local injections of human IL-2 secreting Vero cells after surgical removal of the tumor followed by ^{60}Co-radiotherapy were evaluated. This combined treatment resulted in a considerably higher median survival of 270 days compared to 75 days of the surgery plus radiation controls (n=16, each group). The treatment resulted safe.

An individually targeted autologous *ex vivo* approach for spontaneous canine melanoma involving human GM-CSF gene transfer, was developed by Hogge *et al.* [1998]. In this case, after tumor removal, a suspension of tumor cells was subjected to a gene gun shot with gold particles coated with a plasmid carrying the human GM-CSF gene. After sub-lethal ^{137}Cs irradiation, transgenic cells were delivered as intra-dermal injections in the flank of the patients. As part of a phase I clinical trial, the treatment of 10 canine melanoma bearing patients resulted in 3 objective responses and 1 stable disease, while 3 cases of fibrosarcoma yielded 2 objective responses. No animals have exhibited any signs of local or systemic toxicity. Even though statistically not significant because the low number of cases, survival time of melanoma responders (>300 days) largely exceeded the expected values for surgery treated patients (90-165 days). Furthermore in a preclinical development, Hogge *et al.* [1999] demonstrated in healthy dogs the safety and feasibility of intra-dermal vaccination with genetically engineered human GM-CSF producing allogeneic melanoma cells.

By using intratumoral injections of bacterial superantigen gene (staphylococcal enterotoxin B, SEB) as immune-adjuvant plus immunostimulatory gene canine GM-CSF, Dow *et al.* [1998] informed the objective responses and median survivals for spontaneous canine melanoma as follows: stage I, 3/3-427 days; stage II, 3/5-399 days; stage III 4/12-168 days; stage IV, 0/2-n.d. Median survival (168 days) of stage III patients (n=12) resulted significantly higher than historical surgery controls (105 days). Intratumoral expression of SEB and canine GM-CSF genes carrying plasmid did not induce clinically important toxicity in treated dogs.

Another superantigen gene was assayed to enhance the action of immunostimulant cytokine gene, in this case against the invasive spontaneous canine soft tissue sarcoma that is refractory to most conventional therapies other than surgical excision. Thamm *et al.* [2003] reported the effects of intralesional treatment with a plasmid containing bacterial superantigen gene (staphylococcal enterotoxin A, SEA) plus immunostimulatory canine IL-2 gene before surgical resection or exploration and biopsy of the tumor bed. Median survival of the responders resulted >540 days without experiencing local recurrence or metastasis. Manageable transient adverse effects related to treatment were informed.

Metastatic disease often needs a therapeutic molecule systemic delivery to reach multiple points simultaneously. Osteosarcoma in dogs is a common and highly metastatic tumor that biologically closely resembles osteosarcoma in humans [Vail and MacEwen, 2000; Hansen and Khanna, 2004]. Moreover, dogs with metastatic osteosarcoma do not have other treatment options once adjuvant chemotherapy has failed. Systemic gene delivery by intravenous injection of cationic liposome-DNA complexes carrying canine IL2 gene was assayed in 22 dogs with chemotherapy-resistant osteosarcoma lung metastases, as reported by Dow *et al.* [2005]. The treatment was well tolerated with 3 dogs displaying medium-term objective responses and 4 cases of stable disease. A significant increase of the median survival (82 d) with respect to untreated controls (58 d) was observed.

A totally different approach to promote immunologic "priming" through induction of apoptosis was assayed for canine melanoma by Bianco *et al.* [2003]. Direct intratumoral injections of a plasmid carrying the human FasL gene caused a fast reduction (7 days) of tumor burden that was seen in 3 of 5 treated dogs. At that time, each dog was provided of standard care therapy as indicated for each tumor (surgery, radiation or palliation), and the final result was 4 objective responses with survivals ranging from 168 to 574 days. The treatment did not show any adverse effect.

On the other hand, Bergman *et al.* [2003] found that intramuscular injection of a plasmid containing human tyrosinase gene and its expression as a melanoma xenoantigen considerably prolonged the median survival of canine melanoma bearing patients up to 389 days as compared with historical controls subjected to standard treatments (60-150 days). In addition, Liao *et al.* [2006] reported at least two long-term survivors displaying detectable levels of humoral anti-human tyrosinase antibodies. As reported by Bergman *et al.* [2006] other xenogeneic DNAs were assayed alone or combined, they coded for: murine tyrosinase, murine gp75 and human GM-CSF. Thirty-three stage II–III dogs with locoregionally controlled canine melanoma across the xenogeneic vaccine studies displayed a median survival time of 569 days, largely exceeding the value expected for standard treatments. Minimal to mild pain was noted at vaccination sites.

Gyorffy *et al.* [2005] reported the feasibility of autologous dendritic cells pulsed with adenoviral vector encoding human gp100 were applied as adjuvants of radiotherapy to treat canine melanoma. The 3 treated patients exceed the expected median survival (210 -1440 days), even though one died sooner because of progressive disease. No adverse effects were observed in any of the treated dogs with either the priming or the subsequent vaccine booster doses.

After vaccination with allogeneic cells expressing xenogeneic human gp100 Alexander *et al.* [2006] demonstrated that melanoma bearing dogs experiencing tumor control survived significantly longer than dogs having no response (median survivals: 337 days *vs.* 95 days). Adverse reactions were limited to mild induration and erythema at the site of vaccination.

To enhance the effects of chemotherapy with cyclophosphamide for canine mammary tumors, Winiarczyk *et al.* [2002] proposed the use of encapsulated genetically modified rat cytochrome P450 expressing human cells. However clinical data about the outcome were not published yet.

By adding local HSV thymidine kinase suicide gene bearing plasmid plus ganciclovir, in an approach that included intratumoral injections of xenogeneic hamster cells secreting human IL-2 and human GM-CSF (n=45), Finocchiaro *et al.* [2007] found that dogs presenting local objective responses survived significantly longer than dogs lacking local objective responses (220 days *vs.* 151 days), being both responses considerably higher than those of surgery controls (82 days). As a continuation of these encouraging data, a surgery adjuvant treatment against the minimal residual disease whose rationale appeared to be considerably superior to the previous intra-tumor treatment was assayed [Finocchiaro and Glikin, 2007]. This new treatment consisted of complete or cytoreductive surgery followed by a combination of suicide gene therapy with a subcutaneous vaccine. This vaccine was a mixture of formolized tumor cells and irradiated xenogeneic cells producing human IL-2 and human GM-CSF. The post-surgical margin of the cavity was infiltrated with lipid-complexed thymidine kinase suicide gene co-administrated with ganciclovir. Toxicity was minimal or absent in all patients. With respect to surgery treated controls, this combined treatment significantly increased the fraction of local disease-free patients from 6 to 58% and distant metastases-free patients from 43 to 78%. In addition, the combined treatment significantly improved both overall 78 (23-540) days and metastasis-free survival 112 (0-467) days of surgery treated controls to more than 1312 days (respective ranges: 43-1312 and 0-1312) (Kaplan-Meier analysis). In those patients subjected to partial surgery or presenting local recurrence, the efficacy of the local suicide gene approach was verified by a 49 % of objective responses that averaged 85% of tumor mass loss, while only 22% displayed tumor progression as 94% of the surgery controls did. This study suggested that the most optimal clinical setting is this surgery adjuvant treatment against minimal residual disease, a strong strategy that not only delays or prevents recurrence and distant metastasis, but substantially extends disease-free and overall survival, with a consequent improving in the quality of life.

Two feasibility studies for viral gene transfer to tumors using marker genes were reported. Chauvet *et al.* [1998] demonstrated that intra-arterial (carotid) injection of adenoviral vector could be used to transfer genes to a benign canine meningioma. Dumey *et al.* [2005], using intravesical instillation of retroviral vector were able to selectively transfer genes into canine malignant bladder tumors.

Siddiqui *et al.* [2007] determined the viability of using human sodium iodide symporter with $Na^{99m}TcO_4$ as a reporter gene to study the *in vivo* dynamics of adenoviral transgene expression in a case of canine soft tissue sarcoma.

Even though they did not aimed to fight directly against cancer, Draghia-Akli *et al.* [2002] and Tone *et al.* [2004] successfully contributed in diminishing paraneoplastic symptoms in canine patients with advanced melanoma, sarcoma, carcinoma and lymphoma patients. By *in vivo* electroporation enhanced delivery of a plasmid containing the GHRH gene, they succeeded in normalizing the hematological parameters with a consequent improving of patients quality of life.

FELINE CANCER GENE THERAPY

The pioneering work of Quintin-Colonna *et al.* [1996] also described the effects of the *ex vivo* genetically engineered xenogeneic cell gene therapy approach on the highly invasive feline fibrosarcoma that often presents post-surgical local relapse. There, they evaluated the effects of repeated peritumoral local injections of human IL-2 secreting cells after surgical removal of the tumor followed by ^{192}Ir-brachytherapy. This combined treatment resulted in a significantly longer median survival > of 480 days compared to 240 days of the surgery plus radiation controls (both groups: n=16). Interestingly the combined treatment drastically reduced the relapse rate after 480 days of treatment from 69% in the control group to 31 %.

As adjunct treatment following surgery and ^{192}Ir-brachytherapy for feline fibrosarcoma Jourdier *et al.* [2003] assayed the peritumoral injection of feline IL-2 or human IL-2 genes carried by poxviral vectors. The treatment significantly diminished the rate of recurrence at day 365 from 11/18 (control) to 5/18 (feline IL-2) and 7/18 (human IL-2).

Siddiqui *et al.* [2007] reported the feasibility of combining fractionated radiotherapy, hyperthermia, and heat-inducible intra-tumor adenoviral feline IL-12 gene therapy for feline soft tissue sarcoma as well as they determined the dose-dependent systemic toxicity in a phase I trial.

Equine Cancer Gene Therapy

As far as we know there is only one report on equine cancer gene therapy. Heinzerling *et al.* [2001] treated melanoma metastases in gray horses with a plasmid encoding immunostimulatory human IL-12 (n=7). A mean reduction in tumor size to 41% was observed after one cycle, compared to 88% in the group treated with non-coding control vector and 107 % in untreated animals. This transient volume reduction could be repeated with subsequent human IL-12 plasmid transfer. No side effects of the treatment were observed.

Based on our experience with spontaneous canine melanoma, we assayed the combination of local suicide gene therapy combined with a cancer vaccine following surgical removal of the superficial tumors in a single male gray horse patient with metastatic melanoma [Finocchiaro *et al.*, 2008]. The patient presented multiple grouped superficial lesions on the foreskin and perianally that were surgically removed and some isolated subcutaneous masses in the neck, back and shoulders that were injected with the suicide gene plus pro-drug (HSV-*tk* gene carrying plasmid, ganciclovir). Excised tumors were used to prepare a vaccine that was subcutaneously injected in the flanks as scheduled for canine treatment [Finocchiaro and Glikin, 2007]. No undesirable side effects were observed. One year after starting the six months lasting treatment, the patient recovered its quality of life including its full reproductive function, without local relapse at the surgery areas.

Conclusion

Most of the veterinary cancer gene therapy trials on patients with spontaneous tumors could be classified as immunogene therapy and were performed with non viral vectors. In general terms very slight or no adverse collateral effects were found and most of the times treated animals displayed a better course of the disease (longer survival, delayed or suppressed local or systemic relapse, recovery of the quality of life) suggesting the utility of this sort of approach as standard adjuvant treatment.

Besides, all these trials also demonstrate the utility of spontaneous tumors in companion animals as a valid translational model for the evaluation of novel DNA based therapies.

As it is the case for human patients, usually survival times for those veterinary patients that displayed objectives responses were significantly higher than for non responders, but the molecular basis for these differences has yet to be elucidated. In addition better results were obtained when treating the early stages of the disease and, in the case of advanced disease presenting bulky tumors, previous standard procedures such as surgery, chemotherapy and/or radiotherapy were necessary to obtain the best outcome of the whole treatment.

It is worth to note that the efficacy displayed by plasmid-based non-viral vectors used in 74 % of the trials involving large animals demonstrated their usefulness for present and future gene therapy treatments.

Although intravenous injections of cationic lipid:DNA complexes had some anti-tumor activity against canine STS regardless the transgene carried by the plasmid in the case of angiostatin "therapeutic" or luciferase "reporter" gene [Kamstock *et al.*, 2006], this fact should no be taken as negative. In addition to the immune enhancing effects of complexes carrying non-coding plasmid in a vaccine proposed against hemangiosarcoma [U'Ren *et al.*, 2007], the expression of therapeutic genes displayed specific anti-tumor activity as repeatedly evidenced in many papers listed in table 1. Further work has to be done to ascertain the contribution of each component *in vivo*.

An increasing interest in cancer therapy trials in large animals (especially dogs and cats) including those using gene therapy techniques will serve as concept, safety and effectiveness proofs. This new trend in the research of novel cancer therapies will indeed benefit both companion animals and human patients [Khanna *et al.* 2006, Mack 2006, Waters and Wildasin 2006].

Even though trials in companion animals are shorter in time and at lower costs than in humans, ethical and clinical concerns should be analyzed before involving them in clinical trials [Porrello *et al.*, 2004]. Nowadays, there are conditions for the development of translational research in the oncology field, intending to apply scientific information to solve present problems in relatively brief periods of time. Proper cancer models involving companion animals spontaneously induce the investigators to work in the duality between the veterinary perspective and the potential application to human medicine. However, these are not contradictory objectives, and trials in humans based on the equivalent trials in pets will possibly come soon.

ACKNOWLEDGEMENTS

This work was partially supported by grants from ANPCYT-FONCYT: BID1201/OC-AR PID 2000 - 00161 and BID1728/OC-AR PICT 2002 - 12084. L.M.E.F. and G.C.G. are members of the Consejo Nacional de Investigaciones Científicas y Técnicas (CONICET, Argentina).

REFERENCES

Alexander AN, Huelsmeyer MK, Mitzey A, Dubielzig RR, Kurzman ID, Macewen EG, Vail DM. Development of an allogeneic whole-cell tumor vaccine expressing xenogeneic gp100 and its implementation in a phase II clinical trial in canine patients with malignant melanoma. *Cancer Immunol Immunother.* 2006, *55:* 433-442.

Bergman PJ, Camps-Palau MA, McKnight JA, Leibman NF, Craft DM, Leung C, Liao J, Riviere I, Sadelain M, Hohenhaus AE, *et al.* Development of a xenogeneic DNA vaccine program for canine malignant melanoma at the Animal Medical Center. *Vaccine*. 2006; *24:* 4582-4585.

Bergman PJ, McKnight J, Novosad A, Charney S, Farrelly J, Craft D, Wulderk M, Jeffers Y, Sadelain M, Hohenhaus AE, *et al.* Long-term survival of dogs with advanced malignant melanoma after DNA vaccination with xenogeneic human tyrosinase: a phase I trial. *Clin Cancer Res.* 2003; *9:* 1284-1290.

Bianco SR, Sun J, Fosmire SP, Hance K, Padilla ML, Ritt MG, Getzy DM, Duke RC, Withrow SJ, Lana S, Matthiesen DT, *et al.* Enhancing antimelanoma immune responses through apoptosis. *Cancer Gene Ther.* 2003; *10:* 726-736.

Casal M, Haskins M. Large animal models and gene therapy. *Eur J Hum Genet.* 2006; *14:* 266-272.

Chauvet AE, Kesava PP, Goh CS, Badie B. Selective intraarterial gene delivery into a canine meningioma. *J Neurosurg.* 1998; *88:* 870-873.

Cross D and Burmester JK. Gene Therapy for Cancer Treatment: Past, Present and Future. *Clin Med Res.* 2006; *4:* 218-227.

Dow S, Elmslie R, Kurzman I, MacEwen G, Pericle F, Liggitt D. Phase I study of liposome-DNA complexes encoding the interleukin-2 gene in dogs with osteosarcoma lung metastases. *Hum Gene Ther.* 2005; *16:* 937-946.

Dow SW, Elmslie RE, Willson AP, Roche L, Gorman C, Potter TA. In vivo tumor transfection with superantigen plus cytokine genes induces tumor regression and prolongs survival in dogs with malignant melanoma. *J Clin Invest.* 1998; *101:* 2406-2414.

Draghia-Akli R, Hahn KA, King GK, Cummings KK, Carpenter RH. Effects of plasmid-mediated growth hormone-releasing hormone in severely debilitated dogs with cancer. *Mol Ther.* 2002;*6:* 830-836.

Finocchiaro, LME, Fiszman GL, Karara AL, Glikin GC. Suicide gene and cytokines combined non viral gene therapy for canine spontaneous melanoma. *Cancer Gene Ther.* 2007; *14*: In press.

Finocchiaro, LME, Glikin, GC. Cytokine-enhanced vaccine and suicide gene therapy as surgery adjuvant treatments for spontaneous canine melanoma. *Gene Ther.* 2007; *14*: In press.

Finocchiaro, LME, Riveros, MD, Glikin, GC. Cytokine-enhanced vaccine and suicide gene therapy as surgery adjuvant treatments for metastatic melanoma in a gray stallion". (2008) Submitted.

Gyorffy S, Rodriguez-Lecompte JC, Woods JP, Foley R, Kruth S, Liaw PC, Gauldie J. Bone marrow-derived dendritic cell vaccination of dogs with naturally occurring melanoma by using human gp100 antigen. *J Vet Intern Med.* 2005; *19:* 56-63.

Hansen K, Khanna C. Spontaneous and genetically engineered animal models; use in preclinical cancer drug development. *Eur J Cancer.* 2004; *40:* 858-880.

Heinzerling LM, Feige K, Rieder S, Akens MK, Dummer R, Stranzinger G, Moelling K Tumor regression induced by intratumoral injection of DNA coding for human interleukin 12 into melanoma metastases in gray horses. *J Mol Med.* 2001; *78:* 692-702.

Hogge GS, Burkholder JK, Culp J, Albertini MR, Dubielzig RR, Keller ET, Yang NS, MacEwen EG. Development of human granulocyte-macrophage colony-stimulating factor-transfected tumor cell vaccines for the treatment of spontaneous canine cancer. *Hum Gene Ther.* 1998; *9:* 1851-1861.

Jourdier TM, Moste C, Bonnet MC, Delisle F, Tafani JP, Devauchelle P, Tartaglia J, Moingeon P. Local immunotherapy of spontaneous feline fibrosarcomas using recombinant poxviruses expressing interleukin 2 (IL2). *Gene Ther.* 2003; *10:* 2126-2132.

Kamstock D, Guth A, Elmslie R, Kurzman I, Liggitt D, Coro L, Fairman J, Dow S Liposome-DNA complexes infused intravenously inhibit tumor angiogenesis and elicit antitumor activity in dogs with soft tissue sarcoma. *Cancer Gene Ther.* 2006; *13:* 306-317.

Khanna C, Lindblad-Toh K, Vail D, London C, Bergman P, Barber L, Breen M, Kitchell B, McNeil E, Modiano JF, *et al.* The dog as a cancer model. *Nat Biotechnol.* 2006; *24:* 1065-1066.

Liao JC, Gregor P, Wolchok JD, Orlandi F, Craft D, Leung C, Houghton AN, Bergman PJ. Vaccination with human tyrosinase DNA induces antibody responses in dogs with advanced melanoma. *Cancer Immun.* 2006; *6:* 8.

Mack GS. Clinical trials going to the dogs: canine program to study tumor treatment, biology. *J Natl Cancer Inst.* 2006; *98:* 161-162.

Modiano JF, Breen M, Lana SL, Ehrhart N, Fosmire SP, Thomas R, Jubala CM, Lamerato-Kozicki AR, Eugene J. EJ, Schaack J, *et al.* Naturally occurring translational models for development of cancer gene therapy. *Gene Ther Mol Biol.* 2006; *10:* 31-40.

Porrello A, Cardelli P, Spugnini EP. Pet models in cancer research: general principles. *J Exp Clin Cancer Res.* 2004; *23:* 181-193.

Quintin-Colonna F, Devauchelle P, Fradelizi D, Mourot B, Faure T, Kourilsky P, Roth C, Mehtali M. Gene therapy of spontaneous canine melanoma and feline fibrosarcoma by intratumoral administration of histoincompatible cells expressing human interleukin-2. *Gene Ther.* 1996; *3:* 1104-1112.

Rosenberg SA, Aebersold P, Cornetta K, Kasid A, Morgan RA, Moen R, Karson EM, Lotze MT, Yang JC, Topalian SL, *et al.* Gene transfer into humans--immunotherapy of patients with advanced melanoma, using tumor-infiltrating lymphocytes modified by retroviral gene transduction. *N Engl J Med.* 1990; *323:* 570-578.

Siddiqui F, Barton KN, Stricker HJ, Steyn PF, Larue SM, Karvelis KC, Sparks RB, Kim JH, Brown SL, Freytag SO. Design considerations for incorporating sodium iodide symporter reporter gene imaging into prostate cancer gene therapy trials. *Hum Gene Ther.* 2007; *18:* 312-322.

Siddiqui F, Li CY, Larue SM, Poulson JM, Avery PR, Pruitt AF, Zhang X, Ullrich RL, Thrall DE, Dewhirst MW, Hauck ML. A phase I trial of hyperthermia-induced interleukin-12 gene therapy in spontaneously arising feline soft tissue sarcomas. *Mol Cancer Ther.* 2007; *6:* 380-389.

Tone CM, Cardoza DM, Carpenter RH, Draghia-Akli R Long-term effects of plasmid-mediated growth hormone releasing hormone in dogs. *Cancer Gene Ther.* 2004; *11:* 389-396.

U'Ren LW, Biller BJ, Elmslie RE, Thamm DH, Dow SW. Evaluation of a novel tumor vaccine in dogs with hemangiosarcoma. J Vet Intern Med. 2007; 21:113-120.

Vail DM, MacEwen EG. Spontaneously occurring tumors of companion animals as models for human cancer. *Cancer Invest.* 2000; *18*: 781-792.

Vassaux G, Groot-Wassink T. *In Vivo* Noninvasive Imaging for Gene Therapy. J *Biomed Biotechnol.* 2003: 92-101.

Waters DJ, Wildasin K. Cancer clues from pet dogs. Sci Am. 2006; *295:* 94-101

Winiarczyk S, Gradski Z, Kosztolich B, Gabler C, Konig G, Renner M, Saller RM, Prosl H, Salmons B, Gunzburg WH, Hain J. A clinical protocol for treatment of canine mammary tumors using encapsulated, cytochrome P450 synthesizing cells activating cyclophosphamide: a phase I/II study. *J Mol Med.* 2002; *80:* 610-614.

INDEX

A

B

D

E

F

G

H

I

J

K

Q

R

T

W

X

Y

Z